Burns

Editors

JASON H. KO
BENJAMIN LEVI

HAND CLINICS

www.hand.theclinics.com

Consulting Editor
KEVIN C. CHUNG

May 2017 • Volume 33 • Number 2

ELSEVIER

1600 John F. Kennedy Boulevard • Suite 1800 • Philadelphia, Pennsylvania, 19103-2899

http://www.theclinics.com

HAND CLINICS Volume 33, Number 2
May 2017 ISSN 0749-0712, ISBN-13: 978-0-323-49649-0

Editor: Lauren Boyle
Developmental Editor: Kristen Helm

Hand Clinics (ISSN 0749-0712) is published quarterly by Elsevier Inc., 360 Park Avenue South, New York, NY 10010-1710. Months of publication are February, May, August, and November. Business and Editorial Offices: 1600 John F. Kennedy Blvd., Ste. 1800, Philadelphia, PA 19103-2899. Customer Service Office: 3251 Riverport Lane, Maryland Heights, MO 63043. Periodicals postage paid at New York, NY and at additional mailing offices. Subscription price is $398.00 per year (domestic individuals), $721.00 per year (domestic institutions), $100.00 per year (domestic students/residents), $454.00 per year (Canadian individuals), $839.00 per year (Canadian institutions), $541.00 per year (international individuals), $839.00 per year (international institutions), and $256.00 per year (international and Canadian students/residents). Foreign air speed delivery is included in all *Clinics* subscription prices. All prices are subject to change without notice. **POSTMASTER:** Send address changes to *Hand Clinics*, Elsevier Health Sciences Division, Subscription Customer Service, 3251 Riverport Lane, Maryland Heights, MO 63043. Customer Service (orders, claims, online, change of address): Elsevier Health Sciences Division, Subscription **Customer Service, 3251 Riverport Lane, Maryland Heights, MO 63043. Tel: 1-800-654-2452 (U.S. and Canada); 314-447-8871 (outside U.S. and Canada). Fax: 314-447-8029. E-mail: journalscustomerservice-usa@elsevier.com (for print support); journalsonlinesupport-usa@elsevier.com (for online support).**

Reprints. For copies of 100 or more of articles in this publication, please contact the Commercial Reprints Department, Elsevier Inc., 360 Park Avenue South, New York, New York 10010-1710. Tel.: 212-633-3874; Fax: 212-633-3820; E-mail: reprints@elsevier.com.

Hand Clinics is covered in *MEDLINE/PubMed (Index Medicus), Current Contents/Clinical Medicine, EMBASE/Excerpta Medica,* and *ISI/BIOMED.*

Contributors

CONSULTING EDITOR

KEVIN C. CHUNG, MD, MS
Chief of Hand Surgery, University of Michigan
Health System, Charles B.G. De Nancrede
Professor of Plastic Surgery and Orthopaedic
Surgery, Assistant Dean for Faculty Affairs,
Associate Director of Global REACH,
University of Michigan Medical School,
Ann Arbor, Michigan

EDITORS

JASON H. KO, MD
Assistant Professor, Division of Plastic and
Reconstructive Surgery, Department of
Orthopedic Surgery, Northwestern
University Feinberg School of Medicine,
Chicago, Illinois

BENJAMIN LEVI, MD
Director, Burn/Wound and Regenerative
Medicine Laboratory, Director, Burn
Reconstructive Program, Associate Director
of Burn Surgery, Section of Plastic Surgery,
Assistant Professor, Department of
Surgery, University of Michigan Health
System, University of Michigan, Ann Arbor,
Michigan

AUTHORS

SHAILESH AGARWAL, MD
Section of Plastic Surgery, University of
Michigan, Ann Arbor, Michigan

TANYA BERENZ, MS, OTR/L
Occupational Therapist, Occupational Therapy
Division, Department of Physical Medicine and
Rehabilitation, University of Michigan Health
System, Ann Arbor, Michigan

MILES BICHANICH, BS
Division of Plastic and Reconstructive Surgery,
Washington University School of Medicine,
St Louis, Missouri

MATTHEW BROWN, MD
Division of Plastic Surgery, Department of
Surgery, University of Michigan, Ann Arbor,
Michigan

REUBEN A. BUENO Jr, MD
Chief of Pediatric Plastic Surgery, Department
of Plastic Surgery, Plastic Surgery Residency
Program Director, Monroe Carell, Jr. Children's
Hospital, Vanderbilt University Medical Center,
Nashville, Tennessee

RYAN P. CAULEY, MD, MPH
Resident, Harvard Plastic Surgery Residency
Program, Division of Plastic and
Reconstructive Surgery, Massachusetts
General Hospital, Harvard Medical School,
Boston, Massachusetts

CURTIS L. CETRULO Jr, MD
Assistant Professor of Surgery, Attending
Plastic and Reconstructive Plastic Surgeon,
Division of Plastic Surgery, Massachusetts
General Hospital, Harvard Medical School,
Boston, Massachusetts

DAVID CHOLOK, BS
Section of Plastic and Reconstructive Surgery,
Department of Surgery, University of Michigan,
Ann Arbor, Michigan

KEVIN C. CHUNG, MD, MS
Chief of Hand Surgery, University of Michigan
Health System, Charles B.G. De Nancrede
Professor of Plastic Surgery and Orthopaedic
Surgery, Assistant Dean for Faculty Affairs,
Associate Director of Global REACH,
University of Michigan Medical School,
Ann Arbor, Michigan

DANIEL S. CORLEW, MD, MPH
Formerly CMO, Resurge International,
Sunnyvale, California; CMO, St Thomas
Rutherford Hospital, Murfreesboro, Tennessee

MAURICIO DE LA GARZA, MD
Plastic Surgery Resident, The Institute for
Plastic Surgery, Southern Illinois University,
Springfield, Illinois

MATTHIAS B. DONELAN, MD
Visiting Surgeon, Division of Plastic and
Reconstructive Surgery, Massachusetts
General Hospital, Associate Clinical Professor
of Surgery, Harvard Medical School, Chief of
Staff, Plastic and Reconstructive Surgery,
Shriners Hospital for Children, Boston,
Massachusetts

KYLE R. EBERLIN, MD
Plastic and Reconstructive Surgery, Shriners
Hospital for Children, Assistant Professor of
Surgery, Associate Director, MGH Hand
Surgery Fellowship, Division of Plastic and
Reconstructive Surgery, Massachusetts
General Hospital, Harvard Medical School,
Boston, Massachusetts

GERMANN GÜNTER, MD, PhD
Professor, Department of Hand, Plastic, and
Reconstructive Surgery, Department of Plastic
and Hand Surgery, Burn Center, BG Trauma
Center Ludwigshafen, Plastic and Hand
Surgery, University of Heidelberg,
Ludwigshafen, Germany

LAWRENCE J. GOTTLIEB, MD, FACS
Professor of Surgery, Director of the Burn and
Complex Wound Center, The University of
Chicago Medicine, Chicago, Illinois

DOUGLAS P. HANEL, MD
Professor, Hand and Upper Extremity Surgery,
Department of Orthopedic Surgery,
Harborview Medical Center, University of
Washington, Seattle, Washington

LYDIA A. HELLIWELL, MD
Hand Surgery Fellow, Division of Plastic and
Reconstructive Surgery, Massachusetts
General Hospital, Harvard Medical School,
Boston, Massachusetts

DAVID N. HERNDON, MD, FACS
Director of Burn Services, Professor of Surgery
and Pediatrics, Jesse H Jones Distinguished
Chair in Surgery, University of Texas Medical
Branch, Chief of Staff and Director of
Research, Shriners Hospital for Children,
Galveston, Texas

SHEPARD P. JOHNSON, MBBS
Resident, Department of Surgery, Saint Joseph
Mercy Ann Arbor, Ypsilanti, Michigan

JASON H. KO, MD
Assistant Professor, Division of Plastic and
Reconstructive Surgery, Department of
Orthopedic Surgery, Northwestern University
Feinberg School of Medicine, Chicago, Illinois

PETER O. KWAN, BScE, MD, PhD, FRCSC
Assistant Professor, Department of Surgery,
University of Alberta, Edmonton, Alberta,
Canada

BENJAMIN LEVI, MD
Director, Burn/Wound and Regenerative
Medicine Laboratory, Director, Burn
Reconstructive Program, Associate Director of
Burn Surgery, Section of Plastic Surgery,
Assistant Professor, Department of Surgery,
University of Michigan Health System,
University of Michigan, Ann Arbor, Michigan

SHAWN LODER, BS
Section of Plastic Surgery, University of
Michigan, Ann Arbor, Michigan

MARY CLAIRE MANSKE, MD
Fellow, Hand and Microvascular Surgery,
Department of Orthopedic Surgery,
Harborview Medical Center, University of
Washington, Seattle, Washington

K.A. KELLY McQUEEN, MD, MPH
Professor, Departments of Anesthesiology and
Surgery, Director, Vanderbilt Global
Anesthesia Fellowship, Director, Vanderbilt
Anesthesia Global Health and Development,
Affiliate Faculty, Vanderbilt Institute for Global
Health, Vanderbilt University Medical Center,
Nashville, Tennessee

AMY M. MOORE, MD
Assistant Professor of Surgery, Chief–Hand
Surgery and Trauma, Program Director–Hand
Fellowship, Division of Plastic and
Reconstructive Surgery, Washington
University School of Medicine, St Louis,
Missouri

MICHAEL W. NEUMEISTER, MD
Chair of the Department of Surgery, Chief of
Plastic Surgery, The Institute for Plastic
Surgery, Southern Illinois University,
Springfield, Illinois

WILLIAM B. NORBURY, MD, FRCS(Plast)
Assistant Professor, University of Texas
Medical Branch, Staff Surgeon, Shriners
Hospital for Children, Galveston, Texas

TAM N. PHAM, MD, FACS
Associate Professor, Department of Surgery,
Associate Director, UW Burn Center,
Harborview Medical Center, University of
Washington School of Medicine, University of
Washington, Seattle, Washington

ROBERT C. RUSSELL, MD
Clinical Professor of Plastic Surgery, Heartland
Plastic Surgery Center, Springfield, Illinois

IAN C. SANDO, MD
Section of Plastic Surgery, Department of
Surgery, The University of Michigan Health
System, Ann Arbor, Michigan

MICHAEL SAUERBIER, MD, PhD
Chair, Department of Hand, Plastic, and
Reconstructive Surgery, Burn Center, BG
Trauma Center Ludwigshafen, Plastic and
Hand Surgery, University of Heidelberg,
Ludwigshafen; Department of Plastic and
Hand Surgery, Burn Center, BG Trauma
Center, Frankfurt am Main, Germany

KETAN SHARMA, MD, MPH
Division of Plastic and Reconstructive Surgery,
Washington University School of Medicine,
St Louis, Missouri

DEANA S. SHENAQ, MD
Plastic & Reconstructive Surgery Chief
Resident, The University of Chicago Medicine,
Chicago, Illinois

ASHWIN SONI, MD
Plastic and Reconstructive Surgery Resident,
Division of Plastic Surgery, Department
of Surgery, Harborview Medical
Center, University of Washington, Seattle,
Washington

MICHAEL SORKIN, MD
Section of Plastic and Reconstructive Surgery,
Department of Surgery, University of Michigan,
Ann Arbor, Michigan

EDWARD E. TREDGET, MD, MSc, FRCSC
Professor, Department of Surgery, University
of Alberta, Edmonton, Alberta, Canada

TIFFANY WILLIAMS, MS, OTR/L
Trauma Burn Clinical Specialist, Occupational
Therapy Division, Department of Physical
Medicine and Rehabilitation, University
of Michigan Health System, Ann Arbor,
Michigan

Contents

The hand is extremely susceptible to burn injuries, and hand burns can occur in up to 90% of all major burns. A thorough neurovascular examination of the hand should be performed in the acute setting. Escharotomies are required in patients with full-thickness or circumferential burns, when perfusion of the upper extremity is compromised. The decision for excision and grafting is based on whether the wound will heal in the first 2 to 3 weeks after the burn injury. Acute care and resuscitation are always importance in this patient population; subsequent care leads to optimal hand functionality and cosmetic long-term outcomes.

Worldwide, approximately 500,000 children are admitted to the hospital with burn injuries every year. Referral to an accredited burn center is required for burns that involve the hand regardless of age. As with most burn injuries, a multidisciplinary approach is important; however, in the younger pediatric patient, extra resources such as child life services, pediatric psychotherapy, and music therapy all play major roles alongside the nurse, physical therapists, and psychiatrists so that together with the appropriate support for the family involved, a successful outcome can be achieved.

 Video content accompanies this article at www.hand.theclinics.com.

Upper extremity electrical injuries present with unique pathophysiologic considerations due to the differing mechanisms of injury produced by the electromagnetic field. The initial phase of treatment consists of recognition of other life-threatening injuries, stabilization of patients, and multisystem resuscitation. The second phase of treatment consists of excising devitalized tissue, appropriate wound care to prevent delayed infection, providing temporary and definitive coverage over vital structures, and preventing contracture and joint stiffness via aggressive therapy. The final phase of treatment consists of sensorimotor functional reconstruction via nerve grafting and tendon transfers available based on patients' deficits and available redundant sources.

New treatments of frostbite have led to unprecedented salvage of extremities including fingers and toes. Success is predicated on prompt institution of time-sensitive protocols initiated soon after rewarming, particularly the use of thombolytics. Unfortunately, in the urban setting, most patients are not candidates for these treatment modalities. Triple-phase bone scans have allowed for early determination of devitalized parts that need amputation. Reconstructive surgical techniques are typically used to salvage limb length in these devastating injuries.

The hand is commonly affected in burn injuries. Joints and extensor tendons are vulnerable given their superficial location. Durable coverage that permits relative frictionless tendon gliding and minimizes scar contracture is required to optimize functional outcomes. When soft tissue donor sites are limited, the use of dermal skin substitutes provides stable coverage with minimal scarring, good mobility, and acceptable appearance. A comprehensive review of dermal skin substitutes and their use with burn reconstruction of the hand is provided.

Hypertrophic scar and contracture in burn patients is a complex process. Contributing factors include critical injury depth and activation of key cell subpopulations, including deep dermal fibroblasts, myofibroblasts, fibrocytes, and T-helper cells, which cause scarring rather than regeneration. These cells influence each other via cellular profibrotic and antifibrotic signals, which help to determine the outcome. These cells also both modify and interact with extracellular matrix of the wound, ultimately forming hypertrophic scar. Current treatments reduce hypertrophic scar formation or improve remodeling by targeting these pathways and signals.

Upper extremity burns can result in lifelong complications. A comprehensive occupational therapy program is imperative for restoration of arm function. Edema management, splinting, exercise, scar management, and activities of daily living are key treatment elements to achieve optimal postburn outcomes. Proper patient and family education are essential for therapeutic success. Burn recovery requires a commitment to therapeutic techniques that can progress a patient to their maximal independence.

Burn injury can result in hypertrophic scar formation that can lead to debilitating functional deficits and poor aesthetic outcomes. Although nonoperative modalities in the early phase of scar maturation are critical to minimize hypertrophic scar formation, surgical management is often indicated to restore hand function. The essential tenant of operative scar management is release of tension, which can often be achieved through local tissue rearrangement. Laser therapy has emerged as a central pillar of subsequent scar rehabilitation. These treatment tools provide an effective resource for the reconstructive surgeon to treat hypertrophic hand scars.

Postburn contractures are a common occurrence after severe burn injuries. It is important to understand the pathologic condition and anatomy of specific postburn deformities in order to provide comprehensive surgical care. Postburn contractures can result in a flexion contracture, boutonniere deformity, burn syndactyly, metacarpophalangeal extension contracture, wrist contracture, or claw hand. A patient evaluation is performed before proceeding to the operating room. Surgery sequences require proper incision design, release of the skin, and deeper contracted structures and coverage with an appropriate flap or graft. Postoperative splinting, scar care, and therapy are equally important for a successful outcome.

and rigid contractures may develop that prohibit basic functions of daily living and are often refractory to nonoperative intervention. Surgical intervention is aimed at releasing or excising all pathologic anatomy limiting elbow motion. In patients with proper indications, surgical intervention can result in substantial improvement in elbow motion, allowing patients to return to activities of daily living, employment, and recreational activities.

Accurately assessing function and disability after hand burns is imperative to improving the management of patients. The biological, social, and psychological impact of these injuries should be considered. The International Classification of Functioning Disability (ICF) and Health Core Sets for Hand Conditions provides a guide to what should be measured and reported. Although many outcomes measures instruments are available to assess patients with hand or burn injuries, few are validated in the subpopulation of hand burns. Further efforts are required to investigate the ability of current assessment instruments to evaluate hand burn outcomes within the ICF framework.

Measuring the extent and impact of a health problem is key to being able to address it appropriately. This review uses available information within the framework of the Global Burden of Disease studies to estimate the disease burden due to burn injuries of the hands. The GBD indicates that since 1990 there has been an approximately 30% decrease in the disease burden related to burn injuries. The GBD methods have not been applied specifically to hand burns, but from available data, it is estimated that about 18 million people in the world suffer from sequelae of burns to the hands.

HAND CLINICS

RELATED INTEREST

Critical Care Clinics, October 2016 (Vol. 32, No. 4)
Burn Resuscitation
Kevin N. Foster and Daniel M. Caruso, *Editors*
Available at: http://www.criticalcare.theclinics.com/

THE CLINICS ARE AVAILABLE ONLINE!
Access your subscription at:
www.theclinics.com

Preface

Optimizing the Treatment of Burn Injuries of the Upper Extremity

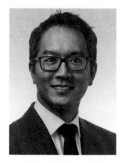 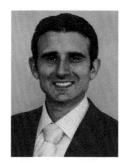

Jason H. Ko, MD   Benjamin Levi, MD

Editors

The current state of burn surgery derives from the vast array of caregivers and researchers who dedicate their lives to improving the outcomes of patients with these devastating and disfiguring injuries. Burn surgery requires a multidisciplinary approach to the patient, so it is only natural that the authors of this issue come from a broad spectrum of expertise, including burn surgeons, hand and upper extremity surgeons, general surgeons, plastic surgeons, scientists, and therapists.

Despite a decrease in large burns in the United States, burn injuries remain a substantial clinical challenge worldwide. In addition, as critical care continues to improve, there are a greater number of patients surviving large burn injuries than previously, thereby increasing the number of burn patients requiring complex reconstruction. One of the most functionally challenging areas of burn care is the treatment and reconstruction of hand and upper extremity burns. Our hands are essential for activities of daily living (and most other activities), and burn injuries to an area of the body that we use constantly can have devastating consequences. Advances in burn care have helped to improve not only the functional outcomes but also the appearance of patients who have survived burn injuries. Burn treatment can range from nonoperative therapy and scar manipulation to complex microsurgical reconstruction, and each technique is a powerful tool to help patients regain and restore function of their upper extremity.

When asked to construct this issue of *Hand Clinics* on "Burns," we strived to create a comprehensive issue on the care and surgery of the burned upper extremity. We were fortunate to have assembled an outstanding group of authors, who have expertly reviewed the core principles and practices of burn injury, including fundamentals of scar biology, nonsurgical therapy, scar rehabilitation, and operative management of conditions caused by burn injuries to the upper extremity.

We are grateful for the incredible contributions and mentorship of esteemed colleagues and friends, who have sacrificed significant time and energy to create a body of work that is both educational and inspiring. We hope that this combined effort by authors and editors provides important insights to expand your knowledge, while encouraging you to continuously improve and innovate in the care of patients with burn injuries.

Jason H. Ko, MD
Northwestern University Feinberg School of Medicine
675 North Saint Clair Street
Suite 19-250
Chicago, IL 60611, USA

Benjamin Levi, MD
University of Michigan
1500 East Medical Center Drive
Tabuman Center 2130
Ann Arbor, MI 48109, USA

E-mail addresses:
Jason.ko@nm.org (J.H. Ko)
blevi@umich.edu (B. Levi)

Hand Clin 33 (2017) xiii
http://dx.doi.org/10.1016/j.hcl.2017.02.001
0749-0712/17/© 2017 Published by Elsevier Inc.

Acute Management of Hand Burns

Ashwin Soni, MD[a], Tam N. Pham, MD[b], Jason H. Ko, MD[c],*

KEYWORDS

- Hand burns • Acute • Wound management • Burn excision • Skin grafting

KEY POINTS

- The hand is extremely susceptible to burn injuries, and it is imperative that one understands the acute management of these burns.
- If perfusion of the upper extremity is compromised, escharotomies or fasciotomies may be required.
- Excision and grafting are often required; the decision often depends on whether the wound will heal in the first 2 to 3 weeks after the burn injury.

INTRODUCTION

The hand is extremely susceptible to burn injuries, and hand burns can occur in approximately up to 90% of all major burns.[1] Burns to the hand can significantly affect one's functional status, as well as quality of life.[2] Thus, the acute management of hand burns is becoming increasingly important; multiple studies have been published to demonstrate the critical nature of early aggressive management with regard to achieving more optimal functional outcomes.[1,3] Restoration and preservation of function is imperative, as well as recognizing the aesthetic components of the hand.[4] For hand burns, admission to a high-volume burn center involving a multidisciplinary team approach is crucial to hand burn management. The multidisciplinary team includes, but is not limited to, burn surgeons, plastic surgeons, nurse practitioners, burn nurses, psychologists, occupational therapists, and physical therapists.

INITIAL EVALUATION OF THE PATIENT

When a patient is admitted to the emergency department, the initial management is implementing the primary survey; ensuring that the patient is stable and that their airway is secure; and guiding fluid resuscitation. One must follow the Advanced Burn Life Support protocols to guide immediate management.[5] Patients with significant hand burns should be transferred to a high-volume burn center to better, and more effectively, manage these more complex upper extremity burns. Hand burns are one of the criteria for referral to a specialized burn facility per the Advanced Burn Life Support Manual.[5] Recognizing that many providers from multiple specialties are often called on to evaluate acute burn injuries, including hand burns, our center has created a video library of resources for providers and patients in the initial assessment, triage, and management of burns.[6]

Disclosure: No relevant disclosures.
[a] Division of Plastic Surgery, Department of Surgery, 7CT70 Harborview Medical Center, University of Washington, 325 9th Avenue, Mailstop #359796, Seattle, WA 98104, USA; [b] Department of Surgery, UW Burn Center, 7CT70 Harborview Medical Center, University of Washington School of Medicine, University of Washington, 325 9th Avenue, Box #359796, Seattle, WA 98104, USA; [c] Division of Plastic and Reconstructive Surgery, Northwestern University Feinberg School of Medicine, 675 North Saint Clair Street, Suite 19-250, Chicago, IL 60611, USA
* Corresponding author.
E-mail address: Jason.ko@nm.org

Hand Clin 33 (2017) 229–236
http://dx.doi.org/10.1016/j.hcl.2016.12.001
0749-0712/17/© 2016 Elsevier Inc. All rights reserved.

Physical examination should be performed during the initial evaluation to estimate the area of the burn, determine the depth of the injury, and evaluate whether or not there is vascular compromise in the upper extremity, along with the extent of the burn. More extensive, high-risk burns include circumferential burns, electrical burns, chemical burns, and crush injuries, which can lead to a compromise in the vascular supply of the upper extremity (**Table 1**).

On examination, one should perform a thorough vascular examination looking specifically for diminished peripheral pulses, slow capillary refill time (normal is less than or equal to 2–3 seconds), decreased skin sensation, and skin that is cool to the touch, which all may suggest vascular compromise. It is also essential to predict burn depth with regard to the thickness of the burn, which can be challenging in acute hand burns,[4] because full-thickness burns can lead to vascular compromise to the hand and digits (**Figs. 1 and 2**). Examination should also involve the use of the Doppler ultrasound probe to elicit where signals are identified in the upper extremity, as well as whether or not there is a change in the pulse in the acute setting. The radial artery, ulnar artery, palmar arch, and digital artery pulses should be checked every hour from the time of admission to detect any change indicating the need for timely escharotomies.[7] However, this practice should not delay surgical management if a compartment syndrome is suspected or if an escharotomy is needed.[8]

A comprehensive history should be elicited from the patient when time permits, which should include the nature and mechanism of injury, hand dominance, patient occupation, and preexisting upper extremity injury. The duration of contact and temperature can determine the depth of tissue damage that the patient sustains.[5]

ESCHAROTOMY

The relationship between extremity burns and the ability to obstruct circulation has been well-knows since the early 1950s. The use of escharotomy for constricting upper extremity burns has been recommended as early as 1951 by Blocker and Moyer.[8,9]

Escharotomies are required in patients with full-thickness or circumferential burns, before vascular compromise. Eschar forms in full-thickness burns when the depth involves both the epidermis and dermis skin layers, producing coagulated, thickened dead skin, known as eschar. This eschar formation leads to an increase in the pressure within the tissue compartments and thus needs to be released. Edema formation also occurs secondary to burn injuries

Table 1
Common mechanisms of acute hand burns and important aspects of their evaluation and management

Mechanism of Hand Burn Injury	Common Age Group, Patient Population	Common Injury Locations	Key Points in Initial Evaluation	Potential Sequelae
Contact with hot surface	Toddlers, at "cruising age"	Volar fingers and palm	Depth of injury	Fingers and palmar contractures
Friction burn	Toddler, children <10 y of age; Adult in MVC or MCC	Volar fingers and palm in treadmill injury	Depth of injury, exposed tendons	Contractures
Electrical burn	Adult worker, more commonly in males	Contact points on fingers, web spaces, palm, and wrists	Assess neurovascular function	Missed compartment syndrome, delayed neurologic symptoms
Grease burn	Adult, cooking in the kitchen	Predominantly dorsal hand	Often difficult to distinguish deep partial thickness from full-thickness	Scarring, decreased hand function
Chemical burn	Adult	Volar or dorsal hand/fingers	Brush off powder, irrigate copiously with water and check pH using litmus paper	Poor healing, chronic wounds, skin sensitivity

Abbreviations: MCC, motor cycle crash; MVC, motor vehicle collision.

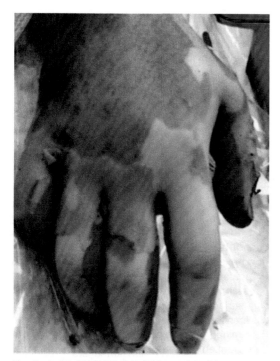

Fig. 1. A third-degree full-thickness hand burn exemplifying the many variations of colors of this degree of hand burn.

and resuscitation, and can also lead to a build up of pressure within fascial compartments of the extremities, resulting in a lack of adequate perfusion. These situations may also necessitate a fasciotomy, depending on the clinical situation.

An escharotomy can be performed at the bedside under sterile conditions with electrocautery or a scalpel, and involves making a full-thickness incision through the eschar to release the pressure within the burned tissues. Care must be taken not to injure underlying structures[4] (**Fig. 3**). The purpose of the escharotomy is to not only release the pressure and allow the tissue compartments to expand, but also to return vascular supply to the hand in a case of compromise. The escharotomy incision does not go through to subcutaneous tissue below, but only through the eschar. The use of digital escharotomies is debated, but can be performed selectively in cases where distal finger perfusion is a concern.[10] The important thing to note here is that one must be mindful not to injure the neurovascular bundles, where the digital nerves and vessels run, when performing this procedure. Midlateral or midaxial incisions will effectively

Fig. 2. A likely fourth-degree burn from contact with electrified wire. This photograph highlights the importance of a thorough hand examination, because it is key to assessing hand and finger neurovascular function on admission.

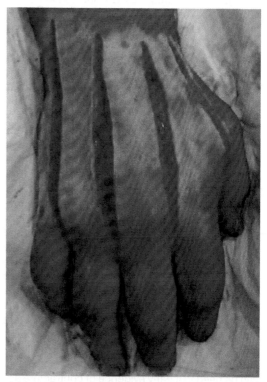

Fig. 3. Escharotomies on the dorsal aspect of the hand in the intermetacarpal spaces. (*From* Sterling J, Gibran NS, Klein MB. Acute management of hand burns. Hand Clin 2009;25(4):455; with permission.)

decompress the fingers while avoiding potential neurovascular compromise.

Fasciotomies are required in cases of electrical injuries or circumferential burns, when a patient has a likely compartment syndrome. In these select cases, fasciotomies are performed with both dorsal and volar incisions to release the pressure within the tissue compartments. At our center, we often perform a prophylactic carpal tunnel release at the time of the fasciotomy and close that skin incision primarily to protect the median nerve.

WOUND MANAGEMENT AT PRESENTATION

Initially, after admission, the burn wounds should be cleaned and debrided to remove any foreign bodies from the wound, in addition to any large, loose blisters that are present. Our center's practice is to completely unroof blisters that are 2 cm or greater, and to aspirate any blisters that are smaller. Once these blisters have been removed, an antibiotic ointment is most commonly applied to the wound. Although silver sulfadiazine has been traditionally the most frequently used topical agent used in the acute burn wounds, many other options exist today. Some are silver-impregnated dressings that do not require daily dressing changes. Other dressings do not contain silver, and are most appropriate in shallow, partial thickness wounds when broad-spectrum antimicrobial activity is not required. For more superficial burns, xeroform and bacitracin can be effective, inexpensive, and allow for more frequent hand washing.[11,12] The advantages of silver sulfadiazine include its antibacterial properties, cost effectiveness, and widespread availability.[13] Small, intact blisters can be left in place if they do not limit the functional ability of the hand.[14] The main goals of all burn dressings and wound care are to prevent infection, decrease fluid loss, and allow reepithelialization.[4,15]

The main goal for hand burn wound management is the ability for patients to participate in early mobilization and hand therapy. Thus, ideal wound care is simple enough to permit the hand to have full passive and active range of motion and to enable stretching at the digits, thumb, palm, and wrist. In all patients, aggressive hand therapy should be initiated to minimize edema and the risk of developing contractures.[11] By prioritizing function, it is important to wrap fingers individually, for instance, so that dressings themselves facilitate instead of limit patient movement. Splinting can be needed if early evidence of contracture appears, or when therapy is not performed sufficiently, with splinting predominantly being used at bedtime.[11]

EXCISION AND GRAFTING OF HAND BURNS

Surgical management for hand burns is often required; however, the timing of this is very much surgeon and center dependent. Initially, conservative management and local wound care are used until the wound demarcates itself to determine what is required surgically. The decision for excision and grafting is based on whether the wound will definitively heal in the first 2 to 3 weeks after the burn injury. In full-thickness burns, when excision will be required, surgical management will be pursued earlier with grafting to follow excision.[11] On the volar hand and fingers, however, a delayed grafting strategy is often prudent given that the specialized function of glabrous skin cannot be replaced adequately by a skin graft. A good example of this strategy is commonly used in pediatric palm burns, where we often wait 1 month to maximize the healing potential of volar skin surfaces (see Long-Term Outcomes).

When the timing of surgical intervention has been determined and the patient is stable, then the patient is taken to the operating room for excision of the hand burn wounds and subsequent grafting. Tourniquets are applied to the upper extremity to minimize the amount of blood lost during excision. A goulian (also known as a weck) blade is used to excise the skin from the hand, occasionally with the use of the Versajet (Smith & Nephew, London, United Kingdom) hydrosurgery system, in areas such as web spaces of the hand. Care must be taken over the hands to not expose underlying structures, including tendons or joints. The use of epinephrine-soaked (concentration 1:10,000) Telfa dressings are used and applied to the wound bed for several minutes, to achieve adequate hemostasis, with an overlying pressure dressing applied. Lap pads or Kerlix are then also soaked in the epinephrine, and placed on top to create the pressure dressing over the wound. Electrocautery is used for any punctate bleeding, and fibrin sealant is often used. Occasionally, burn wounds need multiple debridements before the wound bed is ready for a skin graft. A temporary measure in the form of a skin substitute, such as a xenograft or allograft, can be applied after debridement, allowing the surgeon to test whether the wound bed is ready for definitive skin grafting. If a patient is very edematous—for example, in a patient with a large total body surface area burn—temporizing skin substitutes can also play a role. Once adequate debridement of the wound bed has been performed, and the bed is ready for a graft, then the decision as to what type of graft needs to be made.

Owing to the improved aesthetic appearance, as well as better function and durability, sheet grafts are typically performed in cases of hand and wrist burns and should be considered the standard of care given the cosmetic benefit. Full-thickness grafts in acute hand burns have demonstrated a reduction in the rate of postburn contractures in this patient population.[16] The importance of individualizing each case regarding what type of graft to use should not be underestimated. Factors that should be considered include the size and location of the hand burn, the age and clinical status of the patient, and whether or not there is a paucity of donor sites.[17] At our center, the preferred donor site is the anterolateral thigh given the ease of access in the operating room, the ability for one team to debride the hand while the other team harvests the skin graft, the ability to hide the scar under clothing such as shorts or a skirt, and less discomfort when sitting or lying down compared with posteriorly located donor sites. In younger children, we attempt to use the buttocks, with care taken to ensure that harvest occurs within the confined area of a diaper.

The skin is then harvested using a dermatome, with adequate tension being applied longitudinally and horizontally, to maintain a smooth and even skin graft harvest. Tumescence with 1:1,000,000 epinephrine can also be used to help create more flap donor site and to minimize blood loss. Split-thickness sheet grafts should be harvested slightly thicker than grafts for other sites to maintain durability and elasticity for hand burns. A prospective trial comparing thick versus standard split-thickness skin grafts was performed in 2001 by Mann and colleagues[17] demonstrating no difference in function or patient satisfaction with full-thickness skin grafts. Full-thickness skin grafts can be performed in cases of palm burns or burns in the web spaces, with donor sites in the flank or inguinal crease, because these can be closed easily and primarily. However, there is some debate as to whether the web spaces can be spared to avoid subsequent webbing between digits (see Long-Term Outcomes).

Once the graft has been harvested, it should then be applied to the wound bed and can be affixed to the wound in several ways. The surgeon may choose to place a few absorbable sutures at the corners to affix the graft to the wound bed, and then aerosolized fibrin sealant can be sprayed onto the graft to keep it in place. We also reinforce the edges of the graft with commercially available specialized tape (**Fig. 4**). This type of tape has been shown to help with hemostasis, and reduce the risk of lateral shearing stress, as well as making it easier for dressing changes and reducing operating time as surgeons can avoid placing sutures

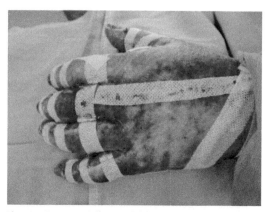

Fig. 4. Commercially available specialized tape fixation reinforcing the skin graft to the hand and digits.

all around the graft.[18] In addition, nonadherent material should be placed over the graft itself, with application of a conforming wrap and resting splint. Grafting should always be performed with the hand in that same position as it will be during postoperative immobilization, and grafts should be inset with the wound bed on maximal stretch. For example, one should place the thumb–index web space as widely as possible to minimize contracture, because this is a common site for this to occur. Grafting the dorsal fingers in slight flexion maximizes the length of graft placed on the wounds, reduces potential for contractures, and helps with postoperative hand therapy. Conversely, grafting the volar fingers and palm in maximal extension will help to minimize scar contractures volarly. When the patient is still anesthetized, we wrap and apply custom-made hand splints to immobilize the grafted hand in the same position to avoid graft dislodgement or shearing.

When sheet grafts are applied, we remove dressings on postoperative day 1 to inspect and examine the graft for underlying seromas or hematomas, which can impair adherence of the graft. We use an #11 blade at the bedside to evacuate any fluid collections that are present to prevent graft loss. If collections are minimal, dressings are reapplied until postoperative day 5, when the graft can then be assessed for graft take and to examine how well it adheres to the wound bed. If the collections underlying the graft on postoperative day 1 are larger, then one would need to inspect the graft in between postoperative day 1 and 5. At postoperative day 5, we then typically apply a lighter dressing and a layer of xeroform and bacitracin overlying the graft so that the graft does not adhere to the overlying dressings. Coban (3M, St Paul, MN), a form of elastic pressure dressing, can be applied if postoperative swelling is present. Hand therapy in the form of active and passive motion should be initiated as early as possible in the healing period, in conjunction with the physical and occupational therapists. At our center, we assess that most grafts are ready for mobilization by postoperative day 3, and progressively increase the range of motion day by day as tolerated by the patient.

Regarding postoperative dressings for the donor site, a number of dressing choices are available; the donor site will heal as a partial-thickness dermal injury. Most recently, we have used silver-impregnated dressings to be left in place for 1 to 2 weeks to permit healing underneath. Mepilex Ag (Mölnlycke Healthcare, Gothenburg, Sweden) is our current dressing of choice. It is a silver sulfate dressing shown to reduce significantly biofilm formation compared with a positive control and, as the literature has demonstrated, biofilm formation is a major contributor to wound colonization and subsequent infection.[19] These dressings should be left in place for approximately 1 to 2 weeks; however, there are other silver-impregnated dressings that lift at the dry edges as the wound bed epithelializes and can be trimmed circumferentially until the donor site healing is complete. For buttock donor sites in infants, silver sulfadiazine can be applied directly into the diaper without a dressing and reapplied after each soiling.

DEEP HAND BURNS AND RECONSTRUCTION

The hand contains relatively thin soft tissue coverage; therefore, any deeper full-thickness hand burns can result in exposed tendons, bones, and neurovascular structures. In these cases, skin grafts are unable to be used because they will not survive if there are exposed "white" structures; thus, flap reconstructive surgery may be necessary. If the burns are deep enough to cause extensor tendon loss, then Kirschner wires (K-wires) can be placed at the time of soft tissue coverage to stabilize the fingers in extension, because these patients will go on to develop severe flexion contractures. This K-wire pinning is useful to prevent subsequent contractures reducing the degree of interphalangeal joint contracture.[10,20] The small finger is especially prone to contracture that is extremely difficult to correct secondarily and, thus, early K-wire fixation can be crucial. This method also allows the patient to start hand therapy with a stable and functionally positioned hand. Early splinting should be used in these deep hand burn cases, with the hand often being maintained in an intrinsic plus position. This position, known as the "safe splinting position," allows for maximal

recovery and less stiffness. In many cases, we work with our therapists to optimize the position of splinting depending on the specific injury pattern.

The type of acute reconstruction depends on the extent and location of the burn injury, as well as the depth of the burn. If a flap donor site is from the ipsilateral upper extremity—for example, a radial forearm fascia or fasciocutaneous flap—it is important to perform an Allen's test to ensure patency of the palmar arch from the ulnar and radial arteries to the hand. Pedicled, tubed flaps can also be taken from the chest, abdomen, flank, or groin if available. The hand and/or digits can be placed under the raised flap at the subfascial level for around 2 to 3 weeks (Crane principle). Subsequently, division of this flap is performed. Alternatively, a free microvascular tissue transfer can also be performed if a local tissue flap is unable to be used in a case of extensive burns. The ideal flap characteristics in this situation would provide a thin, contoured, pliable, and durable coverage for the hand injures. There are many options that can include the contralateral radial forearm flap and the anterolateral thigh flap. Many flap reconstruction procedures will need secondary revisional procedures, including flap debulking, to improve on the contour deformities as a result of thick and bulky flaps. This topic is covered in more extensive detail in Ryan P. Cauley and colleagues' article, "Reconstruction of the Adult and Pediatric Burned Hand," and Mauricio De la Garza and colleagues' article, "Microsurgical Reconstruction of the Burned Hand and Upper Extremity," in this issue.

AMPUTATION

In certain cases of severe hand burns, the extent of burn injury and options regarding management should be evaluated carefully. Realistic and functional expectations should be discussed with the patient, and an assessment of tendon, bone, joint, and neurovascular injury should be performed.

Amputations of digits or the hand are rarely emergent, and time is given to continue to reassess the wound to determine where there is any chance of deep tissue viability and whether or not flap reconstruction in these cases is necessary. Occasionally, the extent of the injury is not salvageable with reconstruction and in these cases amputation must be discussed with the patient, if that is the best option once the tissue viability has declared itself. Deep thermal burns can cause damage to the digital arteries, and this subsequent necrosis may extend deeper than first thought, which can lead to an amputation being warranted.[10] Functional outcome is the overall goal, and if a patient is left with an insensate or immobile digit, then an amputation may be the more optimal choice.

LONG-TERM OUTCOMES

Long-term outcomes can sometimes be foreseen or predicted regarding the hand and digits. A few observations that we have seen in our own practice are stated herein. For deep pediatric palm burns, an option is nonoperative management for the first 3 or more weeks allowing the palm burn wounds to heal without the need for excision and grafting. Sensation may be better after secondary healing than after grafting, and secondary healing maximizes preservation of the palmar–cutaneous ligaments, which provides soft tissue stability and are often excised during surgery. The concern for maintaining these cutaneous–fascial attachments and the Pacinian corpuscles that provide grip and tactile sensation has led to our approach to manage palm burns nonoperatively.[11] However, this management plan requires an emphasis on an aggressive therapy plan and possible extension splinting to maintain adequate range of motion and prevent contraction during the healing process.[11] At the 2- to 3-week mark, one should then assess the wound healing status and whether or not at this point, surgical intervention is warranted. If the wound shows evidence of granulation tissue formation rather than epithelialization, or if the hand has begun to contract in any way, then excision and grafting should be scheduled.

Postburn deformities, such as Boutonniere's deformity, can often be predicted. This deformity can occur after deep hand burns damage the central slip of the extensor apparatus of the digit, displacing the lateral bands as a result.[21] Attempts at grafting may lead to failure of graft adherence over the central slip of the extensor tendon, causing the Boutonniere deformity to result. Subsequent tendon reconstruction in addition to other soft tissue coverage options such as local versus free flaps may need to be considered in these cases when skin grafting is likely to fail.

Another long-term issue is webbing between the web spaces of individual digits after grafting. An option for this management is to spare the webs pace when grafting. Although cosmetically appealing during early healing, a graft over the web space often creates webbing between adjacent fingers. This represents a mild form of syndactyly that can impair independent finger flexion and extension. This restriction is bothersome to patients and may ultimately require release procedures a few months or years after the initial injury. The acute burn surgeon must balance the risk of webbing against delayed healing and hypertrophic scarring at the web space location.

SUMMARY

The management of burn injuries to the hand needs to be approached carefully and thoroughly. A multidisciplinary team is required at a burn center with the capabilities of proficiently managing this patient population. Algorithms and pathways can be in place at certain institutions; however, treatment should be tailored to the individual patient. One should distinguish when surgical intervention is and is not warranted and consider all the various options in a selective manner. The acute care and resuscitation is always of paramount importance in this patient population; however, subsequent attentive care will lead to optimal hand functionality and cosmetic long-term outcomes. This remains to be an area with a large scope for research and more prospective trials are required regarding both nonoperative and operative interventions.

ACKNOWLEDGMENTS

The authors sincerely thank the previous authors of the last edition of this article, Dr Sterling, Dr Gibran, and Dr Klein, as we have learned extensively from their expertise in this area of acute management of hand burns.

REFERENCES

1. Sheridan RL, Hurley J, Smith MA, et al. The acutely burned hand: management and outcome based on a ten-year experience with 1047 acute hand burns. J Trauma 1995;38(3):406–11.
2. Anzarut A, Chen M, Shankowsky H, et al. Quality-of-life and outcome predictors following massive burn injury. Plast Reconstr Surg 2005;116(3):791–7.
3. Kreymerman PA, Andres LA, Lucas HD, et al. Reconstruction of the burned hand. Plast Reconstr Surg 2011;127(2):752–9.
4. Pan BS, Vu AT, Yakuboff KP. Management of the acutely burned hand. J Hand Surg Am 2015;40(7):1477–84.
5. Advanced burn life support course, provider manual. Available at: https://evidencebasedpractice.osumc.edu/Documents/Guidelines/ABLSProviderManual_20101018.pdf.
6. Burn educational videos by UW surgery. Available at: https://www.youtube.com/playlist?list=PLFEMTIzjmLeUC-tONmpxadXa_7rusm_B6.

7. Cartotto R. The burned hand: optimizing long-term outcomes with a standardized approach to acute and subacute care. Clin Plast Surg 2005;32(4):515–27.

8. Saffle JR, Zeluff GR, Warden GD. Intramuscular pressure in the burned arm: measurement and response to escharotomy. Am J Surg 1980;140(6):825–31.

9. Pruitt BA Jr, Dowling JA, Moncrief JA. Escharotomy in early burn care. Arch Surg 1968;96(4):502–7.

10. Schulze SM, Weeks D, Choo J, et al. Amputation following hand escharotomy in patients with burn injury. Eplasty 2016;16:e13.

11. Scott JR, Costa BA, Gibran NS, et al. Pediatric palm contact burns: a ten-year review. J Burn Care Res 2008;29-4:614–8.

12. Yarboro DD. A comparative study of the dressings silver sulfadiazine and Aquacel Ag in the management of superficial partial-thickness burns. Adv Skin Wound Care 2013;26(6):259–62.

13. Heyneman A, Heoksema H, Vandekerckhove D, et al. The role of silver sulphadiazine in the conservative treatment of partial thickness burn wounds: a systematic review. Burns 2016;42(7):1377–86.

14. Sargent RL. Management of blisters in the partial-thickness burn: an integrative research review. J Burn Care Res 2006;27(1):66–81.

15. Greenhalgh DG. Topical antimicrobial agents for burn wounds. Clin Plast Surg 2009;36(4):597–606.

16. Chandrasegaram MD, Harvey J. Full-thickness vs split-skin grafting in pediatric hand burns – a 10-year review of 174 cases. J Burn Care Res 2009; 30(5):867–71.

17. Mann R, Gibran NS, Engrav LH, et al. Prospective trial of thick vs standard split-thickness skin grafts in burns of the hand. J Burn Care Rehabil 2001; 22(6):390–2.

18. Davey RB, Sparnon AL, Lodge M. Technique of split skin graft fixation using hypafix: a 15-year review. ANZ J Surg 2003;73(11):958–62.

19. Halstead FD, Rauf M, Bamford A, et al. Antimicrobial dressings: comparison of the ability of a panel of dressings to prevent biofilm formation by key burn wound pathogens. Burns 2015;41(8):1683–94.

20. Gurusinghe D, Bhandari S, Southern S. Interphalangeal joint K-wiring: a useful adjunct in the acute management of burn injuries to the hand and upper extremity. J Hand Surg Am 2011;36(4):751–2.

21. Grishkevich VM. Surgical treatment of postburn boutonniere deformity. Plast Reconstr Surg 1996; 97(1):126–32.

Management of Acute Pediatric Hand Burns

William B. Norbury, MD, FRCS(Plast)*, David N. Herndon, MD

KEYWORDS

- Pediatric • Hand • Burn • Escharotomy • Fasciotomy

KEY POINTS

- Determination of the burn depth and size is of the utmost importance at the initial examination once the patient has been stabilized from any other life-threatening injuries.
- The pathophysiology of hand burns can be subdivided into those primary effects related to the thermal effects of the injury; these are dependent on the time of contact and the temperature of the heat source involved, and the secondary effects of any ensuing edema, reduced circulation and infection.
- Treating physicians can help to improve any outcome by attenuating each of these effects by adhering to 5 principles: (1) preventing additional propagation of the burn to deeper structures, (2) rapid wound closure, (3) preservation of active and passive range of motion and maintaining elevation, (4) infection control, and (5) early active rehabilitation.

INTRODUCTION

The high frequency of hand burns seen in children is surely a function of their fearless, highly inquisitive nature and developing proprioceptive skills.[1] Within the United States burns are the fourth leading cause of emergency department visits among children less than 1 year of age and represent around 5% of deaths in all children, with a peak between the ages of 1 and 9 years.[2] Worldwide, approximately 500,000 children are admitted to the hospital with burn injuries every year.[3] Referral to an accredited burn center is required for burns that involve the hand regardless of age. As with most burn injuries, a multidisciplinary approach is important; however, in the younger pediatric patient, extra resources such as child life services, pediatric psychotherapy, and music therapy all play major roles alongside the nurse, physical therapists, and psychiatrists so that together with the appropriate support for the family involved, a successful outcome can be achieved.

ETIOLOGY

Whenever a child presents with an injury that does not match the history of the incident, a high degree of suspicion should be sustained and a referral made to social services. Most burns sustained by children are not under any nefarious circumstances; however, if there is any suspicion or further clarification of the details concerning the injury is required, then admission to the burns unit is required until that information is revealed. The reported incidence of nonaccidental injury burns varies wildly from 3.8% to 26%,[4,5] yet burns as a result of neglect outnumber those attributed to abuse to the tune of 9 to 1.[6] Typical patterns of injury that are suspicious include a specific line of demarcation on the forearm depicting a glove like pattern of burn (forced immersion injury), contact burns to the dorsum of the hand (from an iron), and small well-delineated burns on the dorsum of the hand (from a cigarette or lighter).

Most burns sustained by children are accidental; of these, scald burns are generally more

Department of Surgery, Shriners Hospital for Children, 815 Market Street, Suite 718, Galveston, TX 77550, USA
* Corresponding author.
E-mail address: wbnorbur@utmb.edu

Hand Clin 33 (2017) 237–242
http://dx.doi.org/10.1016/j.hcl.2016.12.002
0749-0712/17/© 2017 Elsevier Inc. All rights reserved.

hand.theclinics.com

common in the younger age group (<3 years of age), with flame burns becoming increasingly frequent as children get older. Contact burns to the palmar surface of the hand are common in the very young, as they may lean on hot surfaces (oven doors) while trying to maintain balance. Friction burns are increasingly common in the very young, as they may stumble and fall onto the belt of a moving treadmill, resulting in the hand being caught beneath the machine, causing a friction burn, often to the dorsal surface of the hand. These injuries can be very deep, involving nerves, vessels, and tendons, thereby requiring increasingly complex reconstruction (full-thickness skin grafts or cross-finger flaps). Thankfully frostbite and electrical burns are rare and will be dealt with in other articles of this issue; chemical burns are even less common and should be dealt with in a similar way to adults.

ANATOMY

The anatomy of the hand of a child differs from that of an adult in a few crucial ways. First, the skin of a child is thinner, so it requires less thermal exposure time to result in a full-thickness injury. Second, the subcutaneous adipose tissue in a child is more profuse than an adult, and as such, protects deeper structures such as tendons and nerves and assists in the excision of full-thickness injuries resulting in a layer of soft tissue preservation on the dorsal surface of the hand. This general excess in adipose tissue in the younger child also allows for simpler harvest of full-thickness grafts from the inguinal region, if needed (**Fig. 1**).[1]

The skin on the palmar surface has a thick dermis that is most abundant over the pulp of the finger tips, thinning only for the flexion creases. Grip stability is optimized by the secure attachments between deep fibro-osseous tissue and the surface using the vertical septa of the pulp, along with the ligaments of both Cleland (more dorsal) and Grayson (more volar). Following a burn injury with resulting edema, the compartments of the hand and digit are less able

to expand, resulting in elevated pressure and possibly decreased circulation. The likelihood of the child holding the hand in a dependent position and the relatively small size of the hand both contribute to worsening the situation. Not only the skin but also the nails of the child's hand can be damaged by both the thermal injury and any subsequent compartment syndrome, resulting in a discolored, deviated or notched nail, each of which is difficult to correct surgically.[7]

TREATMENT GOALS

The pathophysiology of hand burns can be subdivided into those primary effects related to the thermal effects of the injury; these are dependent on the time of contact and the temperature of the heat source involved, and the secondary effects of any ensuing edema, reduced circulation, and infection. Treating physicians can help to improve any outcome by attenuating each of these effects by adhering to 5 principles[8]:

1. Preventing additional propagation of the burn to deeper structures
2. Rapid wound closure
3. Preservation of active and passive range of motion and maintaining elevation
4. Infection control
5. Early active rehabilitation

INITIAL EVALUATION

Determination of the burn depth and size is of the utmost importance at the initial examination once the patient has been stabilized from any other life-threatening injuries. As with all trauma and massive burn the appropriate ATLS (Advanced Trauma Life Support) or ABLS (Advanced Burn Life Support) principles should preempt any specific treatment for a hand burn. A clear history of the circumstances surrounding the injury needs to be elicited, from the child if possible, although this will depend on the state of agitation and developmental stage for each patient. If this is not possible, then it should be obtained from a witness to the accident. Specific information that needs to

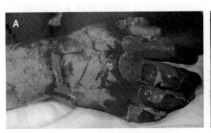
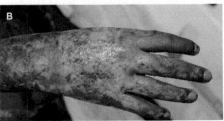

Fig. 1. Full-thickness burns (*A*) at presentation and (*B*) after grafting.

be covered includes time of injury, type of burn (eg, scald, contact, or flame), duration of exposure, and any first aid applied at the time of injury. Before any assessment of the burn depth can be undertaken, a thorough debridement of any loose, blistered tissue needs to be –done; this usually requires strong analgesia at the very least (such as a Fentanyl troche) and occasionally conscious sedation (Ketamine) (**Fig. 2**). Once this has been achieved, a clinical assessment of the burn is undertaken that measures the size and depth of the burn, noting any areas of circumferential injury that may require escharotomy or fasciotomy. Other objective modalities of burn depth assessment are also available including the laser Doppler, which has a large amount of evidence for predicting burn wound outcome.[9,10] Maintaining elevation in a burned extremity is a simple and often underused modality to reduce edema.

ESCHAROTOMY/FASCIOTOMY

The need for escharotomy and/or fasciotomy is most often a clinical judgment based on the history of the injury (eg, electrical or flame), physical examination (circumferentially injured, tense hard tissue), clinical signs (dark urine: myoglobinuria), and laboratory results (raised myoglobin and creatine kinase) (**Fig. 3**).

ESCHAROTOMY

Indications for escharotomy include:
- Circumferential burns of the upper extremity that develop signs of inadequate perfusion (cool to touch, reduced pulse oximetry)
- Circumferential burns of the upper extremity that are likely to lose perfusion with large fluid resuscitation
- Absence of pulse on Doppler distal to injury (presence of a pulse does not rule out need for escharotomy[11]

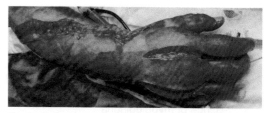

Fig. 3. Escharotomies performed on the upper limb.

Principles include:
- Use electrocautery (scalpel may be used for the digits)
- Full-thickness incisions through burned skin to subcutaneous tissues
- Longitudinal incisions to avoid injury to underlying neurovascular structures, with the limbs in the anatomic position (palms facing forward)
- Commence incision within normal skin, preferably 2 cm from the edge of the burn

The technique is performed as follows:
- With the hand in the anatomic position, longitudinal incisions along both radial and ulnar aspect of the arm and forearm
- Ulnar incision should pass anterior to the medial epicondyle (avoid ulnar nerve injury)
- Continue incisions onto the skin of the hand overlying hypothenar and thenar eminences at the border of glaborous and nonglaborous skin
- Dorsal hand escharotomies overlying second and fourth metacarpals—can be linked to ulnar escharotomy at wrist
- Digital escharotomies can reduce necrosis and should be made between the neurovascular bundle and the extensors (junction of glaborous and nonglaborous skin), avoiding both structures on the radial border of the thumb and ulnar border of all other digits

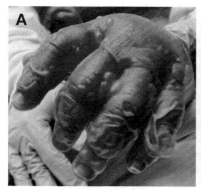
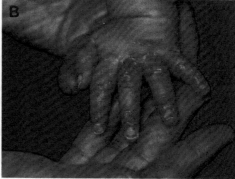

Fig. 2. 2nd degree burns (*A*) before debridement and (*B*) after healing.

FASCIOTOMY

Indications are as per those for escharotomy plus:

- Compartment pressure greater than 30 mm Hg or within 30 mm Hg of systolic blood pressure
- Presence of myoglobinuria
- Inadequate decompression following escharotomy

The technique is as follows:

- Dorsal: longitudinal forearm incision (linked to the dorsal hand incisions). It is important to release all compartments in the hand; this is achieved by retraction of the volar incisions overlying the second and fourth metacarpals to reveal the interossei between the metacarpals. These compartments, both volar and dorsal, can be decompressed via these incisions.
- Volar: Use an "S"-shaped skin incision
  - Starting point: between the hypothenar and thenar eminences
  - Wrist and distal forearm:
  - Decompress the carpal tunnel ± Guyon canal
  - Ensure decompression of pronator quadratus
  - Turn incision to ulnar aspect of wrist and continue along the ulnar border of the distal forearm
  - Midforearm: turn the incision to the radial side of the forearm and then return to the ulnar border radial to the medial epicondyle
  - Recent more limited incision fasciotomies have been described to minimize morbidity of an open wound with nerve exposure
- Proximal forearm and arm: passing volar to the medial epicondyle the incision then passes proximally into the arm along the medial border
- This can be extended into the palm, or a separate incision can be used to release the carpal tunnel

Aims of this procedure include:

- Decompression of medial and ulnar nerves
- Decompression of superficial and deep compartments of forearm
- Exposure and adequate coverage of the median nerve
- Protection of cutaneous nerves and preservation of as many cutaneous veins as possible (**Fig. 4**)

WOUND MANAGEMENT

Initial first aid should include cooling the injured hand with cool, but not cold, running water for

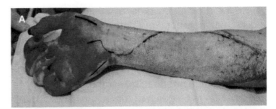
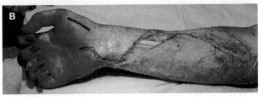

Fig. 4. (A) Forearm markings for volar fasciotomy. (B) following incisional release of volar fasciotomy; thenar and hypothenar eminences not yet released.

about 20 minutes. The use of a basin of water should be discouraged as if this was ever used for a chemical burn this could lead to an increase in the size of the burned area. Elevation of the burned extremity will also assist in the prevention of excessive edema in an otherwise dependent limb.

Superficial partial-thickness burns that are pink, moist, blanching, and painful will generally heal within 2 weeks of injury if a well perfused and infection-free wound environment is maintained. There are many dressings on the market to treat such wounds such as nonadherent paraffin-soaked gauze (Bactigras or Xeroform), which need to be changed daily. There are also dressings that can be left in place for several days allowing for re-epithelialization beneath. Biobrane is one such dressing that allows visualization of the wound as it heals beneath the dressing. Biobrane consists of a semipermeable silicone membrane with nylon fabric overlay into which is incorporated porcine type I collagen. The production of biobrane gloves has especially aided in the use of such dressings on the hand. Reduced number of dressing changes and observation of the wound through the translucent material both aid in the use of this dressing. Biobrane is especially useful in superficial partial-thickness burns. For those partial thickness burns that appear to be extending a little deeper, the use of Suprathel is recommended; it is a polymer of lactic acid that is supplied as a membrane that can be applied directly to the moist burn wound following debridement of any blisters. The benefits of Suprathel are similar to Biobrane but also include a reduction in the pH of the wound and hence reduced infection rates.[12] One of the benefits over and above that of Biobrane is that the membrane degrades over time and can simply be washed off once the dressing is removed.

Deeper dermal and ful- thickness wounds will require definitive debridement and grafting; a temporizing measure prior to surgery is often the use of a topical agent such as either silver sulfadiazine or mafenide acetate.[13] Silver sulfadiazine confers an antibacterial action from the silver ions binding to the DNA of any superficial bacterial organism and inhibiting proliferation of both bacteria and fungi. Sulfadiazine acts by the inhibition of folic acid production necessary for bacterial proliferation. Mafenide acetate is a sulfonamide available as either a solution or cream; it can penetrate deeply into the burn eschar with excellent gram-positive, gram-negative, and *Clostridium* cover. Application of mafenide over a large area can lead to metabolic acidosis due to its conversion by monoamine oxidase to p-sulfamylvanzoic acid, a carbonic anhydrase inhibitor, which prevents the conversion of hydrogen ions to carbonic acid. The use of mafenide on a single hand would be highly unlikely to trigger such an event. In general, these wounds should be changed daily; however, if there are signs of gross infection then this can be increased. When concerned with dressings of the hand, it is of utmost import to keep the dressings as thin as possible to allow early mobilization.

SURGICAL MANAGEMENT

With obvious full-thickness burns, the decision for surgical debridement is an easy one; however, occasionally the decision to debride is delayed for 48 hours to allow areas to delineate so that neither over-resection nor under-resection is carried out. Once in the operating room, debridement is carried out under tourniquet control with a Weck or Goulian knife. In the authors' experience, if the entire upper extremity requires debridement, then it is best to resect the skin overlying the proximal arm, and, following hemostasis, then apply the sterile tourniquet to the resected area. Elevation of the limb for 2 minutes is sufficient; no use of esmarch bandage is made. Debridement is carried out in a tangential fashion until all dermal elements have been removed, thereby reducing the likelihood of inclusion cysts beneath the sheet grafts that will be applied. Once debridement is complete, the hand is raised and the tourniquet is deflated, allowing visualization of a bleeding wound bed and the opportunity for meticulous hemostasis. Dorsal hands burns often require early debridement and grafting, whereas palmar burns will often heal spontaneously with proper splinting and dressing changes.

Grafts placed on the dorsal and palmar surface of the hand differ; traditional thin split-thickness skin grafts (0.01 in) are adequate cover for the dorsal surface of both the hand and digits. These can be harvested from the thigh, back or scalp, trimmed to size and fixed into position with Artiss fibrin sealant (Baxter Healthcare Corporation, Westlake Village, California) and an absorbable suture, such as 5/0 Vicryl rapide or 5/0 chromic. However, less graft contracture is seen in thicker grafts, so a greater thickness of graft is required for the palmar surface—either a thick split thickness graft or full thickness graft must be harvested.[14] In general, more time should be given to allow the palm to heal as grafts placed on the palm will never be as durable as palmar skin and will lack sensation. If needed, the thick split-thickness graft is harvested from the thigh with the dermatome set on 0.015 to 0.018 inch; this is then applied to the palm is the same way as the dorsal surface. Then another thin split-thickness skin graft (0.005 inch) is taken from the area on the thigh adjoining the first donor. This thin graft is then applied to the other donor site as an over-graft to aid in healing, reduce pain, and avoid significant donor site scarring. An alternative is to take a full-thickness graft from the inguinal region and then close the defect directly; this is certainly an option if only small areas on the palm need to be resurfaced rather than the entire palmar surface of both hands. Sheet grafts should always be used in the hands wherever possible; this will reduce both the amount of contracture and the unsightly cosmetic appearance of the meshed pattern on the hands.[15] All patients require splinting postoperatively; in the authors' institute, many hand burns that require grafting have Kirschner wires placed longitudinally to splint the digits in a resting position (flexed 70–90° at the metacarpophalangeal joint [MCPJ], extended at the interphalangeal joints [IPJ]). The splint applied to the hand over the dressing will assist in maintaining this position and also extend up the forearm, positioning the wrist in approximately 30° of extension. Due to the occlusive nature of the sheet grafts placed on the hand, the postoperative management is somewhat different to grafts placed elsewhere. The dressings need to be removed on the first postoperative day and the grafts inspected for any underlying seroma or hematoma. These must be evacuated at the bedside in order to maximize graft take.

In cases where the child presents with fourth-degree burns involving the deepest structures such as tendon, bone, and muscle, a more extensive debridement is required, often several in succession to arrive at a healthy wound bed. Skin grafts alone will not be sufficient cover for such wounds; therefore the use of regional flaps (reversed radial forearm flap or reversed posterior interosseous artery flap), distant (groin flap), or free flaps (temporoparietal fascial flap, lateral arm flap or thinned antero-lateral thigh flap). Amputations are often required in very extensive burns and those involving a high voltage electrical injury; however, they should only be done on dry, mummified tissue. Judicious debridement will allow preservation of length of each digit, increasing functional outcome in the longer term.

EARLY REHABILITATION

Once the grafts have taken to the wound bed, passive range of motion exercises are imperative. Any Kirschner wires need to be removed and should not remain in place longer than 1 week. During the dressing changes, a trained therapist needs to assess the passive and active range of motion of each digit and global hand function. A strict exercise regime needs to be embarked upon, which for the very young can be challenging. The use of a multidisciplinary approach including psychotherapists, occupational therapist, child life specialists, and music therapists, all make for a better outcome. Resting splints often need to be adjusted as the amount of dressing needed is reduced. As with primary grafting, the splints should have 20° to 30° of extension at the wrist, 70° to 90° of flexion at the MCPJs and extended at the IPJs. These should be worn at any time that the child is not actively taking part in therapy, but especially at night when asleep. Once the grafts have started to mature, then compression techniques can be used to reduce the edema further; the use of Coban tape (3M Health Care, St Paul, Minnesota) for the digits and hands helps in the short term until a custom-fitted pressure garment has been made that can be worn 23 hours a day for around 2 years. The gloves will generally need to be changed every 3 months to maintain adequate pressure, as the material will begin to stretch, reducing the beneficial effect.

Hand therapy is required daily not only while an inpatient but also once discharged from the hospital; therefore it is imperative to have sufficient buy-in from a suitably able caregiver, such as a parent or older sibling, so that the regime of scar management including wearing of pressure garments and splint, stretching, and scar massage are all adhered to within a daily routine so as to maximize functional outcome and reduce the need for burn scar contracture release surgery. Most patients still need at least weekly follow-up in the short term to ensure that they are benefiting from the hand therapy, and any deleterious loss of function can be addressed as soon as possible. With a supportive social network, daily hand therapy, regular outpatient clinic attendance, and constant use of pressure garments, the best possible functional outcome can be obtained.

REFERENCES

1. Feldmann ME, Evans J, O SJ. Early management of the burned pediatric hand. J Craniofac Surg 2008; 19(4):942–50.
2. Borse NGJ, Dellinger A, Rudd R, et al. CDC childhood injury report: patterns of unintentional injuries among 0-19 year olds in the United States, 2000-2006. Fam Community Health 2009;32(2):189.
3. Burd A, Yuen C. A global study of hospitalized paediatric burn patients. Burns 2005;31(4):432–8.
4. Hultman CS, Priolo D, Cairns BA, et al. Return to jeopardy: the fate of pediatric burn patients who are victims of abuse and neglect. J Burn Care Rehabil 1998;19(4):367–76 [discussion: 6–7].
5. Ojo P, Palmer J, Garvey R, et al. Pattern of burns in child abuse. Am Surg 2007;73(3):253–5.
6. Chester DL, Jose RM, Aldlyami E, et al. Non-accidental burns in children–are we neglecting neglect? Burns 2006;32(2):222–8.
7. Spauwen PH, Brown IF, Sauer EW, et al. Management of fingernail deformities after thermal injury. Scand J Plast Reconstr Surg Hand Surg 1987; 21(3):253–5.
8. Robson MC, Smith DJ Jr, VanderZee AJ, et al. Making the burned hand functional. Clin Plast Surg 1992;19(3):663–71.
9. Jeng JC, Bridgeman A, Shivnan L, et al. Laser Doppler imaging determines need for excision and grafting in advance of clinical judgment: a prospective blinded trial. Burns 2003;29(7):665–70.
10. La Hei ER, Holland AJ, Martin HC. Laser Doppler imaging of paediatric burns: burn wound outcome can be predicted independent of clinical examination. Burns 2006;32(5):550–3.
11. Saffle JR, Zeluff GR, Warden GD. Intramuscular pressure in the burned arm: measurement and response to escharotomy. Am J Surg 1980;140(6): 825–31.
12. Everett M, Massand S, Davis W, et al. Use of a copolymer dressing on superficial and partial-thickness burns in a paediatric population. J Wound Care 2015;24(7):S4–8.
13. Greenhalgh DG. Topical antimicrobial agents for burn wounds. Clin Plast Surg 2009;36(4):597–606.
14. Jang YC, Kwon OK, Lee JW, et al. The optimal management of pediatric steam burn from electric ricecooker: STSG or FTSG? J burn Care Rehabil 2001; 22(1):15–20.
15. Greenhalgh DG. Management of acute burn injuries of the upper extremity in the pediatric population. Hand Clin 2000;16(2):175–86, vii.

A 3-Phase Approach for the Management of Upper Extremity Electrical Injuries

Ketan Sharma, MD, MPH[a], Miles Bichanich, BS[a],
Amy M. Moore, MD[b],*

KEYWORDS

- Electrical burn • Burn • Electrical injury • Microsurgery • Nerve grafting • Tendon reconstruction
- Amputation

KEY POINTS

- Because of the pathophysiologic mechanism of the electric field, the magnitude and depth of electrical injuries can be far greater than what is superficially visible and can produce additional injury independent from traditional thermal damage.
- In accordance with Ohm's law, electricity will flow through the body simultaneously through different tissue planes according to individual tissue resistance. Resistance increases by tissue type as follows: nerve, vessels, muscle, skin, tendon, fat, and then bone.
- The treatment of electrical injuries of the upper extremity remains firmly grounded on fundamental trauma-relevant principles.
- All patients with high-voltage electrical injuries to the upper extremity warrant early, if not immediate, operative exploration for debridement and compartment releases.
- Reconstruction of the electrical injury demands a systematic approach to restoring sensory and motor function using basic reconstructive principles, including stable soft tissue coverage followed by tendon and nerve transfers and grafting.

 Video content accompanies this article at www.hand.theclinics.com.

INTRODUCTION

Electrical burn injuries constitute a minority of presentations to major burn centers (approximately 4% in the most recent national burn repository[1]). However, they are often described as being "the most devastating of all thermal injuries on a size-for-size-basis,"[2] with high-voltage injuries having been shown to exhibit increased inpatient length of stay, more operations required per patient, and increased mortality when compared with other burns of similar size.[3]

Electrical injuries constitute a unique point along the spectrum of burn disease because of the pathophysiologic mechanism of the electric field, which can produce additional injury independent from traditional thermal damage. These electric field effects are frequency dependent and can

Disclosures: The authors have no financial or conflicts of interest to disclose.
[a] Division of Plastic and Reconstructive Surgery, Washington University School of Medicine, 660 South Euclid Avenue, Campus Box 8238, St Louis, MO 63110, USA; [b] Hand Fellowship, Division of Plastic and Reconstructive Surgery, Washington University School of Medicine, 660 South Euclid Avenue, Campus Box 8238, St Louis, MO 63110, USA
* Corresponding author.
E-mail address: mooream@wustl.edu

Hand Clin 33 (2017) 243–256
http://dx.doi.org/10.1016/j.hcl.2016.12.012

injure biological tissues in completely nonthermal fashions.[4] At a basic conceptual level, the electric flow (or current) between 2 points is a function of the electric potential difference (voltage) and resistance to flow between those points. This concept is quantified as Ohm's law ($I = V/R$, where I is electric flow, V is voltage, and R is resistance to flow). The clinically relevant message is that electricity will flow through the body simultaneously through different tissue planes according to individual tissue resistance. More flow will occur in tissues of lesser resistance and less flow in those of higher resistance. Resistance increases by tissue type as follows: nerve, vessels, muscle, skin, tendon, fat, and then bone. Skin acts initially as a protective barrier; but once its resistance is overcome, current flows freely through underlying deeper tissues.

Electric flow generates increased tissue temperature, which is a key contributor to the magnitude of tissue damage,[5] with most of the heat produced at skeletal muscle because of volume considerations.[6] In addition, nonthermal causes of injury include microvascular and macrovascular thrombotic insult, protein denaturation, and direct cell necrosis due to electroporation.[6–8] Moreover, electric flow can also directly induce cardiac arrhythmia and respiratory muscle spasm.[4] Severity of injury itself is a function of voltage, current, current type (alternating vs direct), and contact time. *In essence, the magnitude and depth of injury can be far greater than what is superficially visible. Therefore, suspicion for concurrent and potentially hidden deeper tissue injury must remain high with any electrical injury of the upper extremity.*

Sources of electrical injury are categorized into high voltage (>1000 V) or low voltage (<1000 V). Most electrical injuries seen at burn centers result from contact with high-voltage power lines. Greater than 90% occur in young men at work-related settings and originate in the upper extremities.[3] The most common location of an electrical injury entry wound is the right hand, followed by the left hand, with the exit wounds most commonly at the left foot.[9]

Low-voltage injuries result almost exclusively from indoor contact with domestic electrical sockets or wires. These injuries typically produce relatively minor superficial skin burns or transient peripheral neurologic symptoms, but complex injuries due to prolonged contact time or oral contact have also been reported. Other less common sources are lightning strikes, with a reported mortality of up to 30%,[4] and arc injuries whereby current induces flash-type thermal injury by passing through air without directly conducting through patients.

Despite these unique and complex considerations, the treatment of electrical injuries of the upper extremity remains firmly grounded on fundamental trauma-relevant principles. Treatment is conceptually divided into 3 phases: initial management consistent with Advanced Trauma Life Support (ATLS) and Advanced Burn Life Support (ABLS) protocols, maintenance therapy to preserve tissue equilibrium, and delayed reconstruction (≥3 months after injury) to restore upper extremity sensory and motor function.

INITIAL MANAGEMENT
Life over Limb

All patients who present with electrical injuries should be initially assessed as trauma patients consistent with ATLS protocols. This critical first phase focuses on recognition of other life-threatening injuries, stabilization of patients, and multisystem resuscitation. These protocols have been described extensively elsewhere,[10] but unique considerations in this patient population are described in detail here.

The importance of managing life over limb at initial assessment of any upper extremity electrical injury cannot be overemphasized because of the chance of other concurrent and potentially life-threatening injuries, which has been estimated to be as high as 15%.[2] Mortality rates from these injuries range from 3% to 14%.[11] In one series, concurrent injuries included myoglobinuria (44%), metabolic acidosis (31%), oliguria (19%), electrocardiogram changes (12.5%), and acute renal failure (4.5%),[12] whereas another study listed loss of consciousness (52%), traumatic brain injury (5%), chest injury (5%), abdominal injury (2%), soft tissue injury (11%), and fractures (11%) in high-voltage patients.[3] Fractures often result from tetanic muscle contractions induced by electrical flow.[2] The index of suspicion for concurrent injury must remain high, especially with high-voltage mechanisms.

A unique consideration in this patient population is the likelihood of current-induced cardiac arrhythmias. Therefore, these patients should receive an initial electrocardiogram (ECG), followed by subsequent 24- to 48-hour cardiac monitoring for any ECG abnormalities, cardiac dysrhythmias, cardiac arrest, or loss of consciousness.[13]

The Secondary Survey

The secondary survey follows the primary survey.[10] Importantly, once adequately stabilized and resuscitated, all patients with electrical burns should be transferred to specialized burn centers, consistent with the American Burn Association's referral criteria.[14] In this population, the secondary survey should also detail burn-specific components, including approximate size and depth of burns; presence of circumferential burns of the torso, abdomen, or extremities; involvement of the face, eyes, ears, hands, genitals, or feet; presence of chemical or electrical injury; as well as potential for abusive or nonaccidental mechanism of injury.

Burn size and depth are critical determinants of overall prognosis[15] as well as key factors in guiding initial therapy. As with all burns, fluid resuscitation should be initiated.[16] Because electrical injuries confer deep tissue injury, fluid requirements tend to be underestimated in this population.[2] Therefore, all fluid given should be titrated to the key end points of resuscitation: normocardia, normotension, and urine output of approximately 1 to 2 mL/kg/h.

Patients with electrical injuries can also present with gross pigmenturia due to hemoglobinuria and myoglobinuria from myonecrosis. These conditions can be confirmed by urine dipstick test. Myonecrosis can also produce elevated creatinine kinase (CK) and lactate dehydrogenase levels, which can serve as helpful diagnostic adjuncts.[17] Myoglobinuria in particular can induce renal failure through several mechanisms.[18] In this setting, fluid should be titrated for a urine output of approximately 200 to 300 mL/h until urine appears grossly visually clear and until plasma CK levels are less than 5000/L.[19]

Surgical Intervention

Circumferential burns of the extremities are likely with electrical burns (in one study, 12% required escharotomy and 12% fasciotomy[20]) and should be addressed in the secondary survey. Any extremity with circumferential or near-circumferential burn should be closely monitored for signs of vascular compromise in the first 48 hours. The indications for formal escharotomy include compartment pressures greater than 40 mm Hg and/or lack of Doppler signals in distal arteries (such as digital vessels or palmar arches).

Compartment syndrome is not uncommon in this patient population given the propensity for deeper tissue damage from electrical flow. Compartment syndrome can be diagnosed clinically, with early findings consisting of pain disproportionate to examination, pain with passive stretch, and firm and tense compartments. Later findings include diminished sensation, paralysis, or absent pulses and objective measures, such as compartment pressures greater than 30 mm Hg or within 30 mm of diastolic pressure.[21] Indications for formal fasciotomy include progressive neurologic dysfunction, vascular compromise,

increased compartment pressures, or systemic clinical worsening from suspected myonecrosis.[2] Fasciotomy should routinely address the superficial and deep flexor compartments, dorsal compartment, and mobile wad, while releasing the intrinsic hand compartments and carpal tunnel on a case-by-case basis.[13,22]

Continued neurovascular monitoring is required either after escharotomy or after fasciotomy to identify inadequate release or recurrence. The consequences of missed or delayed compartment syndrome diagnosis are severe, and prior series have reported amputation rates as high as 40% even with early extensive debridement and compartment release.[22] Therefore, all patients with high-voltage electrical injuries to the upper extremity warrant early, if not immediate, operative exploration for debridement and compartment release.

MAINTENANCE TREATMENT

After the critical first phase, treatment of electrical injuries to the upper extremity enters a maintenance phase to achieve tissue equilibrium with the following specific goals:

1. Excise evolving devitalized tissue.
2. Prevent infection.
3. Provide adequate soft tissue coverage over vital structures.
4. Prevent contracture and joint stiffness.

Excise Devitalized Tissue

Initial operative intervention should be followed by close neurovascular monitoring and subsequent operative exploration. The importance of an early second look cannot be overemphasized, as electrically damaged soft tissue (especially muscle) can often look normal initially but thereafter evolve rapidly.[4] The authors advocate for scheduling serial debridements (every 48 hours) at the time of presentation. At the second look, grossly necrotic tissue should be excised; but tissue of questionable or marginal viability can be retained for subsequent reevaluation. Again, operative exploration with debridement should be continued serially every 24 to 48 hours for reinspection until all devitalized tissue is removed and the wound bed no longer evolves; this typically takes greater than 5 days. Ultimately, debridement should be aggressive enough to remove all necrotic and devitalized tissue resulting from the evolving burn but should also attempt to preserve major sensory or motor nerves as these provide the foundation for later restorative functional efforts. In the senior author's experience, peripheral nerves somewhat paradoxically tend to be spared despite their lesser resistance; patients tend to more commonly present with diffuse neurapraxia involving all extremity nerves; if not initially debrided, nerve function surprisingly recovers with time.

Prevent Infection

Between debridements, daily wound care is critical to preventing development of superimposed infections. Numerous agents are available and have been described.[17] Typically, mafenide acetate (Sulfamylon) provides broad-spectrum coverage with effective eschar penetration and should be applied over thick contact points, whereas silver sulfadiazine provides excellent topical coverage over flash injuries.[2] Depending on the size and extent of wounds, negative pressure therapy can serve as an important adjunct for temporizing soft tissue coverage, although exposure of critical vessels mandates immediate soft tissue coverage and may warrant early free tissue transfer.

Soft Tissue Coverage

Definitive closure should be delayed until the affected extremity is free of all devitalized tissue. In general, it is best to obtain stable soft tissue coverage and allow patients to recover from the significant trauma incurred by the electrical injury. Planning for future functional reconstruction, however, should begin early. Early and ongoing assessment of patients' needs should be considered, and choice of coverage should facilitate future reconstruction.

Plastic surgery offers numerous options depending on the location and size of the wound as well as the structures involved. Defects not involving joint surfaces with underlying vascularized soft tissue can be covered with split-thickness skin grafts (STSGs), whereas defects with underlying vascularized soft tissue over joints may require full-thickness skin grafts (FTSGs) as these are less likely to lead to contracture. Conversely, defects with underlying exposed bone or tendon require either locoregional autologous tissue (if available) or free autologous tissue transfer (most commonly). Notably, exposure of critical vessels requires soft tissue coverage and may mandate free flap transfer before full tissue equilibrium has been reached.

The advent of modern free tissue transfer has revolutionized the variety of options for defect coverage of the upper extremity. Fasciocutaneous flaps are preferred, especially in the distal forearm, wrist, and hand, as they provide smooth gliding surfaces for easier tendon reconstruction and motion, appropriate thinness limiting unaesthetic bulk, and superior cosmesis.[23] A multitude of options for free tissue transfer exists.[24] The choice depends on the availability of tissue (outside of burn involvement) and need for future reconstructive function and form.

Prevent Contracture and Joint Stiffness

Initially, the affected extremity should be splinted in functional position to alleviate pain and prevent contracture: the shoulder abducted, elbow extended, and hand in the intrinsic plus position.[25] Custom splints can be fabricated by occupational therapists. In addition, ongoing physical therapy is paramount to prevent joint stiffness and maintain passive and active range of motion (ROM). Notably, prevention of contracture and joint stiffness is critical as these can significantly impair future functional restorative efforts. If these develop, patients will require future closed or open joint capsulotomy with possible collateral ligament release and/or surgical contracture release via excision and grafting or Z-plasty.

RECONSTRUCTION: RESTORATION OF FUNCTION

Once stable soft tissue coverage has been established and patients have recovered from the traumatic injury (including renal and/or cardiac abnormalities), the final phase of treatment of electrical injuries to the upper extremity begins. This phase usually begins 3 to 6 months after the injury and can last up to 2 to 3 years. The reconstruction phase involves carefully planned restoration of sensory and motor function. It also requires a thorough understanding of previous procedures performed and an accurate assessment of remaining structures and function. Adequate cataloging of intact and/or debrided structures is critical. Standard principles of upper extremity reconstruction must be applied.

Electrical injuries cause devastating wounds resulting in significant soft tissue resection at initial presentation and subsequent debridements. Significant scarring of the soft tissue and flexor tendon sheaths should be expected and makes assessing intact structures difficult (thus, the reason for detailed notes in the initial phase). Even if most wounds are located at the forearm, expect distal scarring to be present as the electrical current disrupts these gliding planes. For example, tenolysis will likely be required with tendon reconstructions, even if passive ROM is present.

In the following illustrative cases, the authors explore surgical options to restore hand function including finger flexion, pinch and grip, and sensation after electrical burn injuries. In the end, as with all upper extremity reconstructive procedures, the priorities of reconstruction should be individualized to each patient.

ILLUSTRATIVE CASE EXAMPLES
Case 1: E.D.

E.D. is a 33-year-old right-hand-dominant electrical lineman who sustained a high-voltage injury to the bilateral upper extremities when grasping a live wire. Phase I and II treatment at an outside hospital resulted in transhumeral amputation of the right; the left upper extremity was salvaged but underwent multiple debridements, including excision of all flexor tendons (except for proximal and distal stumps) and the median and ulnar nerve. The radial artery perfused the hand. The patient received fasciotomies and coverage of the volar hand, wrist, and forearm with a pedicled groin flap (**Fig. 1**). The patient was then referred for evaluation for return of sensation and motor function to his remaining hand (phase III).

At referral, the patient presented with no sensation in ulnar or median nerve distributions, no active finger flexion, limited (~10°–15°) active wrist flexion, scar contracture of the dorsal first web space, and palmar contractures of the index finger (IF) and long finger (LF) metacarpophalangeal (MCP) joints. Notably, the patient had full supple passive ROM of all fingers, approximately 40° of active wrist extension, full active finger extension, and intact radial nerve sensation.

Staged reconstruction was planned based on sensory and motor deficits and available redundant sources for nerve and tendon reconstruction. The patient first underwent flap liposuction for debulking, scar contracture release of the first

web space with transposition of the flap into the first web space, scar contracture release of the palm with FTSG coverage, and Hunter rod placement through the defatted flap to create tunnels for later tendon and nerve graft passage (**Fig. 2**). Following release, the patient exhibited near-full passive ROM of the previously contracted IF and LF MCP. After 1 week postoperatively the patient was started on aggressive therapy to reinstate active and passive ROM of all fingers to alleviate stiffness from immobilization.

The patient later underwent delayed sensorimotor reconstruction. Tendon and nerve reconstruction consisted of extensive tenolysis of all flexor tendons followed by reconstruction using bilateral plantaris tendon and sural nerve autografts. The patient refused consent for toe extensor harvest because he had adapted to using his feet to assist with his activities of daily living. In summary, the patient's flexor pollicis longus was reconstructed with a 12-cm plantaris autograft. The flexor digitorum profundus (FDP) to the LF, ring finger (RF), and small finger (SF) was reconstructed with 14-cm plantaris autografts. The IF suffered the most traumatic injury; given the paucity of tendon autograft, the IF FDP tendon was reconstructed with a 14-cm peroneus longus allograft. Nerve reconstruction consisted of four 15-cm sural nerve autografts from the proximal median nerve stump (which was debrided to healthy fascicular pattern) to the thumb ulnar digital nerve (UDN), second common digital nerve (CDN), third CDN, and SF UDN. To restore sensation to the fourth web space, the fourth CDN was brought end to side to the LF nerve graft (**Fig. 3**).

Postoperatively, the patient was started on passive ROM flexor tendon reconstruction protocol at

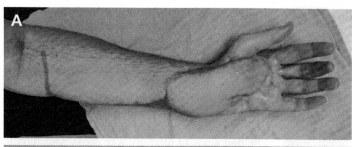
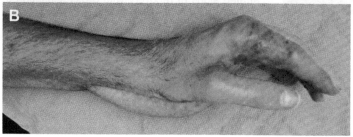

Fig. 1. Preoperative photographs of patient E.D. (*A*) The patient complained of the bulkiness of the volar soft tissue flap and significant first web space contracture. (*B*) The lateral image demonstrates significant scar contraction at the level of the distal palm/metacarpophalangeal joint preventing finger extension. The patient lacked flexion and sensation of all digits.

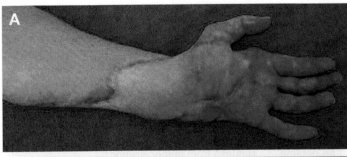

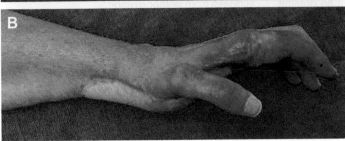

Fig. 2. (*A*) Anterior and (*B*) lateral postoperative photographs of patient E.D. after flap debulking, scar contracture release of the palm, and first web space release.

less than 1 week to prevent stiffness. Over time, the patient exhibited a progressing Tinel sign from the median nerve 4 cm proximal to his incision, increased forearm musculature girth, and active flexion. At the most recent follow-up (~2 years from initial presentation), E.D. exhibited strong active flexion of all digits and intact sensation to gross touch in median nerve distributions (**Fig. 4**, Video 1). The patient reports return of independence and function.

Case 2: D.B.

D.B. is a 20-year-old right-hand-dominant electrical lineman who sustained high-voltage electrical

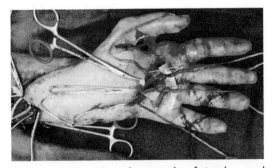

Fig. 3. Intraoperative photograph of tendon and nerve reconstruction. The sural nerve grafts extend distally and are marked by the blue background. They were coapted distally then transferred proximally to the median nerve stump. The tendon grafts were secured distally and then woven with a Pulvertaft weave proximally. Hunter rods were placed at the initial procedure, and separate tunnels were used for the nerves and tendons.

burns to bilateral upper extremities from a power line. He had cardiac arrest requiring cardiopulmonary resuscitation at the scene. Before referral, he had undergone bilateral fasciotomies with numerous upper extremity debridements, finger amputations, and failed skin grafting to bilateral hands and forearms.

On presentation, the patient had significant bilateral wounds. Although his injuries and reconstruction are described separately, they were addressed initially at the same time with multiple debridements (**Fig. 5**). However, throughout this process, the patient's needs and overall function were considered and the reconstruction was tailored to providing the best care per extremity. After the initial debridements, the patient underwent staged reconstructive procedures on either limb every 3 months for 2 years.

On the right side, the patient had a large volar distal forearm wound with exposed flexor tendons, a proximal median nerve neuroma, and a large hand wound involving the first web space with exposed MCP joint of the thumb (see **Fig. 5**C). An angiogram demonstrated perfusion of the hand by the ulnar artery, and the ulnar nerve demonstrated signs of recovery with gross sensation to the RF and SF. After multiple soft tissue debridements, he underwent thumb MCP arthrodesis and definitive soft tissue coverage with free fasciocutaneous anterior lateral thigh (ALT) flap.

Three months after stable soft tissue coverage was achieved, the patient underwent tendon reconstruction with toe extensor tendon autografts (**Fig. 6**). Tenolysis was required for all fingers at time of reconstruction despite passive ROM

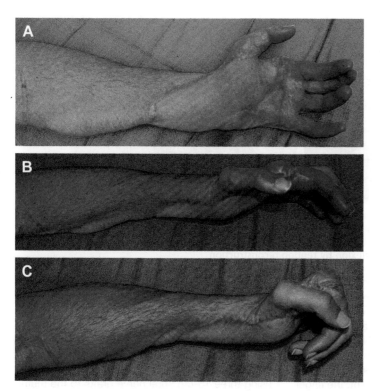

Fig. 4. (A) Anterior and (B, C) lateral photographs of patient E.D. at 2 years postoperatively.

present. There was significant scarring of the flexor tendon sheaths into the fingers. Sensation to the radial aspect of the hand was restored with end-to-side nerve grafting of the fourth web space to the radial digital nerve of the IF using a 5-cm lateral antebrachial cutaneous nerve graft. Subsequent interventions for this extremity included first web space deepening and flap excisions and debulking. All procedures were separated by 3 months to allow for soft tissue stabilization. Postoperative photographs and recover of sensation on Semmes-Weinstein test are presented in **Fig. 7**.

The left upper extremity at presentation had equally devastating wounds. His SF was previously amputated, and his RF although present had a desiccated and exposed MCP joint with no crossing structures. There was also a large distal volar forearm wound with exposed desiccated tendons and nerves (see **Fig. 5B**). An angiogram

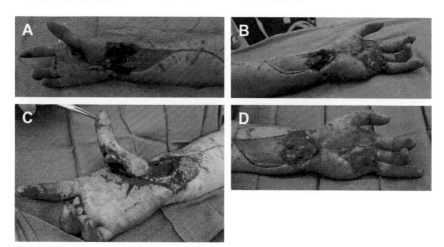

Fig. 5. Photograph of patient D.B.'s (A) right and (B) left hands at presentation. (C) After initial debridement the patient had significant soft tissue wounds and an exposed MCP joint of the thumb on the right and (D) RF on the left (black asterisk).

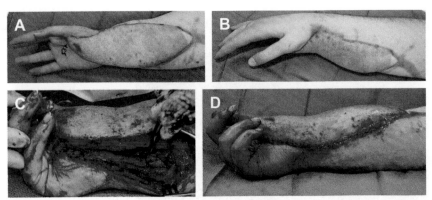

Fig. 6. Tendon and nerve reconstruction of the right hand. (*A, B*) Preoperative photographs of D.B.'s right hand after soft tissue stabilization and full passive ROM of the fingers achieved. (*C*) Intraoperative photograph of the tendon gap of the FDP tendons of IF, RF, and SF (tendon ends are marked with *asterisk*). (*D*) On table, postprocedure photograph of fingers held in flexion by tendon reconstruction.

revealed perfusion via the radial artery. Initial operative debridements included all flexor digitorum superficialis tendons and excision of the desiccated ulnar nerve and artery. Integra (Integra Life Sciences Corporation, Plainsboro, NJ) placement was used initially for coverage. Subsequent procedures included a SF revision amputation; given the exposed and necrotic RF MCP joint, the finger was amputated. A finger filet flap was used to provide soft tissue coverage of the palm (**Fig. 8**). Although STSG over the Integra was attempted, complete coverage of the tendons at the wrist level was not achieved and ultimately required free fasciocutaneous ALT coverage (**Fig. 9**).

Sensorimotor reconstruction was performed on the left hand with multiple staged procedures. Three months after stable soft tissue coverage was achieved, tenolysis of the flexor tendons was performed. The median nerve was also reconstructed using three 15-cm sural nerve grafts to the thumb UDN, the index radial digital nerve and the LF radial digital nerve (**Fig. 10**). Subsequent procedures included an extensor digiti quinti (EDQ) opponensplasty to restore opposition later followed by

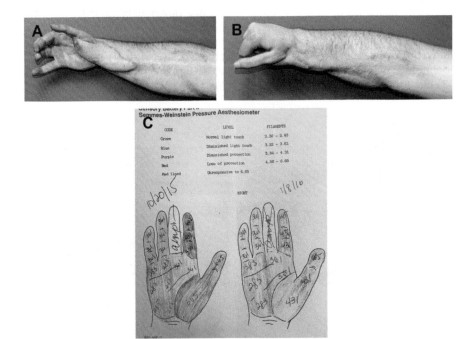

Fig. 7. (*A, B*) Postoperative photographs of right hand function at 2 years. (*C*) Semmes-Weinstein demonstrates improved sensation over time on the radial aspect of the IF after end-to-side nerve transfer from the fourth web space.

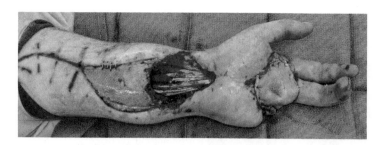

Fig. 8. Finger filet flap was used to cover the volar palm to provide stable soft tissue and avoid scar contracture.

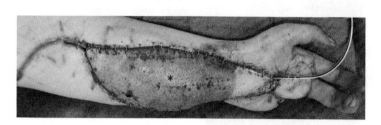

Fig. 9. An ALT fasciocutaneous free flap was used for soft tissue coverage. The hyperemic appearance of the flap (*asterisk*) is from skin graft donor site on the thigh.

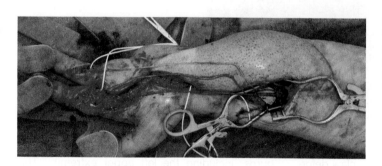

Fig. 10. Sensation to the left hand was restored with 3 long (15 cm) sural nerve grafts from the proximal median nerve to radial digital nerves of the IF and LF and the UDN of the thumb.

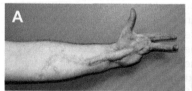
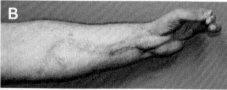
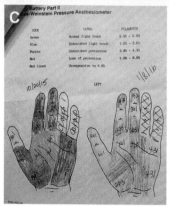

Fig. 11. (*A, B*) Postoperative photographs of the left hand function at 2 years. (*C*) Semmes-Weinstein demonstrates improved protective sensation over time into the fingers and thumb.

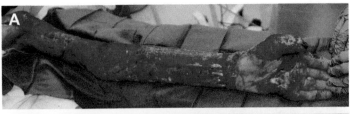

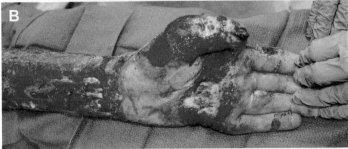

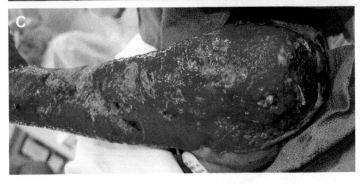

Fig. 12. Photographs of Z.S.'s left upper extremity at presentation. (A) The patient has both electrical and flame burns affecting the arm. Hypergranulation tissue is present throughout due to the prolonged allograft skin application. (B) Multiple exposed desiccated tendons are present at the forearm and hand. The distal phalanx of the thumb is also nonviable. (C) The posterior shoulder has significant soft tissue injury with exposed acromion at the base.

dynamic tendon transfers for an ulnar claw deformity. Specifically, he received a 2-tailed tendon graft transfer of extensor carpi radialis brevis (ECRB) to the lateral bands and pinchplasty from the extensor indicis proprius (EIP) to thumb adductor insertion to restore pinch. Lastly, the patient underwent forearm flap debulking and excision. At the most recent follow-up, the patient exhibited significant return of motor and sensory function of his bilateral hands (see **Fig. 7**; **Fig. 11**, Video 2).

Case 3: Z.S.

Z.S. is a 25-year-old farmer who sustained severe (~65% total body surface area [TBSA])

burns, including the left upper extremity. This injury was sustained when a farming machine ran through a power line and caught on fire. Unaware of the electrical component to the fire, the farmer jumped onto the equipment to reach the fire extinguisher. In addition to a flame injury, the patient had an electrical injury with entry at the left volar palm and exit via the bilateral lower extremities and left posterior shoulder. Before referral, the patient underwent bilateral lower extremity amputations, extensive skin grafting to the entire body, multiple debridements of the left upper extremity including much of the shoulder girdle, and temporary coverage with

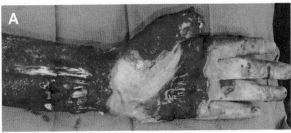

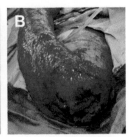

Fig. 13. Multiple excisional debridements are necessary to clean the wound beds in preparation for reconstruction. Photographs of the (A) hand, forearm, and (B) shoulder after multiple debridements.

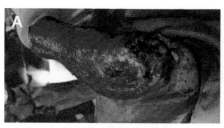
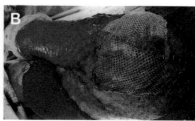

Fig. 14. (A) Preoperative and (B) postprocedure coverage of the left posterior shoulder with a pedicled latissimus dorsi muscle flap and STSG.

cadaveric allograft to the left upper extremity. The patient was referred for potential salvage of the left arm.

On arrival, the patient had devastating injuries to the left upper extremity including necrotic soft tissue of the shoulder with desiccated acromion. His left arm had exposed and grossly nonviable flexor tendons both in the distal forearm and in the palm with complete thumb degloving. He exhibited lack of finger flexion and sensation to the hand (**Fig. 12**).

Initially, the patient underwent irrigation and sharp debridement of the nonviable tissue of the hand, forearm, and shoulder (**Fig. 13**). The left exposed shoulder joint was definitively covered with a pedicled latissimus dorsi flap and STSG (**Fig. 14**). Once the volar forearm, hand, and thumb were debrided, all wounds were

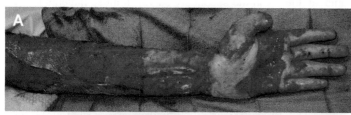

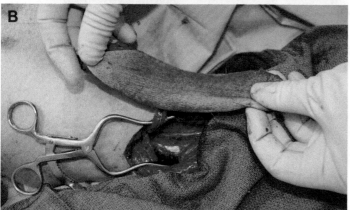

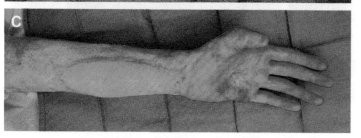

Fig. 15. Soft tissue coverage of the volar forearm tendons was provided by a contralateral lateral arm flap. (A) Preoperative photographs of left arm with intact Integra dermal matrix to forearm and hand. (B) Elevation of the right lateral arm fasciocutaneous free flap. (C) Postoperative photographs of the left arm 3 months after free tissue transfer and STSG.

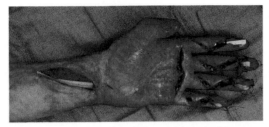

Fig. 16. Intraoperative photograph of first-stage flexor tendon reconstruction with Hunter rods.

Hunter rod was placed to the base of the LF proximal phalanx to be used as a tunnel for subsequent median nerve grafting to the fingers. Of note, the ulnar nerve appeared desiccated at the time of presentation; however, it was left in continuity and over time has recovered providing motor but not sensory function (**Fig. 17**). The patient underwent second-stage tendon reconstruction with the use of allograft tendons. At time of publication, he awaits tenolysis to improve active finger flexion (**Fig. 18**).

temporarily covered with Integra. After several subsequent debridements and STSG to the left arm, a contralateral free lateral arm flap was harvested for definitive soft tissue coverage over the volar tendons to provide the soft tissue bed for future tendon and nerve reconstruction (**Fig. 15**).

Roughly 8 months from injury, functional reconstruction began. Because of significant scarring of the flexor tendon sheath and distal tendons, first-stage flexor tendon reconstruction using Hunter rods attached distally to FDP remnants at the DIP level was performed (**Fig. 16**). A second

SUMMARY

Electrical injuries of the upper extremity present with unique pathophysiologic considerations because of the differing mechanisms of injury produced by the electromagnetic field. Despite the daunting nature of these injuries, fundamental trauma principles apply and sensorimotor reconstruction is possible. Treatment can be conceptually organized into 3 phases (**Table 1**). The initial critical phase consists of recognition of other life-threatening injuries, stabilization of patients, and multisystem resuscitation. Notable unique points in the secondary survey in these patients include current-induced cardiac arrhythmias, higher fluid

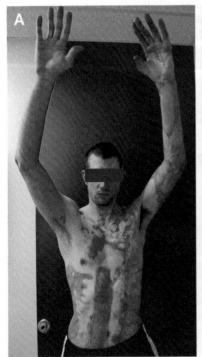
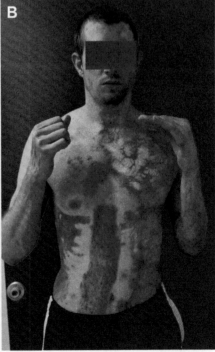

Fig. 17. Postoperative photographs of Z.S. demonstrate active (*A*) shoulder function and (*B*) ulnar nerve function of the hand.

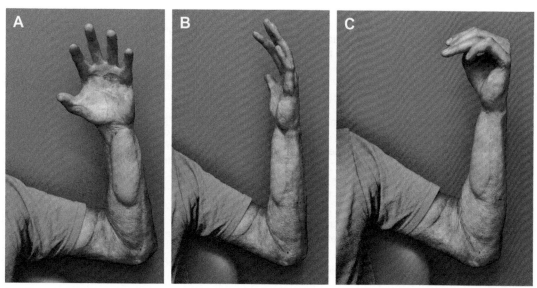

Fig. 18. Postoperative photographs (at time of publication) of Z.S. demonstrate (*A*) stable soft tissue coverage (*B*) finger extension and (*C*) finger flexion before tenolysis.

requirements, possible myoglobinuria, and potential deeper tissue injury. All high-voltage injuries mandate early operative exploration to assess or release compartments. The second phase is a maintenance phase and involves excision of evolving devitalized tissue, appropriate wound care to prevent delayed infection, providing temporary and then definitive coverage over vital structures, and preventing contracture and joint stiffness via aggressive therapy. Lastly, the third phase consists of sensorimotor functional reconstruction via the myriad of nerve and tendon grafting and nerve and tendon transfers available based on the patients' initial deficits and available redundant sources. If a systematic approach is applied, functional reconstruction and salvage of the limbs after a devastating electrical injury is possible.

Table 1
Summary of the 3 phases of management of electrical injury

Phase	Timing	Goals
Initial: ATLS and ABLS	Immediate to 48 h	<ul><li>Stabilization</li><li>Multisystem resuscitation</li><li>Recognition of potential life-threatening injuries</li><li>Initial operative exploration with debridement and possible escharotomies/fasciotomies for compartment syndrome</li></ul>
Maintenance	48 h to 3 mo after injury	<ul><li>Serial debridements to excise evolving devitalized tissue</li><li>Wound care to prevent infection</li><li>Soft tissue coverage of vital structures</li><li>Therapy and splinting to prevent joint contracture</li></ul>
Reconstruction	3 mo to 2–3 y	<ul><li>Sensorimotor functional reconstruction via nerve grafting, tendon grafting, tendon transfers, and adjunctive procedures to improve aesthetic and functional use of the limb</li></ul>

SUPPLEMENTARY DATA

Supplementary data related to this article can be found online at http://dx.doi.org/10.1016/j.hcl.2016.12.012.

REFERENCES

1. American Burn Association. 2012 national burn repository. Chicago (IL): American Burn Association; 2012. Available at: http://www.ameriburn.org/2012NBRAnnualReport.pdf.

2. Arnoldo BD, Purdue GF. The diagnosis and management of electrical injuries. Hand Clin 2009; 25(4):469–79.

3. Arnoldo BD, Purdue GF, Kowalske K, et al. Electrical injuries: a 20-year review. J Burn Care Rehabil 2004; 25(6):479–84.

4. Lee R. Injury by electrical forces: pathophysiology, manifestations, and therapy. Curr Probl Surg 1997; 34(9):677–764.

5. Hunt JL, Mason AD Jr, Masterson TS, et al. The pathophysiology of acute electric injuries. J Trauma 1976;16(5):335–40.

6. Chen W, Lee RC. Altered ion channel conductance and ionic selectivity induced by large imposed membrane potential pulse. Biophys J 1994;67(2):603–12.

7. Lee RC, Zhang D, Hannig J. Biophysical injury mechanisms in electrical shock trauma. Annu Rev Biomed Eng 2000;2:477–509.

8. DeBono R. A histological analysis of a high voltage electric current injury to an upper limb. Burns 1999;25(6):541–7.

9. Guntheti BK, Khaja S, Singh UP. Pattern of injuries due to electric current. J Indian Acad Forensic Med 2012;34:44–8.

10. The American College of Surgeons. Committee on Trauma, A.C.o.S. ATLS: advanced trauma life support program for doctors. 8th edition. Chicago: 2008. Available at: https://www.amazon.com/Atls-Student-Course-Manual-Advanced/dp/1880696029/ref=pd_sim_14_1?_encoding=UTF8&pd_rd_i=1880696029&pd_rd_r=2BSXQ7KXJQ1805SA0HC2&pd_rd_w=9zPUx&pd_rd_wg=dl3s8&psc=1&refRID=2BSXQ7KXJQ1805SA0HC2.

11. Esses SI, Peters WJ. Electrical burns; pathophysiology and complications. Can J Surg 1981;24(1): 11–4.

12. Hanumadass ML, Voora SB, Kagan RJ, et al. Acute electrical burns: a 10-year clinical experience. Burns Incl Therm Inj 1986;12(6):427–31.

13. Arnoldo B, Klein M, Gibran NS. Practice guidelines for the management of electrical injuries. J Burn Care Res 2006;27(4):439–47.

14. Carter JE, Neff LP, Holmes JHT. Adherence to burn center referral criteria: are patients appropriately being referred? J Burn Care Res 2010;31(1): 26–30.

15. Saffle JR, Davis B, Williams P. Recent outcomes in the treatment of burn injury in the United States: a report from the American Burn Association Patient Registry. J Burn Care Rehabil 1995; 16(3 Pt 1):219–32 [discussion: 288–9].

16. Anjaria DJ, Deitch EA. Burn fluid resuscitation, in encyclopedia of intensive care medicine. Springer; 2012. p. 404–8. Available at: http://link.springer.com/referenceworkentry/10.1007%2F978-3-642-00418-6_376.

17. Choi M, Armstrong MB, Panthaki ZJ. Pediatric hand burns: thermal, electrical, chemical. J Craniofac Surg 2009;20(4):1045–8.

18. Chatzizisis YS, Misirli G, Hatzitolios AI, et al. The syndrome of rhabdomyolysis: complications and treatment. Eur J Intern Med 2008;19(8):568–74.

19. Palevsky PM. In: Prevention and treatment of heme pigment-induced acute kidney injury (acute renal failure). UpToDate; 2015. Available at: https://www.uptodate.com/contents/prevention-and-treatment-of-heme-pigment-induced-acute-kidney-injury-acute-renal-failure.

20. Rai J, Jeschke MG, Barrow RE, et al. Electrical injuries: a 30-year review. J Trauma 1999;46(5): 933–6.

21. UpToDate. Acute compartment syndrome of the extremities. 2014. Available at: https://www.uptodate.com/contents/acute-compartment-syndrome-of-the-extremities.

22. Achauer B, Applebaum R, Vander Kam VM. Electrical burn injury to the upper extremity. Br J Plast Surg 1994;47(5):331–40.

23. Woo SH, Seul JH. Optimizing the correction of severe postburn hand deformities by using aggressive contracture releases and fasciocutaneous free-tissue transfers. Plast Reconstr Surg 2001;107(1): 1–8.

24. Ofer N, Baumeister S, Megerle K, et al. Current concepts of microvascular reconstruction for limb salvage in electrical burn injuries. J Plast Reconstr Aesthet Surg 2007;60(7):724–30.

25. Kwan MW, Ha KW. Splinting programme for patients with burnt hand. Hand Surg 2002;7(2):231–41.

Cold Injuries

Deana S. Shenaq, MD, Lawrence J. Gottlieb, MD*

KEYWORDS

- Frostbite • Limb salvage • Thrombolytics • Bone scan • Urban

KEY POINTS

- Cold injuries can be divided into the following spectrum: frostnip, superficial frostbite, and deep frostbite.
- Under ideal circumstances, severely frostbitten extremities are rapidly warmed and treated with thrombolytic therapy within 6 to 24 hours.
- Many victims of cold injury, particularly those in urban environments, do not meet inclusion criteria for thrombolytic administration.
- Technetium-99m bone scans or single-photon emission computed tomography/computed tomography can predict tissue demarcation within 48 hours, allowing for determination of level of amputation or limb salvage.
- Limb salvage or maximizing limb length with grafts and flaps play a leading role in management.

INTRODUCTION

The populations affected by cold injuries are diverse. Historically, the first cases of frostbite were seen in soldiers on military campaigns. Cold-related injuries almost completely destroyed Napoleon's army during the Russian invasion of 1812 to 1813, and more than a million people succumbed to the condition during World Wars I and II and the Korean Wars.[1] Within the last 20 to 30 years, an increased interest in outdoor sports and recreation led to frostbite injuries within the civilian population, in particular, skiers or mountaineers and others who venture outdoors in cold weather for work. Civilians are also affected by frostbite in the inner cities, hence the term, *urban frostbite*. In an urban environment, most patients who suffer frostbite injuries present in a delayed fashion and sustain repeated cold injuries as a result of psychological issues, intoxication, or homelessness. These social aspects present unique barriers to treatment. Frostbite can also be categorized as experimental, when injuries are inflicted on anesthetized experimental animals'

ears and paws in an attempt to elucidate mechanism of injury and test therapeutic modalities.

Irrespective of the population affected by frostbite, the early management of cold injuries relied primarily on the principles of rapid rewarding, watchful waiting and delayed amputation,[2,3] following the adage "freeze in January, amputate in July."[4] The treatment of frostbite then remained stagnant until the 1980s and 1990s, when a paradigm shift in management occurred based on the recognition that the pathogenesis of progressive dermal ischemia was related to the arachidonic acid cascade and the introduction of thrombolytic therapies for attempted limb salvage.[5] Previous investigations into adjuvant treatments such as antiplatelet agents, digital sympathectomies, and hyperbaric oxygen therapy are discussed in this article but have not proven as effective as prostacyclin analogs and thrombolytics in the clinical arena. To appreciate the mechanism by which these various modalities function in frostbite management, it is imperative first to understand the pathophysiology of cold injuries.

Financial Disclosure: The authors have nothing to disclose.
Funding Support: None.
The University of Chicago Medicine, 5841 South Maryland Avenue, MC 6035, Chicago, IL 60637, USA
* Corresponding author.
E-mail address: lgottlie@surgery.bsd.uchicago.edu

hand.theclinics.com

PATHOPHYSIOLOGY

Most frostbite occurs when tissues freeze slowly and form ice crystals. The temperatures necessary to produce this injury are typically less than 28.4°F (−2°C). Injuries are circumferential, progress distal to proximal, and are potentially reversible. Local tissue damage is influenced by the susceptibility of specific body tissues to cold, the cooling rate, the lowest tissue temperature achieved, the duration of the cold exposure and ischemia time, and the rewarming conditions. Skin will freeze faster at lower temperatures but the degree of tissue disruption depends mainly on the duration of the freezing process. Cellular damage occurs as the tissue freezes and when it thaws (during and after rewarming).

Tissue Freezing

Cold exposure of an extremity causes vasoconstriction, which leads to reduced peripheral blood flow and cooling of the skin. This cooling then results in further vasoconstriction. In an attempt to rewarm the extremity and protect against freezing, the body responds with cycles of vasodilation and vasoconstriction transiently every 5 to 10 minutes. This reaction is called the *hunting response*.[6] Unfortunately, this vasodilation then brings cold blood back to the main circulation, which causes the core temperature to drop. At very cold temperatures, the hunting response is blunted to allow maintenance of core temperature at the expense of extremity rewarming. As the extremity is cooled, skin blanches, producing a burning, heat sensation. Once the core temperature decreases, arteriovenous shunting occurs, which shifts blood flow away from the skin. Sensory nerve dysfunction occurs at 10°C, and the digits become stiff and numb. As the skin cools further, blood viscosity increases, producing microvasculature constriction with transendothelial plasma leakage.

During rapid freezing, intracellular ice crystals can form. Except in accidental injuries, such as liquid nitrogen emersions, rapid freezing generally only occurs in experimental conditions. Typically, with slower freezing as seen clinically, ice crystals form initially in the extracellular space.[7,8] Increased extracellular osmotic pressure draws free water across the cell membrane, producing intracellular water loss, hyperosmolality, and decreased cell volume. Extracellular and intracellular electrolyte and acid-base disturbances ensue with a resultant destruction of enzymes. Growing ice crystals can also damage cells and their membranes directly. Endothelial injury leads to microvascular damage, which harms tissues indirectly. This disruption of the microvasculature, along with ice crystal formation in plasma and sludging of red blood cells, results in eventual cessation of the microcirculation.[9]

Tissue Thawing/Rewarming

Most of the tissue damage sustained from frostbite injury is caused by the damaging effects during and soon after rewarming. Once the extremity is rewarmed, the damaged capillary endothelium leaks fluid and protein into the interstitial space, which is manifested by swelling and leads to blister formation. Occasionally, blisters do not form, which signifies either a very superficial injury or an extremely deep injury. Typically, blisters are filled with straw-colored or blood-tinged fluid.[10] The most significant injuries are most likely caused by reperfusion injury with the generation of oxygen free radical formation and initiation of the arachidonic acid cascade with prostaglandin-induced vasoconstriction, leukocyte adherence, and aggregation of red and white blood cells and platelets.[7,11] This mechanism is hypothesized because prostaglandin F_{2a} and thromboxane A_2, which have been implicated in vasoconstriction, platelet aggregation, and thrombosis, are found in the blister fluid.[12] Although the exact timing and sequence of events are not clear, it is evident that these changes will lead to significant tissue loss if no intervention is initiated in the crucial first 24 to 48 hours after rewarming.

CLASSIFICATION

Cold injuries have been classified in a variety of different ways. The simplest is to separate prefreezing and freezing injuries. The prefreezing injuries include trench foot and chilblains or pernio. Trench or immersion foot mainly affects military personnel with prolonged exposure to damp conditions at freezing temperatures. The affected feet may become numb, erythematous, or cyanotic as a result of poor circulation. Chilblain (pernio) occurs in response to repeated cold, nonfreezing temperatures in dry conditions. Symptoms include: 189 burning, pruritus, swelling, erythema, and blistering that can progress to ulceration. Usually, the lesions resolve within 2 weeks but can lead to chronic problems such as vasculitis, typically seen in young, middle-aged women.[6]

Historically, frostbite injuries were classified like burns as a range of first to fourth degree injuries. These categories can be difficult to assess in the field, as often the still-frozen part is hard, pale, and anesthetic. Thus, the previous system was tough to apply and led to confusion among providers. A simpler scheme by Mills and Whaley[13] divides tissue injury into the following spectrum: frostnip, superficial frostbite, and deep frostbite. The severity of frostbite can vary within an extremity with some areas exhibiting superficial injury, whereas others can be deeper.[14]

Frostnip is a very superficial form of local freezing with symptoms such as numbness and tingling that typically resolve after rewarming. There is intense vasoconstriction resulting in the affected areas appearing hyperemic. Digits can exhibit pallor but do not blister. There is no ice crystal formation or microvascular injury; therefore, no irreversible tissue damage seems to occur. Frostnip is a harbinger for frostbite and should signal one to take appropriate measures to prevent reinjury.

Superficial frostbite presents with numbness, erythema (reactive hyperemia), and skin vesicles. It is characteristically supple when depressed and painful after thawing. Clear or milky fluid is present within the blisters with surrounding edema. There is no or minimal anticipated tissue loss. Good prognostic indicators include clear blisters located distally on warm hyperemic limbs with intact sensation.[15]

Deep frostbite results in hemorrhagic blisters, indicating that the injury has extended into the reticular dermis and beneath the dermal vascular plexus. The necrosis can extend to muscle or bone, and tissue loss is anticipated.[16] Signs indicating a poor prognosis include hemorrhagic blebs located proximally on the limb, with distal tissue that remains cold, ischemic, and insensate. The tissue has a firm, woody feel with a blue-gray appearance and, unlike superficial injuries, remains anesthetic after thawing.[15]

An even simpler grading system based on the extent of digital cyanosis after rewarming was proposed by Cauchy and colleagues[17] in 2001. The accuracy of this classification scheme was verified with dual-phase bone scans and was recently found to be helpful in guiding treatment in austere environments.[18]

RISK FACTORS

Survival in cold environments is contingent on insulation with adequate protective clothing and gear. Venturing out in cold weather without appropriate clothing and protective wear is clearly the leading risk factor for frostbite. Although occasionally people might find themselves in this situation accidentally, typically, in the urban environment, most frostbite victims are compromised by psychiatric illness or intoxication.[19–21] The malnourished or chronically ill are also more susceptible to cold-induced injuries because of decreased capacity for normal thermoregulation. Similarly, patients with Raynaud's disease and peripheral vascular disease are at higher risk for cold injuries. One may think that smokers would also be at an increased risk, as nicotine elevates plasma catecholamine levels and other chemicals in smoke reduce the synthesis of nitric oxide, a vasodilator.[22] Smoking also increases fibrinogen and platelet levels, which can lead to thrombosis. Interestingly, the literature has not been able to show a definitive increased risk of frostbite with smoking.[23,24]

TREATMENT
Hypothermia

Life-threatening conditions such as hypothermia require urgent treatment. Hypothermia causes peripheral vasoconstriction that will impair blood flow to the extremities; thus, these conditions should be treated effectively before addressing the frostbite injury. There are many ways to warm patients, depending on the degree of hypothermia, and each method varies in invasiveness as follows: extracorporeal membrane oxygenation or venovenous perfusion for the most severe; warm peritoneal or pleural irrigations, warming intravenous fluids, and gastric lavage for moderate hypothermia; and truncal immersion in water at 104°F (40°C) for correction of mild-to-moderate hypothermia. Frozen extremities should not be rewarmed until the core temperature reaches 95°F (35°C), when immersion of a single extremity at a time should be performed.[25] If the extremities are submerged before core rewarming, a phenomenon called *afterdrop*[26] can transpire, which results from the cold peripheral blood returning to the core, causing the central temperature to plummet. If the returning blood is acidic and high in potassium, cardiac dysrhythmia and vascular collapse may result, known as *rewarming shock*.[27,28]

Rewarming

Although it is accepted that the severe injuries are linked to a longer duration of the freezing process, it is not clear if, once the tissue is frozen, whether there is a critical time for when it should be rewarmed. Because refreezing a thawed extremity is far worse than keeping it frozen, in recreational or wilderness frostbite, it is generally recommended to not rewarm frozen extremities if transport to medical care is less than 2 hours.[26] However, limiting uncontrolled, slow spontaneous thawing while attempting to keep people warm is difficult. If thawing begins, it is paramount to prevent the thawed tissues from refreezing, which can lead to further tissue damage.

Field rewarming by warm water bath immersion can be performed if the proper equipment and methods are available and definitive care is more than 2 hours away. Water should be heated to 37°C to 39°C (98.6–102.21°F).[29] When the involved part develops a red or purple appearance and becomes soft and pliable, this signifies the completion of rewarming, which is usually accomplished in approximately 30 minutes. The affected tissues should be allowed to air dry or gently dried with blotting motions to minimize further damage. Under appropriate circumstances, this method of field rewarming is the first definitive step in frostbite treatment.[16]

There is no evidence for or against administering prophylactic antibiotics or adding any antimicrobial or antiseptic solution to rewarming baths. Rewarming is also generally very painful and may require opioid analgesics or regional anesthetic block. As with most extremity injuries, dependent edema should be prevented by elevation of the extremity. If tetanus prophylaxis is not up to date, then it should be administered.

HOSPITAL MANAGEMENT

All patients with any injury more than the most superficial frostbite should be admitted to the hospital and ideally treated at a specialized facility, usually a burn center. After rapid rewarming, there are a few interventions that alter the natural history of frostbite. Many treatments have been beneficial in experimental animal models and possess only anecdotal advantages in clinical settings. The goals of postthaw care are aimed at preserving viable tissue, preventing progression of disease or injury from superficial to deep, and avoiding infection. Good animal experimental studies, observational clinical studies, and one nonrandomized controlled study show a benefit of topical thromboxane inhibition with aloe vera and nonsteroidal anti-inflammatory treatment with either aspirin or ibuprofen to address both the arachidonic acid cascade and platelet aggregation.[4,24,30–32]

There are a few retrospective studies and case reports that suggest a decreased incidence of amputation when tissue plasminogen activator (tPA) is used in the first 24 hours after rewarming.[3,33,34] One prospective study found a decreased amputation rate with rapid rewarming, aspirin, thrombolysis, and prostacyclin analogues with the most impressive results in the prostacyclin analog group.[35] Unfortunately, the prostacyclin analog used, iloprost, is not available in intravenous form in the United States.

Local Wound Care

There is clinical controversy, without good evidence, as to the treatment of blisters in cold-related injuries. As previously discussed, clear or cloudy blister fluid contains prostaglandin F_{2a} and thromboxane A_2, which have been implicated in platelet aggregation and thrombosis and may be damaging to underlying tissue. Therefore, most clinicians will either aspirate clear blister fluid or debride the blister to avoid fluid accumulation. Hemorrhagic blisters signify deeper tissue damage and are commonly left intact.[6,30,31,36] Some clinicians debride all blisters, regardless of whether they are hemorrhagic or clear. The main concern for debriding blisters is the potential desiccation of the underlying wound bed, yet the major reason for debriding blisters is to avoid the interference with radionucleotide scans and infection. There are clinical data to support the routine use of topical aloe vera, a thromboxane inhibitor, on frostbitten tissue.[24,32]

Triple-Phase Bone Scanning

Despite the variation in populations affected by frostbite, one fact remains universal across all subsets of patients—the initial clinical assessment of cold injuries is notoriously unreliable. As stated previously, hospital treatment guidelines once followed the widely accepted adage, "freeze in January, amputate in July."[4] Historically, patients suffered frostbite injuries during the winter and waited 1 to 6 months to allow the injured areas to demarcate and determine the need for and level of amputation.[37–40] However, with the popularization of technetium-99m (^{99m}Tc) pertechnetate triple-phase bone scanning, there has been a paradigm shift in the management of frostbite injuries (**Fig. 1**). This shift is primarily because bone scans can reliably predict the likelihood and level of amputation as early as 2 to 3 days after rewarming.[37] Mehta and Wilson[15] advocate for triple-phase bone scans 48 hours after admission and found 3 patterns of frostbite injury:

1. Hyperemic flow with an increased blood-pool phase and normal delayed scans of the skeleton and soft tissues
2. Absent blood flow, with no blood-pool images, but normal depiction of bone uptake in delayed scans
3. Absent blood pool with absent bone uptake in delayed images

According to their report, delayed images were most useful in accurately defining the line of tissue demarcation. They advocated nonoperative

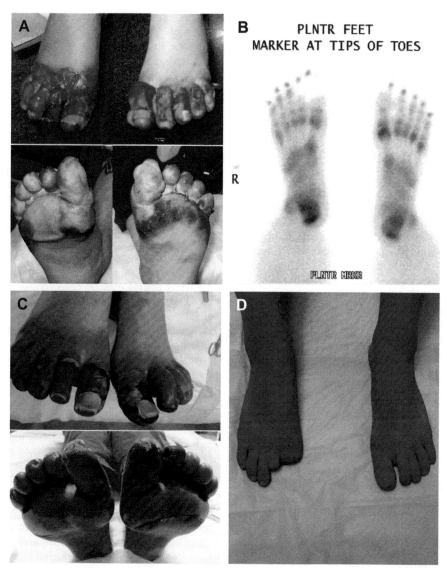

Fig. 1. Predictive value of bone scan. (*A*) A 22-year-old woman got frostbite after hiking for 11 hours. She presented 2 weeks after injury. Note, the right great and second toe are more purple than the left. (*B*) Bone scan shows no flow in right great toe and second toe. (*C*) Toe demarcation is consistent with bone scan results. (*D*) After amputation of nonviable tissue. (*Courtesy of* L.J. Gottlieb, MD, FACS, Chicago, IL.)

management if the delayed images were normal. If the delayed images were absent, indicating no radioisotope uptake in bone, then prognostication for amputation could be made by 3 days after rewarming. Greenwald and colleagues[41] used triple-phase isotope bone scanning to determine if patients with severe frostbite injuries were candidates for attempted salvage rather than amputations.

Although clinical studies found that bone scans could reliably forecast the microvascular condition of limbs affected by frostbite, the predictive value varies with the time after injury.[15,37,42–44] Cauchy and colleagues[37] found that the predictive value of 99mTc bone scans varied with the time obtained after rewarming. The accuracy at 48 hours after rewarming was 84%, which then increased to almost 100% correlation between abnormal 99mTc dual-phase bone scans and amputation by the end of first week.

There is no evidence that validates the predictive value of 99mTc bone scans in the first 24 hours after rewarming, especially when making decisions on the early phases of the scans. Despite this fact, 99mTc scanning obtained within hours of presentation has become part of routine protocols at some institutions and are used to guide management decisions, including the use of thrombolytic therapy for limb salvage.[15,45,46]

Magnetic resonance angiography (MRA) is another modality used to evaluate perfusion in digits with frostbite to identify unsalvageable digits.[47,48] MRA is used to distinguish blood vessels from the surrounding tissue related either to detected flow through the vessels or injected contrast.[49] These images can accurately detail blood flow and identify areas in which there is no flow. MRA can be used in patients with frostbite to identify patent blood vessels versus vasculature destroyed by frostbite to determine what areas have no deep blood flow and to determine the level of required amputation.[47] Barker and colleagues[48] argue that MRA is superior to ^{99m}Tc-methylene diphosphonate bone scans because it allows for direct visualization of vessels and a more obvious line of demarcation between viable and nonviable tissue. However this must be further studied for a definitive comparison. MRA may also be useful for detailing the efficacy of tPA administration.[50]

Single-photon emission computed tomography/computed tomography (SPECT/CT) is an imaging modality that was recently described as an option for the evaluation of frostbite extent and the ability of tissue to be salvaged.[51,52] SPECT/CT is a combination of a ^{99m}Tc-methylene diphosphonate bone scan and a computed tomography scan for improved anatomic localization of the radiotracer uptake.[23] This imaging modality allows for improved localization of deep-tissue necrosis in frostbite patients and allows for more rapid amputation of unsalvageable digits without compromising digits that will heal. SPECT/CT is able to provide clinically and surgically relevant information via anatomic landmarks beyond what is provided by a conventional bone scan alone.

Sympathectomy

Surgical sympathectomies have also been suggested as an adjunctive treatment. Surgical sympathectomies have been shown to shorten the time to resolution of pain and to demarcation of tissue necrosis but may not reduce the extent of tissue loss.[10] When performed immediately, surgical sympathectomy may increase edema, but some resolution of this swelling has been seen when performed 24 to 48 after thaw. Bouwman and colleagues[53] conducted a clinical trial in which chemical sympathectomy was attempted with reserpine starting 3 hours after rewarming and combined with surgical sympathectomies at an average of 3 days later. The only benefit noted was protection from recurrent cold injury, as there was no reduction in pain or edema or evidence of tissue preservation. Distal sympathectomies performed at the level of the individual digital vessels have been shown to alleviate frostbite-induced chronic vasospasm. Results in a series of 3 patients included improvement in pain, elevation in skin temperature by 1.5°C to 2.5°C, and healing of chronic ulcers.[54]

Hyperbaric Oxygen

Many wounds unrelated to frostbite show accelerated healing after hyperbaric oxygen therapy.[55] Therefore, the application of hyperbaric oxygen for the treatment of frostbite injuries, first described by Ledingham in 1963,[56] was a natural progression. Increasing the amount of dissolved oxygen in plasma promotes angiogenesis and neovascularization and down-regulation of the inflammatory response.[57] Other purported benefits include bacteriologic control, decreased edema in postischemic tissues, and increased erythrocyte flexibility.[58] However, with frostbite in particular, the blood supply to the distal tissues may be compromised; therefore, some argue that hyperbaric therapy may not be as effective. Anecdotal case reports describe improvement with hyperbaric oxygen starting 5 to 10 days after injury.[59,60] But, in the absence of controlled clinical trials, it is hard to recommend hyperbaric oxygen therapy as a routine protocol, and it should be considered on a case-by-case basis.

Thrombolytics

The basis of frostbite management has relied on fluid resuscitation and rapid rewarming, followed by local wound care and watchful waiting, as previously discussed. Rapid rewarming, however, addresses primarily the ice crystal phase of tissue damage and does not improve already thrombosed or injured vessels, nor does it alter the course of progressive necrosis and thrombosis from free radicals and reperfusion injury that may continue many hours after rewarming.[13,34] Therefore, adjunctive treatments have been proposed, aimed at optimizing blood flow by inhibiting vasoconstriction and clotting. Some of these modalities include surgical lumbar sympathectomy, brachial plexus blockade, intra-arterial reserpine, oral nifedipine, ibuprofen, and clopidogrel. These treatments, however, are limited to case reports, retrospective reviews, or animal models. Thrombolytic therapy as a means to reverse cold injuries was introduced in a small pilot study in the 1992,[45] and a few centers around the country have been successful at instituting protocols to implement this modality,[3,33,34,46] showing a marked reduction in amputations of affected hands and feet.

Under ideal circumstances, severely frostbitten extremities are rapidly warmed and treated with thrombolytic therapy within 6 to 24 hours (**Box 1**). Although thrombolytic therapy for frostbite injury

Box 1
Recommendations for intravenous thrombolytic administration

- tPA dose: 0.15 mg/kg intravenous bolus followed by 0.15 mg/kg/h over 6 hours (up to a total 100 mg).

- After tPA completion, give 3000 units intravenous heparin.

- Heparin infusion is then continued to reach desired partial thromboplastin time of 2 times control and continued for 3 to 5 days.

Adapted from Johnson AR, Jensen HL, Peltier G, et al. Efficacy of intravenous tissue plasminogen activator in frostbite patients and presentation of a treatment protocol for frostbite patients. Foot Ankle Specialist 2011;4(6):344–8.

Box 2
Patient criteria for thrombolytic therapy

Criteria for tPA Use

- No improvement on rapid rewarming in tepid water (38° to 42°C for 15–20 min)

- Absent Doppler pulses in limbs or digits

- Limited perfusion on ^{99m}Tc triple-phase bone scan

- Less than 24 hours since rewarming completed

Exclusion Criteria

- Severe hypertension

- Recent trauma, stroke, or bleeding

- Pregnancy

- Mental incapacity

- Repeated freeze-thaw cycles

- More than 24 hours after rewarming

Adapted from Johnson AR, Jensen HL, Peltier G, et al. Efficacy of intravenous tissue plasminogen activator in frostbite patients and presentation of a treatment protocol for frostbite patients. Foot Ankle Specialist 2011;4(6):344–8.

has been implemented successfully using streptokinase or urokinase, these treatments have not yet been validated by randomized controlled trials, and current studies are now using tPA or prostacyclin derivatives. Twomey and colleagues[33] found that early administration of tPA can result in complete avoidance of proximal amputation, with digital salvage rates of up to 80%. In this study, 6 of 19 severely frostbitten patients met criteria for intra-arterial tPA administration, and 13 received intravenous tPA. Of the 174 digits at risk for amputation (ie, no perfusion on ^{99m}Tc early bone scans), only 19% were amputated. No patients had complications with intravenous tPA administration, but 2 patients suffered from bleeding diathesis with intra-arterial use. Massachusetts General Hospital also instituted a protocol in 2012 in which patients with severe frostbite were treated with intra-arterial tPA based on clinical evidence of decreased perfusion from emergent angiography.[34] Ibrahim and colleagues[34] reported successful salvage of bilateral lower extremities in a case series of 3 patients after intra-arterial tPA administration, which was delivered via a brachial or femoral artery catheter placed by interventional radiology. Bruen and colleagues[3] published a case series of 7 severely frostbitten patients who were treated with intra-arterial tPA within 24 hours of exposure and compared outcomes with those of historical controls who received conservative treatment. In their series, the amputation rate of the tPA cohort was 10%, compared with 41% in the non–tPA-treated group. An intraperitoneal hematoma developed in a patient who received tPA that resolved without intervention.

However, the proposed inclusion criteria for the use of tPA is strict, and many patients do not always meet these guidelines (**Box 2**). Intravenous thrombolytic therapy is only effective if given in the first hours after rewarming,[33] and intra-arterial administration works for up to 24 hours. Thrombolytics are generally ineffective for patients with cold injuries presenting greater than 24 hours from exposure and for those who have suffered multiple freeze-thaw cycles.[33] They are also contraindicated in alcoholics because of the risk of concomitant head injuries or internal bleeding, which may be difficult to determine in the incapacitated patient. Because our patient population has not historically qualified for tPA administration, our protocol has focused on salvaging limb length with early local or free flap coverage (see later discussion).

SURGICAL TREATMENT

Surgical intervention in patients with frostbite can be grouped into 3 categories: acute, subacute, and delayed.

Acute Surgery

Other than surgically debriding blisters (usually done at the bedside) and occasionally having to perform decompressive fasciotomies in the hand or foot, surgical intervention is rarely required or indicated in the acute setting after rewarming.

Subacute Surgery (First Week)

All patients with deep frostbite injuries should undergo triple-phase bone scans[41] 2 to 3 days after rewarming regardless of the postrewarming protocol. The importance of this scan is to determine whether there is any blood flow to the bone by radioisotope uptake. If there is normal uptake, the patient will recover and no surgery is indicated. With decreased uptake, a repeat scan should be performed 3 to 4 days later. If the repeat scan continues to demonstrate bone uptake, then the affected digits will likely survive. If either scan shows no uptake in the bone, one can predict the level of demarcation, with the natural progression leading to the development of dry gangrene by day 10 to 14 and subsequent amputation. In situations in which the amount of tissue loss would be devastating to hand function, such as anticipated loss of complete thumb, multiple digits or extensive hand involvement, limb salvage techniques should be considered.[41] Salvage surgery should proceed before the development of dry, leathery eschar, usually before 10 days after injury.

Delayed Surgery

We define delayed surgery as any surgery after clinical demarcation, which is generally after 2 weeks rewarming. This surgery may include soft tissue debridement of demarcated or infected tissue, bony amputation guided by bone scans, and skin grafts or flaps to close wounds (**Fig. 2**) and preserve length (**Fig. 3**).

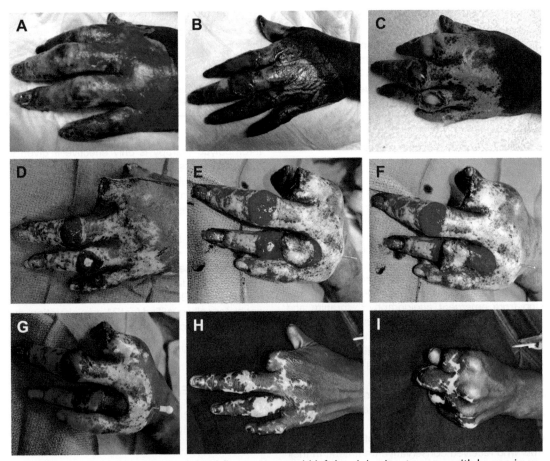

Fig. 2. Subacute frostbite treated with local flap. A 50-year-old left-hand dominant woman with human immunodeficiency virus presented with subacute frostbite injury that occurred 9 days before presentation while waiting for a bus outdoors. She was admitted to an outside hospital for 3 days and discharged. (*A*) On presentation: increased drainage and concern for infection. (*B*) One week later: Integra placed over proximal interphalangeal joints of index, middle, and ring fingers. (*C*) Two weeks later: distal phalanges of index and thumb demarcated. Integra becomes infected. (*D*) Index and thumb amputated; Integra removed with exposed extensor tendon. (*E*) Propeller flap elevated, ring finger. (*F*) Propeller flap transposed, ring finger. (*G*) Donor site and middle finger closed with full-thickness skin graft. (*H*) Healed wounds 6 months later. (*I*) Good range of motion. (*Courtesy of* L.J. Gottlieb, MD, FACS, Chicago, IL.)

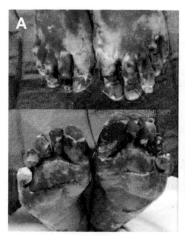
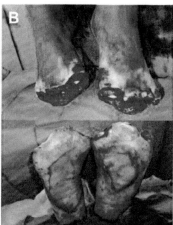
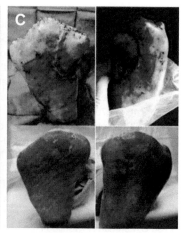

Fig. 3. Delayed frostbite treated with local flap. A 43-year-old homeless man was transferred from an outside hospital with frostbite on his feet after about 4 weeks of living outside. The patient was protecting his feet with boots, which were frozen to his feet at presentation. (*A*) Demarcated toes bilaterally. (*B*) Amputation of toes at metatarsophalangeal joints. (*C*) V-Y plantar flap to preserve metatarsal head (lower panel at 3-month follow-up). (*Courtesy of* L.J. Gottlieb, MD, FACS, Chicago, IL.)

PROGNOSIS AND SEQUELAE

It is rare for frostbitten tissues to recover completely.[27] Long-term complications include cold sensitivity (75%), sensory loss (68%), hyperhidrosis (75%), and chronic pain (67%).[21,61] Treatment measures and agents include sympathetic nerve blocks, vasodilators, and α-blockers. An increased susceptibility to future cold injuries is common because of impaired circulation in affected areas.[6] Electrodiagnostic studies of patients with cold exposure injury to the extremities have detected decreased motor and sensory nerve conduction velocities, especially in lower extremity injuries.[62] Eventually, nerve decompressions, such as carpal tunnel release, may be required.

Frostbite can also cause musculoskeletal issues such as localized osteopenia, subchondral bone loss, or joint contractures.[63,64] Children have an increased potential for bony abnormalities, even without initial soft tissue loss.[10] Articular cartilage damage is evident on radiographs 6 to 12 months after cold injury.[65] Visible deformities include dwarfing of the middle and distal phalanges, degenerative arthritis, and poor alignment of the proximal and distal interphalangeal joints. Bony growth arrest with shortening has also been reported if the epiphyseal plates are damaged.[66]

SUMMARY

Since the beginning of time, man has battled the elements, and the cold, in particular, has proven a lethal opponent throughout history. Human adaption to frigid temperatures is minimal, and survival depends on insulation with protective gear. The most common risk factors associated with frostbite injury are alcohol and drugs, mental illness, and homelessness. Of all the proposed protocols for frostbite treatment, rapid rewarming is the most universally accepted.

Historically, watchful waiting and delayed amputation were the tenets of cold injury management. However, triple-phase bone scans can now predict at-risk tissues at earlier time points, and there is currently a role for reversal of injuries with thrombolytic administration. Findings suggest that the early administration of tPA may result in avoidance of proximal amputation and digital salvage rates between 80% and 90%. Prostacyclin analogs are another promising treatment that have less risk than thrombolytics and can be administered up to 48 hours after rewarming. There remain patients who are either not candidates or who will not respond to these treatments. These patients may be candidates for salvaging limb length with free and local flaps.

REFERENCES

1. Orr KD, Fainer DC. Cold injuries in Korea during winter of 1950-51. Medicine (Baltimore) 1952;31(2):177–220.
2. Petrone P, Kuncir E, Asensio JA. Surgical management and strategies in the treatment of hypothermia and cold injury. Emerg Med Clin North Am 2003; 21(4):1165–78.
3. Bruen KJ, Ballard JR, Morris SE, et al. Reduction of the incidence of amputation in frostbite injury with thrombolytic therapy. Arch Surg 2007;142(6): 546–51 [discussion: 551–3].

4. Britt LD, Dascombe WH, Rodriguez A. New horizons in management of hypothermia and frostbite injury. Surg Clin North Am 1991;71(2):345–70.

5. Gross EA, Moore JC. Using thrombolytics in frostbite injury. J Emerg Trauma Shock 2012;5(3):267–71.

6. Golant A, Nord RM, Paksima N, et al. Cold exposure injuries to the extremities. J Am Acad Orthop Surg 2008;16(12):704–15.

7. Mazur P. Cryobiology: the freezing of biological systems. Science 1970;168(3934):939–49.

8. Meryman H. Tissue freezing and local cold injury. Physiol Rev 1957;37(2):233–51.

9. Weatherley-White RC, Sjostrom B, Paton BC. Experimental studies in cold injury II: the pathogenesis of frostbite. J Surg Res 1964;4:17–22.

10. Su C, Lohman R, Gottlieb LJ. Frostbite of the upper extremity. Hand Clin 2000;16:235–47.

11. Manson PN, Jesudass R, Marzella L, et al. Evidence for an early free radical-mediated reperfusion injury in frostbite. Free Radic Biol Med 1991;10(1):7–11.

12. Robson MC, Heggers JP. Evaluation of hand frostbite blister fluid as a clue to pathogenesis. J Hand Surg Am 1981;6(1):43–7.

13. Mills WJ, Whaley R. Frostbite: experience with rapid rewarming and ultrasonic therapy. 1960-1. Wilderness Environ Med 1998;9(4):226.

14. Zafren K. Frostbite: prevention and initial management. High Alt Med Biol 2013;14(1):9–12.

15. Mehta RC, Wilson MA. Frostbite injury: prediction of tissue viability with triple-phase bone scanning. Radiology 2005;170(2):511–4.

16. McIntosh SE, Opacic M, Freer L, et al. Wilderness medical society practice guidelines for the prevention and treatment of frostbite: 2014 update. Wilderness Environ Med 2014;25(Suppl 4):S43–54.

17. Cauchy E, Chetaille E, Marchand V, et al. Retrospective study of 70 cases of severe frostbite lesions: a proposed new classification scheme. Wilderness Environ Med 2001;12(4):248–55.

18. Cauchy E, Davis CB, Pasquier M, et al. A new proposal for management of severe frostbite in the austere environment. Wilderness Environ Med 2016;27(1):92–9.

19. Valnicek SM, Chasmar LR, Clapson JB. Frostbite in the prairies: a 12-year review. Plast Reconstr Surg 1993;92(4):633–41.

20. Pinzur MS, Weaver FM. Is urban frostbite a psychiatric disorder? Orthopedics 1997;20(1):43–5.

21. Koljonen V, Andersson K, Mikkonen K, et al. Frostbite injuries treated in the Helsinki area from 1995 to 2002. J Trauma 2004;57(6):1315–20.

22. Ervasti O, Juopperi K, Kettunen P, et al. The occurrence of frostbite and its risk factors in young men. Int J Circumpolar Health 2004;63(1):71–80.

23. Daanen HAM, van der Struijs NR. Resistance Index of Frostbite as a predictor of cold injury in arctic operations. Aviat Space Environ Med 2005;76(12):1119–22.

24. Heil K, Thomas R, Robertson G, et al. Freezing and non-freezing cold weather injuries: a systematic review. Br Med Bull 2016;117(1):79–93.

25. Ahrenholz DH. Frostbite. Probl Gen Surg 2003;20(1):129–37.

26. Zafren K, Giesbrecht G. State of Alaska cold injuries guidelines. State of Alaska; 2014.

27. Jurkovich GJ. Environmental cold-induced injury. Surg Clin North Am 2007;87(1):247–67.

28. Wittmers LE. Pathophysiology of cold exposure. Minn Med 2001;84(11):30–6.

29. Malhotra MS, Mathew L. Effect of rewarming at various water bath temperatures in experimental frostbite. Aviat Space Environ Med 1978;49(7):874–6.

30. Imray C, Grieve A, Dhillon S, Caudwell Xtreme Everest Research Group. Cold damage to the extremities: frostbite and non-freezing cold injuries. Postgrad Med J 2009;85(1007):481–8.

31. McCauley RL, Hing DN, Robson MC, et al. Frostbite injuries: a rational approach based on the pathophysiology. J Trauma 1983;23(2):143–7.

32. Heggers JP, Robson MC, Manavalen K, et al. Experimental and clinical observations on frostbite. Ann Emerg Med 1987;16(9):1056–62.

33. Twomey JA, Peltier GL, Zera RT. An open-label study to evaluate the safety and efficacy of tissue plasminogen activator in treatment of severe frostbite. J Trauma 2005;59(6):1350–5.

34. Ibrahim AE, Goverman J, Sarhane KA, et al. The emerging role of tissue plasminogen activator in the management of severe frostbite. J Burn Care Res 2015;36(2):e62–6.

35. Cauchy E, Cheguillaume B, Chetaille E. A controlled trial of a prostacyclin and rt-PA in the treatment of severe frostbite. N Engl J Med 2011;364(2):189–90.

36. Reamy BV. Frostbite: review and current concepts. J Am Board Fam Pract 1998;11(1):34–40.

37. Cauchy E, Marsigny B, Allamel G, et al. The value of technetium 99 scintigraphy in the prognosis of amputation in severe frostbite injuries of the extremities: a retrospective study of 92 severe frostbite injuries. J Hand Surg Am 2000;25(5):969–78.

38. Christenson C, Stewart C. Frostbite. Am Fam Physician 1984;30(6):111–22.

39. Page RE, Robertson GA. Management of the frostbitten hand. Hand 1983;15(2):185–91.

40. Knize DM, Weatherley-White RC, Paton BC, et al. Prognostic factors in the management of frostbite. J Trauma 1969;9(9):749–59.

41. Greenwald D, Cooper B, Gottlieb L. An algorithm for early aggressive treatment of frostbite with limb salvage directed by triple-phase scanning. Plast Reconstr Surg 1998;102(4):1069–74.

42. Lisbona R, Rosenthall L. Assessment of bone viability by scintiscanning in frostbite injuries. J Trauma 1976;16(12):989–92 [Internet]. Available at: http://eutils.ncbi.nlm.nih.gov/entrez/eutils/elink.fcgi?dbfrom=pubmed&id=1003589&retmode=ref&cmd=prlinks.

43. Ristkari SK, Vorne M, Mokka RE. Early assessment of amputation level in frostbite by 99mTc-pertechnetate scan. Case report. Acta Chir Scand 1988; 154(5–6):403–5.

44. Salimi Z, Vas W, Tang-Barton P, et al. Assessment of tissue viability in frostbite by 99mTc pertechnetate scintigraphy. AJR Am J Roentgenol 1984;142(2): 415–9.

45. Skolnick AA. Early data suggest clot-dissolving drug may help save frostbitten limbs from amputation. JAMA 1992;267(15):2008–10.

46. Johnson AR, Jensen HL, Peltier G, et al. Efficacy of intravenous tissue plasminogen activator in frostbite patients and presentation of a treatment protocol for frostbite patients. Foot Ankle Spec 2011;4(6):344–8.

47. Raman SR, Jamil Z, Cosgrove J. Magnetic resonance angiography unmasks frostbite injury. Emerg Med J 2011;28:450.

48. Barker JR, Haws MJ, Brown RE, et al. Magnetic resonance imaging of severe frostbite injuries. Ann Plast Surg 1997;38:275–9.

49. Edelman RR. Basic principles of magnetic resonance angiography. Cardiovasc Intervent Radiol 2013;15:3–13.

50. Wagner C, Pannucci CJ. Thrombolytic therapy in the acute management of frostbite injuries. Air Med J 2011;30:39–44.

51. Kraft C, Millet JD, Agarwal S, et al. SPECT/CT in the Evaluation of Frostbite. J Burn Care Res 2016. [Epub ahead of print].

52. Millet JD, Brown RK, Levi B, et al. Frostbite: spectrum of imaging findings and guidelines for management. Radiographics 2016;36(7):2154–69.

53. Bouwman DL, Morrison S, Lucas CE, et al. Early sympathetic blockade for frostbite–is it of value? J Trauma 1980;20(9):744–9.

54. Flatt AE. Digital artery sympathectomy. J Hand Surg Am 1980;5(6):550–6.

55. Thom SR. Hyperbaric oxygen: its mechanisms and efficacy. Plast Reconstr Surg 2011;127(Suppl 1): 131S–41S.

56. Ledingham IM. Some clinical and experimental applications of high pressure oxygen. Proc R Soc Med 1963;56:999–1002.

57. Haik J, Brown S, Liran A, et al. Deep frostbite: the question of adjuvant treatment. Isr Med Assoc J 2016;18(1):56–7.

58. Mohr WJ, Jenabzadeh K, Ahrenholz DH. Cold injury. Hand Clin 2009;25(4):481–96.

59. Ward MP, Garnham JR, Simpson BR, et al. Frostbite: general observations and report of cases treated by hyperbaric oxygen. Proc R Soc Med 1968;61(8): 787–9.

60. Heimburg von D, Noah EM, Sieckmann UP, et al. Hyperbaric oxygen treatment in deep frostbite of both hands in a boy. Burns 2001;27(4):404–8.

61. Blair J, Schatzki R, Orr K. Sequelae to cold injury in one hundred patients; follow-up study four years after occurrence of cold injury. J Am Med Assoc 1957; 163(14):1203–8.

62. Arvesen A, Wilson J, Rosén L. Nerve conduction velocity in human limbs with late sequelae after local cold injury. Eur J Clin Invest 1996;26(6):443–50.

63. Chalmers IM, Bock GW. Cold injury in 2 patients with connective tissue disease–frostbite arthritis plus. J Rheumatol 2000;27(10):2526–9.

64. Kahn JE, Lidove O, Laredo JD, et al. Frostbite arthritis. Ann Rheum Dis 2005;64(6):966–7.

65. Vogel JE, Dellon AL. Frostbite injuries of the hand. Clin Plast Surg 1989;16(3):565–76.

66. Selke AC. Destruction of phalangeal epiphyses by frostbite. Radiology 1969;93(4):859–60.

The Use of Dermal Skin Substitutes for the Treatment of the Burned Hand

Ian C. Sando, MD, Kevin C. Chung, MD, MS*

KEYWORDS

- Hand • Burn • Reconstruction • Graft • Skin substitute

KEY POINTS

- Early débridement and soft tissue coverage are necessary to minimize scar contracture and maximize functional recovery after hand burns.
- Dermal skin substitutes are excellent alternatives to local or regional flaps when donor sites are limited.
- For partial-thickness wounds, xenografts and bioengineered collagen-nylon matrices expedite healing and minimize patient discomfort.
- For full-thickness wounds, application of dermal matrices followed by a second-stage autograft provides durable coverage that permits free articular movement with excellent scar quality.
- As with any skin substitute, adequate débridement, attention to sterility, and meticulous hemostasis are keys to success.

INTRODUCTION

The hands are the most commonly affected area in burn injuries and are involved approximately 80% of the time.[1,2] Hand burns account for a disproportionate amount of disability after burn injuries due to their critical role in daily activities. Burn injuries frequently occur on the dorsum of the hand, and joint and scar contractures are common because of the thinness of the skin and superficial location of critical structures.[3] Adequate treatment is crucial for rapid functional recovery and good aesthetic outcomes.[4–9]

Traditional surgical management for hand burns includes early escharectomy and autologous skin grafting. Split-thickness sheet grafts are commonly used in superficial hand burns to minimize excessive scarring and prevent desiccation in the interstices of meshed grafts.[10] For full-thickness injuries, flaps or thick autografts that contain all dermal layers are used to obtain pliable coverage and to minimize scar hypertrophy, joint and soft tissue contractures, and an unsatisfactory appearance.[5] Such options may be limited in patients with large total body surface area burns, however, when few donor sites are available.

In recent years, dermal skin substitutes have been used as an alternative to conventional skin grafting techniques for reconstruction of partial-thickness and full-thickness burn wounds.[11–16] Dermal substitutes comprise a 3-D collagen matrix

Research reported in this publication was supported by the National Institute of Arthritis and Musculoskeletal and Skin Diseases of the National Institutes of Health under Award Number 2K24 AR053120-06. The content is solely the responsibility of the authors and does not necessarily represent the official views of the National Institutes of Health.
Disclosure: None of the authors has a financial interest to declare in relation to the content of this article.
Section of Plastic Surgery, Department of Surgery, The University of Michigan Health System, 2130 Taubman Center, SPC 5340, 1500 East Medical Center Drive, Ann Arbor, MI 48109-5340, USA
* Corresponding author.
E-mail address: kecchung@umich.edu

Hand Clin 33 (2017) 269–276
http://dx.doi.org/10.1016/j.hcl.2016.12.008

that serves as a structural template to facilitate generation of a neodermis. They have been shown to optimize healing and improve the quality of scar tissue.[17] Because they serve only to replace the dermal layer, however, epidermal coverage in the form of thin split-thickness skin grafts is still required. Dermal matrices provide many benefits, including the ability to expedite healing,[18,19] decrease length of stay,[20] and provide coverage that is flexible, supple, and mobile.[21–23] Although dermal substitutes have clear advantages in burn reconstruction, they are associated with high cost and may never completely replace autologous tissue transfer. This article reviews the use of various dermal skin substitutes for management of partial-thickness and full-thickness hand burns.

SKIN SUBSTITUTES FOR SUPERFICIAL BURN INJURIES
Acellular Products

Among the numerous xenograft wound care products available, several porcine-based bioengineered dermal substitutes are available to treat superficial burn injuries. These products also provide temporary coverage of skin graft donor sites or widely meshed autografts. Xenoderm (Medical Biomaterial Products, Berlin, Germany) is a newly developed product derived from porcine dermis used for the treatment of second-degree burns.[24] The product is secured to the wound bed after débridement and covered with a temporary dressing. The dressing is removed after 24 hours and the graft is allowed to detach over the following 2 weeks to 5 weeks as re-epithelialization occurs. Although there are theoretic risks of disease transmission from donor animals to patients,[24] the benefits of Xenoderm are its adherence to wounds and the prevention of evaporative water and protein loss.[25] In addition, Hosseini and colleagues[25] found that Xenoderm decreased the number of dressing changes, minimized patient discomfort, and lessened infection rate and length of hospital stay compared with silver sulfadiazine (SSD) when used for the management of partial-thickness burns. EZ Derm (Brennan Medical, St. Paul, Minnesota) is a processed porcine dermal graft that can be stored at room temperature and has a shelf life of approximately 18 months. It promotes epithelialization by acting as an epidermal barrier[26,27]; however, the major disadvantage with EZ Derm is that the pigskin hardens as it dries out and may have deleterious effects on function and range of motion during the healing process.[27] OASIS (Healthpoint, Fort Worth, Texas) is an acellular matrix derived from porcine small intestine submucosa that is processed to remove the serosa, smooth muscle, and mucosa, rendering a collagen scaffold with glycosaminoglycans, fibronectin, proteoglycans, and growth factors.[27] OASIS promotes healing by absorbing, retaining, and protecting bioactive molecules from the wound environment.[28] As with the other porcine-based skin substitutes, it is contraindicated in those with a history of reactivity to porcine products or third-degree burns.[29]

Synthetic Products

Biobrane (Smith & Nephew, United Kingdom) was the first biologically based wound dressing approved by the Food and Drug Administration and is one of the most widely used biosynthetic wound dressings used in the treatment of superficial partial-thickness burns. It is also used to promote healing of skin graft donor sites and meshed autografts. Biobrane is a bilaminate skin substitute consisting of a silicone film bounded to type 1 porcine collagen within a nylon cross-linked fabric.[30] The outer silicone layer reduces evaporative water loss and the nylon matrix becomes anchored to the wound by the blood and serum clot. The porosity of the silicone layer permits drainage of exudates and provides permeability to topical antibiotics, while resisting the ingress of bacteria, providing a vapor barrier, and preventing wound desiccation.[31] Compared with typical dressings, Biobrane has been shown to decrease total healing time, pain, fluid and electrolyte losses, hypothermia, and length of hospitalization.[32–35] It should be applied to burn wounds with no eschar and low bacterial counts.[36] Biobrane gloves are available to treat partial-thickness hand burns once débrided. The fabric is placed sterilely and should be gently stretched to remove all wrinkles, then wrapped in an absorptive dressing, which is left in place for 24 hours to 48 hours.[37] Biobrane is transparent, which facilitates visualization of the wound bed and monitoring for fluid accumulation, which should be drained under sterile conditions to minimize infection.[38] With any dermal substitute, a clean, hemostatic wound that has been properly débrided is a prerequisite to avoid infection and ensure incorporation. Biobrane remains in place for the life of the wound; once adherent, no further dressings are needed and the fabric should be trimmed as it becomes loose. When re-epithelialization is complete, the Biobrane acquires an opaque appearance and may be removed.[37]

Advanced Wound Bioengineered Alternative Tissue (AWBAT) (Aubrey, Carlsbad, California) is a next-generation Biobrane approved by the Food and Drug Administration in 2009. AWBAT has continuity of the 3-D nylon structure and larger pores than those of Biobrane (8.8 mm² vs 6.2 mm²), making it approximately 500% more porous.[39] The increased porosity is expected to result in improved egress of fluid and exudate and theoretically decrease rates of infection, improve acute adherence, and shorten healing time. Although studies comparing Biobrane to AWBAT are limited, Greenwood[40] described his experience with both products and found that AWBAT was easier and less painful to remove but was less elastic. Both products had comparable times to full healing and levels of discomfort at rest and during therapy.

TransCyte (Advanced Tissue Sciences, La Jolla, California) is a temporary biosynthetic covering composed of a semipermeable silicone membrane and newborn human fibroblast cells cultured on a porcine collagen-coated nylon mesh.[41] It is indicated for coverage of excised burns prior to autografting or partial-thickness burns that do not require grafting.[41] TransCyte is thawed at 37°C prior to use and then applied to the burn using adhesive strips or surgical adhesives. A bulky, compression dressing or elastic wrap is applied to maintain contact with the wound until the product is adherent. Once the product is adherent, dressings are removed and the site is left open to the air.[42,43] A splint may be used for temporary immobilization. If the product is nonadherent after 24 hours, or exudate is visualized under the product, the exudate is evacuated, the outer dressing is replaced, and the site is evaluated a day later. TransCyte may be trimmed when it begins to peel as the burn heals (7–14 days).

ACELLULAR DERMAL SUBSTITUTES FOR DEEP INJURIES

Integra (Johnson and Johnson, Hamburg, Germany; Integra LifeSciences, Plainsboro, New Jersey) is a bilaminate membrane consisting of a bovine collagen-based dermal analog of glycosaminoglycans and chondroitin-6-sulphate and a temporary epidermal substitute layer of semipermeable silicone. It is the most widely used dermal substitute for burn reconstruction.[12,13] Its large pore size maximizes the in-growth of cells, and the high degree of cross-linking as well as the glycosaminoglycan composition is designed to control the rate of degradation.

Numerous studies cite Integra's effectiveness in the treatment of acute full-thickness and partial-thickness burn injuries.[5,11,12,44,45] In one of the largest studies, Heimbach and colleagues[46] assessed the safety and effectiveness of Integra when used to treat 216 burn patients. They noted a 3.1% incidence of invasive infection, a mean take rate of Integra of 76.2%, and a mean take rate of epidermal autograft of 87.7%. The investigators conclude that Integra is a valuable, effective, and safe treatment modality for managing challenging patients with extensive burns. In addition to its established role in the acute management of severely burned patients, it is useful in postburn reconstructive procedures to resurface areas after release of burn scar contractures.[11,47,48]

Integra requires a 2-stage process. After débridement, the dermal matrix is meshed 1:1 and secured to the wound. A sterile, moist dressing is applied to keep the matrix hydrated. The dressing is a removed after 5 days and a regimen of moist dressings is instituted several times a day to prevent desiccation. Alternatively, negative pressure therapy may be used to expedite incorporation.[49] This may be uncomfortable, however, for some patients and the infrequency of sponge changes does not permit close monitoring for pockets of infection, which should be drained and sent for culture. After 2 weeks to 3 weeks, the silicone layer is removed and an ultrathin (0.003–0.006 in) split-thickness autograft is applied to the neodermis. **Figs. 1** and **2** illustrate the use of Integra for coverage of palmar and dorsal hand burns, respectively.

Dantzer and colleagues[22,45] have detailed their experience using Integra for management of hand burns. They describe a 100% rate of take in the hand and note that wound coverage is durable enough for the use of prostheses. When used over extensor tendons, engraftment is complete and supple, and the Integra does not adhere to the deeper layers, thus permitting free articular and with good function. The use of Integra also provides acceptable scar quality with respects to mobility, softness, sensation, and appearance.[5,22,44,48,50–52]

The disadvantages of Integra include the risk of infection and the necessity for 2 operations, which may delay the initiation of active range of motion.[37] Nonetheless, Integra has many advantages, including its immediate availability, the simplicity and reliability of its application, its pliability, and potential for good cosmetic appearance.

MatriDerm (Dr. Suwelack, Billerbeck, Germany) is a highly porous, 1-mm thick membrane consisting of a native bovine collagen fiber template coated with elastin hydrolysate that is designed to support dermal regeneration by providing a structure for the invasion of native cells. Compared with other dermal substitutes, MatriDerm has shown success when used simultaneously with thin split-thickness autografts in 1-stage

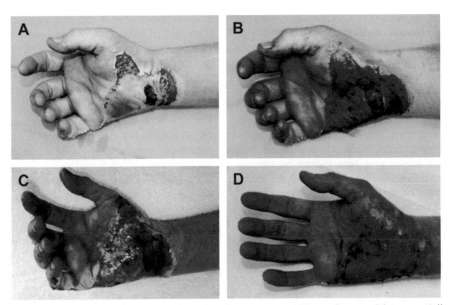

Fig. 1. (A) Full-thickness burn injury to the right palm of an 11-year-old boy who was (B) tangentially débrided down to healthy tissue. (C) Day 4 after application of Integra. (D) One week after second-stage application of a thin autograft demonstrating good graft take.

procedures. The ability to obviate a second operation has the potential to expedite healing, decrease costs, and improve functional outcomes by minimizing the need for immobilization. Take rates are reported to be greater than 95%[53,54] and do not depend on whether meshed or unmeshed skin grafts are applied.[55–57] Long-term results show excellent appearance, pliability, and hand function[58–60] with similar elasticity and protective properties compared with normal skin.[59] Currently, MatriDerm is unavailable for use in the United States; however, Integra LifeSciences has developed an ultrathin version (Integra Single Layer 1.3 mm) that may be used in conjunction with autografts in single-staged reconstruction. Bottcher-Haberzeth and colleagues[61] compared Integra Single Layer to MatriDerm, 1 mm, in an animal model and showed that the 2 performed similar

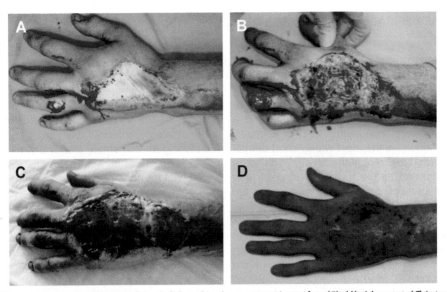

Fig. 2. (A) Burn injury to the dorsum of the left hand in the same patient after (B) débridement, (C) Integra placement, and (D) autografting.

with regard to graft take, neodermal thickness, collagen deposition, vascularization, and inflammatory response. Although clinical experience with MatriDerm, 1 mm, is limited,[62] its potential for use in conjunction with autografting in a 1-stage procedure could have great implications.

AlloDerm (LifeCell, Branchburg, New Jersey) is an acellular dermal matrix engineered from banked, human cadaver skin. During proprietary processing, epidermal and cellular components are removed and the product is freeze-dried. On rehydration, AlloDerm regenerates into a viable dermis. Similar to MatriDerm, it has been used concurrently with autograft in 1-stage procedures with reported reductions in wound contracture rates compared with autograft alone.[63] Rates of autograft take exceed 80% as long as a thin, 0.010 in-thick graft is used, which allows for more frequent recropping of donor sites.[64] Lattari and colleagues[18] described the use of AlloDerm with thin autografts on the hand in 2 patients with full-thickness burns. Range of motion, grip strength, fine motor coordination, and functional performance were considered excellent. Bhavsar and Tenenhaus[65] used meshed AlloDerm to cover exposed joints, tendons, and neurovascular structures in deep hand burns when flaps were unavailable. Fingers and joints were gently moved, and at approximately 2 weeks' postapplication, thin sheet grafts were applied. The investigators describe good soft tissue coverage in 19 of the 26 treated digits. Despite good outcomes reported with AlloDerm, its use in the management of burn injuries has been limited compared with other dermal substitutes.

COST

Although the high costs of dermal skin substitutes remain a concern, accumulating data have shown that they expedite healing, decrease scarring, and minimize patient discomfort compared with traditional burn care.[5,20,22,41–44,50] For example, compared with SSD, TransCyte and Biobrane decrease healing time, minimize the need for pain medication, and decrease the number of dressing changes.[42] Lukish and colleagues[20] found that TransCyte decreases length of stay and use of nursing care and is a significant economic benefit. In addition, Noordenbos and colleagues[43] compared TransCyte-treated wounds to SSD-treated wounds and found that TransCyte-treated wounds healed more rapidly (11 days vs 18 days) with less hypertrophy. Taken together, dermal skin substitutes seem to decrease the overall cost of burn care despite their high individual costs; however, it is difficult to draw

definitive conclusions from these studies due to their limited design. The lack of rigorous multicenter, prospective clinical burn trials across product types leads to individualized practice patterns and methods of burn care.[66] There remains a need for studies to evaluate the financial implications of dermal skin substitutes on burn care.

SUMMARY

Managing hand burn injuries is complex and requires careful planning to provide stable coverage by the safest and least invasive method. The ability to obtain supple, soft tissue reconstruction is paramount to optimizing functional and aesthetic outcomes. Technological advancements in bioengineered skin substitutes have added to the armamentarium of the reconstructive hand surgeon, particularly in the setting of large total body surface area burns when donor sites are limited. Skin substitutes have proved beneficial both in the acute setting and for delayed reconstruction. It is important for surgeons to be aware of the indications, advantages, and disadvantages of each. The most commonly used skin substitutes include Biobrane for temporary coverage of superficial burn injuries and Integra followed by staged placement of thin split-thickness autograft for deeper injuries. Although currently unavailable in the United States, excellent results have been obtained with MatriDerm when used in conjunction with autografts in single-staged reconstructions. As with any skin substitute, adequate débridement, attention to sterility, and meticulous hemostasis are keys to success. Although the use of dermal skin substitutes seems to improve hand function compared with traditional grafting techniques, patient-reported outcomes are limited and there remains a need for studies that use validated tools to assess hand function. Lastly, the financial implications of dermal skin substitutes on the health care system are not well defined in the literature and clinicians must be cognizant of the ultimate cost of the various products and weigh their advantages with respect to patient comfort, hand function, and appearance.

REFERENCES

1. Pruitt BA. Burns of the upper extremity. Epidemiology and general considerations. Major Probl Clin Surg 1976;19:1–15.
2. Luce EA. The acute and subacute management of the burned hand. Clin Plast Surg 2000;27(1): 49–63.
3. Tredget EE. Management of the acutely burned upper extremity. Hand Clin 2000;16(2):187–203.

4. Braithwaite F, Watson J. Some observations on the treatment of the dorsal burn of the hand. Br J Plast Surg 1949;2(1):21–31.

5. Sheridan RL, Hurley J, Smith MA, et al. The acutely burned hand: management and outcome based on a ten-year experience with 1047 acute hand burns. J Trauma 1995;38(3):406–11.

6. Tanigawa MC, O'Donnell OK, Graham PL. The burned hand: a physical therapy protocol. Phys Ther 1974;54(9):953–8.

7. Omar MT, Hassan AA. Evaluation of hand function after early excision and skin grafting of burns versus delayed skin grafting: a randomized clinical trial. Burns 2011;37(4):707–13.

8. Tambuscio A, Governa M, Caputo G, et al. Deep burn of the hands: Early surgical treatment avoids the need for late revisions? Burns 2006;32(8):1000–4.

9. Pereira C, Gold W, Herndon D. Review paper: burn coverage technologies: current concepts and future directions. J Biomater Appl 2007;22(2):101–21.

10. Waymack P, Duff RG, Sabolinski M. The effect of a tissue engineered bilayered living skin analog, over meshed split-thickness autografts on the healing of excised burn wounds. The Apligraf Burn Study Group. Burns 2000;26(7):609–19.

11. Lorenz C, Petracic A, Hohl HP, et al. Early wound closure and early reconstruction. Experience with a dermal substitute in a child with 60 per cent surface area burn. Burns 1997;23(6):505–8.

12. Burke JF, Yannas IV, Quinby WC Jr, et al. Successful use of a physiologically acceptable artificial skin in the treatment of extensive burn injury. Ann Surg 1981;194(4):413–28.

13. Fitton AR, Drew P, Dickson WA. The use of a bilaminate artificial skin substitute (Integra) in acute resurfacing of burns: an early experience. Br J Plast Surg 2001;54(3):208–12.

14. Jaksic T, Burke JF. The use of "artificial skin" for burns. Annu Rev Med 1987;38:107–17.

15. Groos N, Guillot M, Zilliox R, et al. Use of an artificial dermis (Integra) for the reconstruction of extensive burn scars in children. About 22 grafts. Eur J Pediatr Surg 2005;15(3):187–92.

16. Lamy J, Yassine AH, Gourari A, et al. The role of skin substitutes in the surgical treatment of extensive burns covering more than 60 % of total body surface area. A review of patients over a 10-year period at the Tours University Hospital. Ann Chir Plast Esthet 2015;60(2):131–9 [in French].

17. Yannas IV, Burke JF. Design of an artificial skin. I. Basic design principles. J Biomed Mater Res 1980;14(1):65–81.

18. Lattari V, Jones LM, Varcelotti JR, et al. The use of a permanent dermal allograft in full-thickness burns of the hand and foot: a report of three cases. J Burn Care Rehabil 1997;18(2):147–55.

19. Tsai CC, Lin SD, Lai CS, et al. The use of composite acellular allodermis-ultrathin autograft on joint area in major burn patients–one year follow-up. Kaohsiung J Med Sci 1999;15(11):651–8.

20. Lukish JR, Eichelberger MR, Newman KD, et al. The use of a bioactive skin substitute decreases length of stay for pediatric burn patients. J Pediatr Surg 2001;36(8):1118–21.

21. Verolino P, Casoli V, Masia D, et al. A skin substitute (Integra) in a successful delayed reconstruction of a severe injured hand. Burns 2008;34(2):284–7.

22. Dantzer E, Queruel P, Salinier L, et al. Dermal regeneration template for deep hand burns: clinical utility for both early grafting and reconstructive surgery. Br J Plast Surg 2003;56(8):764–74.

23. Pan Y, Liang Z, Yuan S, et al. A long-term follow-up study of acellular dermal matrix with thin autograft in burns patients. Ann Plast Surg 2011;67(4):346–51.

24. Hosseini SN, Mousavinasab SN, Fallahnezhat M. Xenoderm dressing in the treatment of second degree burns. Burns 2007;33(6):776–81.

25. Hosseini SN, Karimian A, Mousavinasab SN, et al. Xenoderm versus 1% silver sulfadiazine in partial-thickness burns. Asian J Surg 2009;32(4):234–9.

26. Still J, Donker K, Law E, et al. A program to decrease hospital stay in acute burn patients. Burns 1997;23(6):498–500.

27. Capo JT, Kokko KP, Rizzo M, et al. The use of skin substitutes in the treatment of the hand and upper extremity. Hand 2014;9(2):156–65.

28. Nihsen ES, Zopf DA, Ernst DM, et al. Absorption of bioactive molecules into OASIS wound matrix. Adv Skin Wound Care 2007;20(10):541–8.

29. Bello YM, Falabella AF, Eaglstein WH. Tissue-engineered skin. Current status in wound healing. Am J Clin Dermatol 2001;2(5):305–13.

30. Ehrenreich M, Ruszczak Z. Tissue-engineered temporary wound coverings. Important options for the clinician. Acta Dermatovenerol Alp Pannonica Adriat 2006;15(1):5–13.

31. Whitaker IS, Prowse S, Potokar TS. A critical evaluation of the use of Biobrane as a biologic skin substitute: a versatile tool for the plastic and reconstructive surgeon. Ann Plast Surg 2008;60(3):333–7.

32. Barret JP, Dziewulski P, Ramzy PI, et al. Biobrane versus 1% silver sulfadiazine in second-degree pediatric burns. Plast Reconstr Surg 2000;105(1):62–5.

33. Phillips LG, Robson MC, Smith DJ, et al. Uses and abuses of a biosynthetic dressing for partial skin thickness burns. Burns 1989;15(4):254–6.

34. Gerding RL, Imbembo AL, Fratianne RB. Biosynthetic skin substitute vs. 1% silver sulfadiazine for treatment of inpatient partial-thickness thermal burns. J Trauma 1988;28(8):1265–9.

35. Lal S, Barrow RE, Wolf SE, et al. Biobrane improves wound healing in burned children without increased

risk of infection. Shock 2000;14(3):314–8 [discussion: 318–9].

36. Frew Q, Philp B, Shelley O, et al. The use of Biobrane(R) as a delivery method for cultured epithelial autograft in burn patients. Burns 2013;39(5):876–80.

37. Lou RB, Hickerson WL. The use of skin substitutes in hand burns. Hand Clin 2009;25(4):497–509.

38. Yang JY, Tsai YC, Noordhoff MS. Clinical comparison of commercially available Biobrane preparations. Burns 1989;15(3):197–203.

39. Woodroof EA. The search for an ideal temporary skin substitute: AWBAT. Eplasty 2009;9:e10.

40. Greenwood JE. A randomized, prospective study of the treatment of superficial partial-thickness burns: AWBAT-S versus biobrane. Eplasty 2011;11:e10.

41. Pham C, Greenwood J, Cleland H, et al. Bioengineered skin substitutes for the management of burns: a systematic review. Burns 2007;33(8): 946–57.

42. Kumar RJ, Kimble RM, Boots R, et al. Treatment of partial-thickness burns: a prospective, randomized trial using Transcyte. ANZ J Surg 2004;74(8):622–6.

43. Noordenbos J, Dore C, Hansbrough JF. Safety and efficacy of TransCyte for the treatment of partial-thickness burns. J burn Care Rehabil 1999;20(4): 275–81.

44. Moiemen N, Yarrow J, Hodgson E, et al. Long-term clinical and histological analysis of Integra dermal regeneration template. Plast Reconstr Surg 2011; 127(3):1149–54.

45. Dantzer E, Braye FM. Reconstructive surgery using an artificial dermis (Integra): results with 39 grafts. Br J Plast Surg 2001;54(8):659–64.

46. Heimbach DM, Warden GD, Luterman A, et al. Multicenter postapproval clinical trial of Integra dermal regeneration template for burn treatment. J burn Care Rehabil 2003;24(1):42–8.

47. Hunt JA, Moisidis E, Haertsch P. Initial experience of Integra in the treatment of post-burn anterior cervical neck contracture. Br J Plast Surg 2000;53(8): 652–8.

48. Chou TD, Chen SL, Lee TW, et al. Reconstruction of burn scar of the upper extremities with artificial skin. Plast Reconstr Surg 2001;108(2):378–84 [discussion: 385].

49. Molnar JA, DeFranzo AJ, Hadaegh A, et al. Acceleration of Integra incorporation in complex tissue defects with subatmospheric pressure. Plast Reconstr Surg 2004;113(5):1339–46.

50. Nguyen DQ, Potokar TS, Price P. An objective long-term evaluation of Integra (a dermal skin substitute) and split thickness skin grafts, in acute burns and reconstructive surgery. Burns 2010;36(1):23–8.

51. Danin A, Georgesco G, Touze AL, et al. Assessment of burned hands reconstructed with Integra((R)) by ultrasonography and elastometry. Burns 2012; 38(7):998–1004.

52. Weigert R, Choughri H, Casoli V. Management of severe hand wounds with Integra(R) dermal regeneration template. J Hand Surg Eur Vol 2011;36(3): 185–93.

53. Heckmann A, Radtke C, Rennekampff HO, et al. One-stage defect closure of deperiosted bone and exposed tendons with MATRIDERM(R) and skin transplantation. Possibilities and limitations. Unfallchirurg 2012;115(12):1092–8 [in German].

54. Haslik W, Kamolz LP, Nathschlager G, et al. First experiences with the collagen-elastin matrix Matriderm as a dermal substitute in severe burn injuries of the hand. Burns 2007;33(3):364–8.

55. De Vries HJ, Mekkes JR, Middelkoop E, et al. Dermal substitutes for full-thickness wounds in a one-stage grafting model. Wound Repair Regen 1993;1(4):244–52.

56. Hansbrough JF, Dore C, Hansbrough WB. Clinical trials of a living dermal tissue replacement placed beneath meshed, split-thickness skin grafts on excised burn wounds. J Burn Care Rehabil 1992; 13(5):519–29.

57. Ryssel H, Gazyakan E, Germann G, et al. The use of MatriDerm in early excision and simultaneous autologous skin grafting in burns–a pilot study. Burns 2008;34(1):93–7.

58. Ryssel H, Germann G, Kloeters O, et al. Dermal substitution with Matriderm((R)) in burns on the dorsum of the hand. Burns 2010;36(8):1248–53.

59. Min JH, Yun IS, Lew DH, et al. The use of matriderm and autologous skin graft in the treatment of full thickness skin defects. Arch Plast Surg 2014;41(4): 330–6.

60. Haslik W, Kamolz LP, Manna F, et al. Management of full-thickness skin defects in the hand and wrist region: first long-term experiences with the dermal matrix Matriderm. J Plast Reconstr Aesthet Surg 2010;63(2):360–4.

61. Böttcher-Haberzeth S, Biedermann T, Schiestl C, et al. Matriderm 1 mm versus Integra Single Layer 1.3 mm for one-step closure of full thickness skin defects: a comparative experimental study in rats. Pediatr Surg Int 2012;28(2):171–7.

62. Koenen W, Felcht M, Vockenroth K, et al. One-stage reconstruction of deep facial defects with a single layer dermal regeneration template. J Eur Acad Dermatol Venereol 2011;25(7): 788–93.

63. Wainwright D, Madden M, Luterman A, et al. Clinical evaluation of an acellular allograft dermal matrix in full-thickness burns. J Burn Care Rehabil 1996; 17(2):124–36.

64. Callcut RA, Schurr MJ, Sloan M, et al. Clinical experience with Alloderm: a one-staged composite dermal/epidermal replacement utilizing processed cadaver dermis and thin autografts. Burns 2006; 32(5):583–8.

65. Bhavsar D, Tenenhaus M. The use of acellular dermal matrix for coverage of exposed joint and extensor mechanism in thermally injured patients with few options. Eplasty 2008;8:e33.

66. Dorsett-Martin WA, Persons B, Wysocki A, et al. New topical agents for treatment of partial-thickness burns in children: a review of published outcome studies. Wounds 2008;20(11):292–8.

Biological Principles of Scar and Contracture

Peter O. Kwan, BScE, MD, PhD, FRCSC[a], Edward E. Tredget, MD, MSc, FRCSC[b],*

KEYWORDS

- Burns • Hypertrophic scar • Wound healing • Contracture • Cicatrix

KEY POINTS

- Burn hypertrophic scars result from deep burns that take longer to heal and may be related to activation of deep dermal fibroblasts.
- The extracellular matrix of a hypertrophic scar is significantly different from that of normal skin and normotrophic scar, and influences dermal fibroblast behavior.
- Multiple interconnected pathways contribute to hypertrophic scar formation after a burn injury.
- Various treatments for hypertrophic scar can be demonstrated to affect known pathways in hypertrophic scar formation.

INTRODUCTION

As the primary means of physical interaction with the environment, our hands often bear the brunt of burn injury, and therefore hand burns are quite common.[1] In children and toddlers, scald burns frequently occur as they explore the environment,[2] whereas adults tend to suffer flame and flash burns during occupational and recreational activities.[3] Unfortunately, hypertrophic scarring (HSc) and contractions in the hands result in thick, rigid scars that impair function,[4] and can be very disfiguring[5] (**Fig. 1**). This potential for significant morbidity makes hand burns one of the American Burn Association criteria for mandatory burn center referral.[6] This article aims to improve understanding of the underlying pathophysiology of HSc and contracture after a burn injury of the hand, with the hope that this will lead to new treatments and research that improve patient outcomes.

The factors leading to HSc formation are components of an integrated and complex wound healing process that has become dysregulated

or dysfunctional. The net result is a pathologic pro-fibrotic environment that produces excessive scar and contracture. To better understand the processes leading to HSc and contracture, we first examine the factors leading to scarring or regeneration, the underlying signaling molecules involved, the local cell populations involved, and the systemic immune response. Finally, we discuss some of the therapies available and their mechanisms of action.

CRITICAL INJURIES PRODUCE SCARS AND CONTRACTURES

The formation of scar and HSc after a burn injury is tied intimately to the depth of injury, and the time it takes for healing and reepithelialization to occur. It is well-established that superficial burn wounds healing within 2 weeks regenerate and reepithelialize with minimal deformity[7]; deeper burn wounds taking longer than 3 weeks to heal will form a scar, often require excision and skin grafting, and are prone to HSc and contractures.[8] The key difference between superficial and deep

Disclosure Statement: Nothing to disclose.

[a] 2A Plastic Surgery, Kaye Edmonton Clinic, University of Alberta, 11400 University Avenue, Edmonton, Alberta T6G 1Z1, Canada; [b] Department of Surgery, University of Alberta, 2D2.28 WMHSC, 8440-112 Street Northwest, Edmonton, Alberta T6G 2B7, Canada
* Corresponding author.
E-mail address: etredget@ualberta.ca

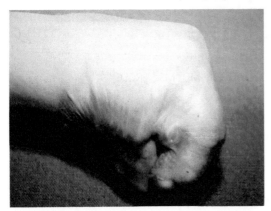

Fig. 1. Hypertrophic scarring and scar contractures of the hand impair function and appearance. (*From* Kwan P, Hori K, Ding J, et al. Scar and contracture: biological principles. Hand Clin 2009;25(4):512; with permission.)

burn wounds relates to the degree of damage, and the predominant fibroblast subpopulation present. This concept of a critical depth of injury is best demonstrated by the linear scratch model of Dunkin and colleagues,[9] where a wound of increasing depth was made through the skin, and the superficial portion regenerated, whereas those areas deeper than 0.56 mm produced scar. This idea of a critical depth for scarring correlates with multiple studies demonstrating that dermal fibroblasts can be divided into superficial (papillary) and deep (reticular) based on their location within the dermis, and that these subpopulations have very different responses to injury[10,11] (**Fig. 2**).

A number of studies have demonstrated that the fibroblasts in HSc most closely match those of the deep dermis in behavior, appearance, and extracellular matrix (ECM) production,[12] and this suggests 2 major hypotheses of HSc formation:

1. Selective proliferation of profibrotic deep dermal fibroblasts in response to fibrogenic cytokines, and
2. Destruction of regenerative superficial dermal fibroblast by deep burn injuries, leaving deeper dermal fibroblasts to repopulate the wound and form HSc.[13]

EXTRACELLULAR MATRIX PROPERTIES INFLUENCE PHYSICAL SCAR AND CELLULAR BEHAVIOR

The ECM formed during the wound closure and the proliferation phase is remodeled over time as wound healing and scarring occur. However, the local wound environment and ECM persist in a significantly altered fashion in HSc as compared with normal skin. Conceptually, the dermal ECM contains 2 main constituents: fibrillar collagen, which provides mechanical strength, and glycosaminoglycans and proteoglycans, which contribute to hydration.[13] On a clinical level, HSc is raised, erythematous, and firm.[14] Histologically, HSc ECM is also thicker, hyperhydrated, and has a thicker epidermis, as compared with normal skin[13] (**Fig. 3**). Morphologically, this is reflected by a change from the basket weave pattern of thick collagen bundles seen in normal skin, to dense nodules or whorls of poorly organized and thin collagen fibrils in HSc[15] (see **Fig. 3**). This is a result of alterations in both collagen and glycosaminoglycan content.

In normal skin, the ECM is composed primarily of type I collagen (80%), type III collagen (10%–15%), and minimal type V collagens, whereas HSc is quite different with more type III (33%) and type V (10%) collagens.[16,17] Because type III and type V collagens alter the fibrillar diameter of type I collagen bundles, these different ratios in HSc likely account for some of the morphologic changes seen.[18,19]

In addition to these major changes in collagen composition, the glycosaminoglycan content of HSc is significantly different from that of normal skin.[20] There is a 2-fold increase in glycosaminoglycan content, which leads to HSc hyperhydration and is clinically manifested as firmness.[13] In normal skin, decorin (DCN), a small leucine-rich proteoglycan, is the predominant proteoglycan, whereas in HSc DCN levels are markedly and significantly reduced.[20] This finding is significant because DCN is not only an ECM structural component that modulates collagen fibril formation,[21] but it also regulates transforming growth factor-β (TGF-β),[22] reduces fibrosis,[23] and reduces contraction.[24] In contrast, 2 other

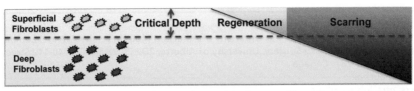

Fig. 2. Superficial skin injuries regenerate, whereas deeper injuries scar. (*From* Kwan P, Hori K, Ding J, et al. Scar and contracture: biological principles. Hand Clin 2009;25(4):513; with permission.)

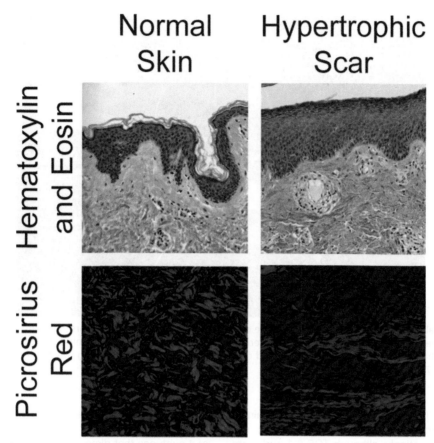

Fig. 3. Histologic comparison of normal skin and hypertrophic scar.

proteoglycans—versican and biglycan—are upregulated in HSc.[20] Versican, which is increased by 6-fold in HSc, is a large proteoglycan that is interposed between collagen fibrils and contributes to tissue turgor and expands the ECM framework and, thus, contributes to the increased scar volume of HSc.[13]

Cytokines and Signaling Molecules

The overall goal of wound healing is wound closure, whether it results in scarring or regeneration, and this is achieved by many cells acting together in concert. The signaling and communication required to achieve this occurs through a balance of various profibrotic and antifibrotic cytokines. This balance has a significant impact on the final outcome, and an imbalance leads to hyperactivity and HSc. The signaling networks are complex, with various cytokines and signaling molecules acting not only on cell surface receptors and intracellular receptors, but on each other as well. Although we review these signals individually, one should remember that it is the balance and interplay of these signals that influences cellular behavior (**Fig. 4**).

Profibrotic Cytokines and Molecules

Transforming Growth Factor-β

One of the most studied prototypic profibrotic cytokines is TGF-β, which is a member of a larger superfamily of cytokines that share a conserved cysteine knot structure.[25,26] TGF-β has 3 mammalian isoforms—1, 2, and 3[26]—that are produced from multiple sources, including keratinocyte, fibroblasts, platelets, macrophages, T lymphocytes, and endothelial cells.[27] TGF-β also plays multiple roles in numerous cell signaling networks, and is not exclusively a profibrotic cytokine. In skin and wound healing environments, TGF-β is secreted in an inactive form, bound to an associated latent TGF-β–binding protein. TGF-β becomes activated when this bond is cleaved by one of several enzymes present in the blood or released during cell injury, including matrix metalloproteinase-2 (MMP-2), MMP-9, and plasmin.[28] TGF-β 1 and 2 are monocyte chemoattractants,[29] and also upregulate fibroblast ECM production[30] via the Smad pathway.[31] In burn patients with HSc, TGF-β is upregulated both in local HSc tissue and systemically in serum.[32]

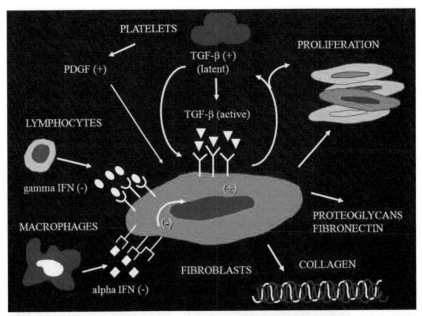

Fig. 4. Signaling pathways in scarring. A balance of profibrotic and antifibrotic factors in wound healing affect the outcome. IFN, interferon; PDGF, platelet-derived growth factor; TGF, transforming growth factor. (*From* Scott PG, Ghahary A, Tredget EE. Molecular and cellular aspects of fibrosis following thermal injury. Hand Clin 2000;16(2):271–87; with permission.)

Thus, TGF-β is crucial in initiating or maintaining the profibrotic environment in which HSc develops. Interestingly, although TGF-β 1 and 2 are profibrotic, the isoform TGF-β3 seems to be antifibrotic and can improve wound healing[33] by reducing ECM deposition,[34] and is upregulated in the later stages of wound healing.[34] Multiple studies demonstrate that modulating TGF-β using antibodies[35] or DCN reduces its profibrotic activities.[22] Thus, TGF-β is the main profibrotic cytokine in most fibrotic pathways.

Connective tissue growth factor/CCN2

Connective tissue growth factor (CTGF) is a prototypical member of the CCN cytokine family,[36] and a well-studied downstream regulator of fibrosis.[37] It is induced by TGF-β, and although TGF-β or CTGF alone induce transient fibrosis, they combine synergistically to promote prolonged fibrosis,[38] which CTGF then sustains when TGF-β levels decrease.[37] It has similar effects to TGF-β, such as stimulating fibroblasts to increase ECM production, and is upregulated in fibrotic diseases such as HSc, scleroderma, and others.[39] Also, studies demonstrate that blocking TGF-β stimulation of CTGF via the ras/MEK/ERK pathway using iloprost reduces fibrosis,[40] as do anti-CTGF antibodies, and CTGF small interfering RNA.[41] Thus, CTGF plays a role in promoting prolonged fibrosis.

Platelet-derived growth factor

Platelet-derived growth factor (PDGF) consists of 4 subtypes that dimerize to activate 2 structurally related cell surface tyrosine kinase receptors,[42] causing cellular proliferation and actin reorganization, inducing fibroblasts to transform into myofibroblasts.[43] PDGF also increased ECM production and inhibits myofibroblast apoptosis.[44] In wounds, PDGF is released from platelets, which leave damaged capillaries in the wound bed and stimulate resident fibroblasts. Dermal fibroblasts can also produce PDGF, resulting in an autocrine loop.[45] PDGF upregulates TGF-β receptors,[45] and its effects are magnified in HSc fibroblasts.[46] Thus, PDGF plays a role both in initiating and in sustaining HSc.

Insulinlike growth factor 1

In skin, insulinlike growth factor 1 (IGF-1) is sequestered in epidermal sweat and sebaceous glands, where dermal fibroblasts are not exposed to it until it is released by injury,[47] such as burns. Once released, IGF-1 modulates the effects of various growth hormones on dermal fibroblasts and other cell types,[48] and has multiple profibrotic effects. These include stimulation of TGF-β production,[49] induction of collagen production, and suppression of collagenase.[50] It is also a fibroblast[51] and endothelial cell[52] mitogen. IGF-1 is increased in postburn HSc as compared with normal skin,[47] reflecting its role in fibrosis, whereas in normally healing wounds it decreases over time.[53] Thus, IGF-1 release plays a role in initiating, and potentially sustaining fibrosis.

Antifibrotic Cytokines and Molecules

Interferon
There are a number of interferons that have been demonstrated to be antifibrotic, including interferon-α2b (IFN-α2b), and IFN-γ. IFN-α is produced by leukocytes and fibroblasts, and IFN-γ is produced by Th1 T-helper cells,[54] which all play key roles in wound healing. IFNs decrease fibroblast ECM production,[13] increase collagenase production, and decrease tissue inhibitor of MMP 1 (TIMP-1), which blocks remodeling MMPs.[55] These effects have been observed clinically in a trial where IFN-α2b reduced HSc volume, normalized TGF-β levels, and reduced scar angiogenesis in burn patients.[32]

Tumor necrosis factor
Tumor necrosis factor-α (TNF-α) is produced by macrophages,[43] and TNF-α–producing cells are decreased in HSc.[56] Fibroblasts treated transiently with TNF-α have decreased collagen production, and TNF-α suppressed α-smooth muscle actin expression by fibroblasts and the transformation into myofibroblasts.[57] However, other studies seem to demonstrate TNF-α inducing fibrosis,[58] suggesting that it may have a biphasic or combinatorial response.

Decorin
DCN, and several other small leucine-rich proteoglycans, serve dual roles as both structural and signaling molecules. As a direct signaling molecule, DCN binds to receptors, including epidermal growth factor receptor,[59] IGF-1R,[60] and hepatocyte growth factor receptor,[61] with the effect of blocking or downregulating fibroblast activation. DCN also blocks the profibrotic signaling molecules TGF-β,[22] and CTGF[62] by binding them and preventing their interaction with their cell receptors. Multiple studies have used DCN to reduce fibrosis[23] and contraction,[63] and improve wound healing and regeneration.[64]

MicroRNA
An additional level of regulation occurs involving microRNA (miRNA), short RNA strands of 22 nucleotides that regulate the translation of messenger RNA into proteins via several pathways.[65] The upregulation or downregulation of various miRNA, thus, has direct effects on multiple intracellular signaling pathways. Studies demonstrate that miRNA 181b,[66] miRNA 21,[67] miRNA

133,[68] and others[69] all play significant roles in modulating wound healing, fibrosis, and HSc formation, with some being profibrotic and others antifibrotic, depending on their targets.

CELLS INVOLVED IN WOUND HEALING

There are significant local and systemic components to wound healing (**Fig. 5**), which both play roles in HSc formation and contracture. On a local level, the main cell types involved in wound healing are keratinocytes and resident fibroblasts, of which there are several potential subtypes. On a systemic level, it seems that the cells involved are bone marrow derived and fall into the category of either fibrocytes, or various components of the systemic immune system.

Local Cells

Keratinocytes
Although the tensile strength of skin comes primarily from the dermis, it is the keratinocytes that produce the epithelial barrier that is ultimately responsible for protection. Wound inflammation continues until the burn wound has reepithelialized, at which time wound healing can progress to the proliferation and maturation phases. Thus, prolonged inflammation and an extended time to reepithelialization is a known risk factor for HSc.[70] Keratinocytes from HSc demonstrate increased production of TIMP1.[71] An extensive cross-talk network exists between keratinocytes and fibroblasts, with each being able to modulate the other's behavior.[72] Keratinocytes suppress fibroblast production of TGF-β and CTGF,[73] and also secrete stratifin which decreases ECM production via upregulation of MMP1, while simultaneously increasing fibroblast proliferation.[74] Although it is unclear to what degree HSc results from abnormal keratinocytes or abnormal fibroblasts, or some other factor, it is clear that keratinocytes isolated from HSc are abnormal.[75] HSc-derived keratinocytes induce fibroblasts to produce larger quantities of ECM as compared with normal skin keratinocytes,[75] suggesting that abnormal keratinocyte–fibroblast cross-talk contributes to HSc formation and maintenance.

Dermal fibroblasts
Fibroblasts play a key role in wound healing, scar formation, and wound contraction. Fibroblasts alter the physical wound by producing and remodeling ECM.[76] The heterogeneity of dermal fibroblasts follows an ordered structural pattern with divergent behavior between superficial (papillary) and deep (reticular) fibroblasts.[11] Compared with

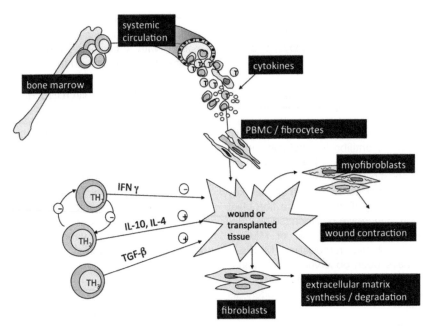

Fig. 5. Cellular interactions in wound healing. Role of T-helper (TH) cells and bone marrow-derived cells in the healing wound. IFN, interferon; IL, interleukin; PBMC, Peripheral Blood Mononuclear Cell; TGF, transforming growth factor. (*Modified from* Armour A, Scott PG, Tredget EE. Cellular and molecular pathology of HTS: basis for treatment. Wound Repair Regen 2007;15:S13; with permission.)

superficial fibroblasts, the deeper fibroblasts produce more collagen,[10] cause greater gel contraction,[77] produce less DCN,[66] proliferate more slowly,[78] induce irregular keratinocyte behavior,[11] and do not support capillary formation.[79] This difference in the layers of dermal fibroblasts helps to account for the different patterns of wound healing seen with varying depths of dermal injury. This pattern has been demonstrated in a mouse model of human skin injury, where deep dermal fibroblasts closed experimental wounds and then superficial dermal fibroblasts remodeled them.[80] Thus, it may be that in extensive deep burns there are insufficient numbers of superficial dermal

fibroblasts to remodel scar as it forms, thus leading to HSc.

Hypertrophic scar fibroblasts

HSc fibroblasts share many properties with deep dermal fibroblasts (**Table 1**), and studies suggest that it is from this deep dermal population that HSc fibroblasts arise.[12] Both TGF-β and CTGF are produced in greater quantities by deep dermal fibroblasts and HSc fibroblasts, as compared with superficial dermal fibroblasts.[12] Deep dermal and HSc fibroblasts also produce more collagen and less DCN, and respond to cytokine stimulation in a similar manner.[10,66] Again, this suggests that

Table 1
Comparison between superficial dermal, deep dermal, and hypertrophic scar fibroblasts

Factor	Normal Skin Superficial Fibroblasts	Deep Fibroblasts	Hypertrophic Scar Fibroblasts
Collagen	↓	↑	↑
Collagenase	↑	↓	↓
Transforming growth factor-β	↓	↑	↑
Connective tissue growth factor	↓	↑	↑
Decorin	↑	↓	↓

Data from Wang J, Dodd C, Shankowsky HA, et al. Deep dermal fibroblasts contribute to hypertrophic scarring. Lab Invest 2008;88(12):1278–90.

HSc fibroblasts are derived from deep dermal fibroblasts.

Myofibroblasts

HSc fibroblasts also share several similar features with myofibroblasts. Myofibroblasts are a terminally differentiated fibroblast phenotype expressing α-smooth muscle actin[81] and widely associated with scar contraction.[82] They also produce more collagen and less collagenase,[12] and are quite numerous in HSc as compared with normal scar.[83] Myofibroblasts in HSc are also resistant to apoptotic signaling, and this property may contribute to HSc formation and persistence.[84]

Systemic Cells

The human body mounts a significant systemic response to burn injury, and this response is not limited to clinically apparent large fluid shifts, cardiac depression, acute renal failure, and other clinical findings, but also includes various components of the innate and adaptive immune systems involved in both inflammation and scarring. Clinically, it seems that injuries with a prolonged immune response, such as burns or infection, are at increased risk of fibroproliferative scar, with recent research demonstrating that it is the type of immune response that is most crucial. The best characterized aspects of this response that impact wound healing are fibrocytes (a peripheral blood mononuclear cell derivative), and various T helper cell subpopulations. Recent research suggests that it is not simply the degree of inflammation, but rather the type of immune response that predisposes to HSc formation.[85]

Macrophages, neutrophils, and mast cells

Macrophages, neutrophils, and mast cells play a significant role in the initial inflammation that occurs during early wound healing,[86] with macrophages driving the shift from inflammation to proliferation.[43] This occurs through the proinflammatory cytokines: interleukin-1 (IL-1), IL-6, and TNF-α, which stimulate keratinocyte and fibroblast proliferation.[43] Macrophages also produce multiple profibrogenic factors, including TGF-β, PDGF, and IGF-1.[87] The importance of macrophages in wound healing is demonstrated in a knockout mouse model of impaired macrophage migration that showed impaired wound healing.[88] There are 2 subtypes of macrophages involved in wound healing, the M1 subtype, which appears early during wound healing, and the M2 macrophage subtype, which becomes predominant after several weeks and is associated with HSc formation,[89] and depletion of this M2 population in an animal model of HSc formation significantly improved the resulting scars.[90] Thus macrophages are crucial for the transition from inflammation to proliferation, and likely play a role in initiating HSc formation.

Fibrocytes

Fibrocytes are a bone marrow-derived peripheral blood mononuclear cell, identifiable by their double staining for procollagen I and leukocyte-specific protein 1.[91] Fibrocytes home to burn wounds, which release stromal cell–derived factor 1 into the circulation via their CXCR4 receptors,[92] or home to wounds where injured endothelium releases secondary lymphoid chemokines into the circulation via their CCR7 receptors.[93] Fibrocytes then differentiate from a leukocyte subpopulation, into a fibroblastlike cell under TGF-β stimulation.[93] This leads to large numbers of fibrocytes in HSc burn scars,[94] where profibrotic cytokine stimulation causes them to secrete ECM and transdifferentiate into myofibroblasts.[95] Fibrocytes also regulate resident fibroblasts in the wound through production of TGF-β and CTGF.[91] In addition, fibrocytes express Toll-like receptors,[96] and are also antigen presenting cells allowing them to prime naïve T-helper cells.[97] This ability to respond as part of the innate immune system to invading bacteria in burn wounds provides an additional link between the immune system and wound fibrosis.

T-helper cells

The cytokines and signaling molecules previously discussed are serve not only as modulators of wound healing, but also as controls of differentiation in the adaptive immune system, specifically T-helper cells (CD4+). These T-helper cells also produce various cytokines that direct the wound healing process.[98] Once naïve T-helper cells are activated by antigen-presenting cells (eg, macrophages[99] or dendritic cells[100]), they become polarized toward a Th1 or Th2 subtype and produce a corresponding specific cytokine profile.[101] HSc dermis contains a high level of infiltrating CD4+ T lymphocytes compared with normal skin.[102] Of the 2 subtypes, Th1 cells are primarily part of cell-mediated immunity, and produce a number of antifibrotic cytokines (IL-2, IFN-γ, and IL-12). They also induce proapoptotic genes and collagenase expression in fibroblasts.[103] In contrast, Th2 cells are part of antibody-mediated immunity, and produce a number of profibrotic cytokines (IL-4, IL-5, and IL-13). Th2 responses include upregulated ECM production including procollagens I, III, and V, and TIMP-1 production.[104] Serum from burn patients demonstrates elevation of Th2 cytokine levels (IL-4 and IL-10), and reduced Th1 cytokine levels (IFN-γ and IL-12) for more than 1 year after the burn injury.[105,106] Exposing fibroblasts to serum from burn patients also results in Th2 polarized responses including cellular proliferation, TGF-β upregulation, and myofibroblast transformation.[102] This demonstrates the significant degree to which the immune system influences and regulates fibrosis and HSc formation.

WOUND CONTRACTION, SCAR CONTRACTURES, AND FORCES CAUSING SCARRING

A key distinction must be made between wound contraction, which forms a significant part of the initial wound closure and healing process, and subsequent scar contracture that occurs as the scar matures. In this context, wound contraction occurs as the open wound edges are pulled together by forces intrinsic to the wound healing process.[107] In contrast, scar contractures result from shrinkage occurring in an already healed scar.[107]

Current research into contraction and contracture is guided and limited by available models. Wound contraction is frequently modeled by the use of standardized wounds on the backs of animals, or in vitro fibroblast-populated collagen lattices (FPCL),[108] which are photographed and analyzed at varying time points. The main limitation is that wound contraction plays a more significant role in wound healing in animals as compared with in humans.[109] In contrast, scar contractures result from HSc over joints and mobile surfaces that contract secondarily, but because HSc only occurs in humans[107] there are currently only limited animal models available.[110]

There are 2 main theories regarding the relative roles of fibroblasts and myofibroblasts in wound contraction and scar contracture. The first theory is that contraction occurs through myofibroblast cell shortening via α-smooth muscle actin, and that surrounding ECM is then remodeled, and excess ECM is produced by these myofibroblasts.[107,111] The second theory is that fibroblasts exert a traction force as they move through the ECM.[112] This theory is supported by the finding that myofibroblasts are not predominant until 1 week after the majority of contraction has already occurred,[107] suggesting that myofibroblasts do not cause contraction but rather maintain the equilibrium already established in tissue.[113] This concept is also supported by experiments demonstrating that the external application of force or tension on normal skin or scars leads to myofibroblast differentiation.[83]

Fibroblasts primarily cause wound contraction and are influenced by the same wound healing factors discussed previously, such as TGF-β.[114] Modeling of wound contraction, using FPCL, demonstrates this process is accelerated by higher numbers of fibroblasts, and decreased by higher collagen concentrations.[115] Fibroblast morphology studies in FPCL demonstrate that myofibroblast like cells appear in the periphery, whereas bipolar fibroblasts are found predominantly in the center and exert greater contractile forces.[107] TGF-β increases the rate of contraction,[114] whereas, IFN-α2b decreases it,[116] and early wound closure, such as with skin grafts, is also effective in inhibiting wound contraction.[117] This finding suggests that reducing wound contraction can be achieved by reducing inflammation and fibroblast stimulation.

Myofibroblasts primarily cause scar contraction, with HSc being a major risk factor.[54] This is due in part to altered ECM in HSc, which has much more type III collagen than normal skin, with FPCL composed of collagen isolated from HSc[113] or with high levels of type III collagen having greater contraction rates.[118] Similarly, DCN reduces FPCL contraction, but HSc ECM has low levels of DCN,[66] thus suggesting its absence also promotes scar contracture. By comparing fibroblasts and myofibroblasts isolated from HSc, Shin and Minn demonstrated that myofibroblasts are responsible for scar contracture.[82] In addition, HSc is more common over areas of higher tension such as joints and mobile surfaces,[107] and studies show that these forces also reduce myofibroblast apoptosis.[119] This suggests that modulating myofibroblast transdifferentiation and apoptosis is likely crucial in reducing scar contractures.

In addition to the forces created by contraction and contracture, external forces on wounds can also increase scarring and promote HSc formation. Just as mesenchymal cells alter ECM structure, so too forces on the ECM cause changes in cellular behavior. Aarabi and colleagues[120] demonstrated that mechanical stress applied to a murine wound model caused HSc formation and proposed that this occurred via a decrease in cellular apoptosis. In addition, Wong and colleagues[121] demonstrated that a murine focal adhesion kinase knockout model had significantly less inflammation and fibrosis by decoupling the effects of mechanical forces from expression of monocyte chemoattractant protein-1. This mechanism was then confirmed using an monocyte chemoattractant protein-1 knockout mouse, which also developed less fibrosis, and by using small molecular focal adhesion kinase inhibitors that reduced scar formation and attenuated monocyte chemoattractant protein-1 signaling.[121] This finding suggests that the forces applied to wounds as they heal increase fibrosis, and that relieving these forces can reduce scarring and contractures.

PATHOPHYSIOLOGY OF CURRENT TREATMENTS

Although not all the mechanisms by which treatments affect HSc and contractures are known, they generally involve the previously discussed signaling pathways. Here we discuss only those treatments that have been clinically investigated or used, and avoid theoretic treatments or those studied only in animal models. For simplicity, treatments have been divided into mechanical, immunologic and biomolecular, and surgical options.

Mechanical Treatments

Pressure garments

A mainstay of HSc treatments since the 1970s, pressure garments are worn continuously for 23 hours per day until the scar is mature, generally 2 to 3 years.[122] Opinion varies on the pressure required, but recommendations are for 24 to 30 mm Hg. Pressure garments are believed to accelerate scar maturation, reduce contractures, and also reduce the pain and pruritus associated with active HSc. Although a reduction in scar height has been demonstrated, there seem to be no effects in terms of scar pigmentation, vascularity, pliability, or color,[123] and improvements seem to be limited to those patients with moderate or severe scarring.[124] The mechanism of action seems to be via reduced collagen production, and improved realignment of collagen bundles.[122] This may be due to increased myofibroblast apoptosis, ischemic cell damage, and increased MMP-9 activity.[85]

Silicone gel sheets

Silicone gel sheets, composed of a cross-linked dimethylsiloxane polymer, have been used to improve scar remodeling since 1982.[125] Sheets are kept in place for at least 12 hours per day for 3 to 6 months during scar remodeling. They seem to accelerate scar maturation, improve pigmentation, vascularity, pliability, and the pruritus associated with HSc.[126] Again, the mechanism of action is unclear, but may involve an increase of scar temperature, development of a static electrical field, hydration of the stratum corneum, decreased fibroblast contraction, increased fibroblast apoptosis, decreased mast cells, and decreased TGF-β2 levels.[85] Pressure gloves and silicone gel sheets or conformers are frequently

combined when treating scars and contractures of the hand.

Massage

Massage of burn scars has been studied in a large, randomized, controlled trial and demonstrated significant improvement in scar thickness and appearance,[127] similar to findings in an animal model.[128] This improvement can be attributed to reductions in CTGF, which occur with cyclical cell stretching,[129] and alterations in cytoskeletal structure,[130] although this remains an area with minimal conclusive research.

Splinting

As with other types of hand injury, optimal splinting is crucial to avoiding the intrinsic-minus position[131] that results from fluid accumulation in the joint capsules, swelling of the collateral ligaments, and subsequent ligament contracture.[132] By optimally splinting the hand, subsequent contractures can be avoided, which accelerates physiotherapy and preserves function. Splinting can also be useful in deep burns with injury to or exposure of the extensor tendon apparatus, to help avoid rupture and allow tissue coverage.[131]

Dressings

Tension on healing wounds leads to increased scarring and HSc formation, and measures that reduce the tension on healing wounds, such as surgical incisions, can significantly improve the resulting scars. Although surgeons frequently reinforce healing wounds with dressings that relieve tension, such as adhesive surgical tape, these are generally used for a short period of time, on the order of weeks. A randomized, controlled trial of the prolonged use of paper tape on cesarean section scars for multiple months demonstrated a significant improvement in the resulting scars.[133] Similarly, another randomized, controlled trial of a tension-relieving dressing on abdominoplasty scars also demonstrated a significant improvement in the resulting scars.[134] These studies suggest that counteracting the tension placed on linear scars over a significant portion of the scar proliferation and remodeling phases improves the resulting scars significantly.

Immunologic and Biomolecular Treatments

Corticosteroids

Since the 1960s corticosteroids, most commonly triamcinolone acetonide, have been injected into pathologic scars, and are considered a first-line treatment.[135] Side effects include hypopigmentation and subcutaneous atrophy.[136] Although the precise mechanism is unclear, it seems to involve the inhibition of fibroblast proliferation and contraction, suppression of inflammation resulting from leukocyte and monocyte migration and phagocytosis, increased collagenase production via α2-macroglobulin inhibition, and inhibition of TGF-β and IGF-1,[85,136,137] which all play key roles in fibrosis.

5-Fluorouracil
Uses for 5-fluorouracil, a pyrimidine analog antimetabolite chemotherapy agent, range from treating glaucoma[138] and basal cell carcinoma,[139] to pathologic scars such as keloids and HSc.[140] Injections are intralesional, and can be combined with corticosteroids or pulsed-dye laser, and both decrease scar volume and improve softening.[141] 5-Fluorouracil targets rapidly proliferating fibroblasts and inhibits this proliferation while also reducing collagen production.[142]

Interferon
Systemic subcutaneous IFN-α2b treatment of postburn patients with HSc for 24 weeks significantly improved scar appearance and volume.[32] This seems to be due to multiple factors, including decreased collagen and increased collagenase,[54,143] reduced TGF-β levels,[144] reduced vascular endothelial growth factor–mediated angiogenesis,[145] decreased fibrocytes[146] likely due to decreased CXCR4-SDF1 trafficking,[92] and enhanced myofibroblast apoptosis.[147]

Transforming growth factor-β modulators
Because TGF-β 1 and 2 are primary cytokines in the fibrotic process, multiple therapies targeting this pathway have been proposed as treatments for scars, including inhibitors such as DCN,[22] proteolytic inhibitors such as mannose-6-phosphate,[148] and neutralizing antibodies.[35] Clinically, however, only TGF-β3 injection into surgical wounds has been used to modulate the TGF-β pathway, demonstrating significant improvement in scar appearance in a randomized, controlled trial.[149] Unfortunately, further clinical trials of TGF-β3 did not prove to be effective and attempts to use it as an antifibrotic agent have ceased.

Surgical Treatments

Laser
The use of lasers for the treatment of burn scars and contractures is an evolving field. The 2 major categories currently used are ablative nonselective lasers (eg, CO_2) and nonablative selective lasers (eg, pulsed dye, and neodymium:yttrium-argon-garnet). The CO_2 laser has a high affinity for water, and causes thermal necrosis, which promotes wound contraction and collagen remodeling.[150] This can improve the texture and quality

of skin grafts and HSc, as shown in a randomized, controlled trial.[151] Pulsed-dye lasers cause selective photothermolysis of oxyhemoglobin causing coagulation necrosis, and can improve scar texture, redness, size, and pliability.[152] This effect seems to be related to TGF-β1 downregulation, collagenase upregulation,[153] and suppression of fibroblast proliferation.[154] Greater detail of these methods is discussed in the article on "Scar Management of the Burned Hand" by Drs Sorkin, Cholok, and Levi in this issue.

Cryosurgery
Cryotherapy involves multiple sessions of spray or freeze–thaw cycles induced either through surface contact,[136] which can cause hypopigmentation,[137] or using an intralesional cryoprobe.[155] The low temperatures lead to blood stasis, which decreases vascularity causing cell anoxia, and subsequent necrosis and apoptosis of fibroblasts.[136] This leads to reduced scar volume and increased softness.

Surgical prevention
In deep burns at high risk of HSc formation,[8] the optimal solution is frequently to tangentially excise the wound and skin graft it to prevent HSc. Burn depth and the predicted resulting scars can be determined with laser Doppler imaging,[156] thus helping to guide early surgical intervention. In **Fig. 6**, one can see the difference in motion between the hands of a patient who had similar burns

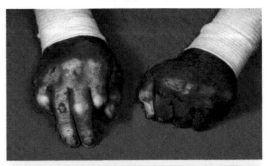

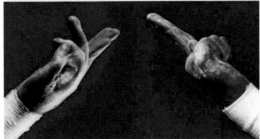

Fig. 6. Prevention of scarring by tangential burn excision and skin grafting. Note that the ungrafted right hand has significant impairment of flexion as compared with the grafted left hand.

but received grafting only to 1 side, illustrating the impact of preventing scarring through early surgical intervention.

Scar revision

Scar revision has 2 main mechanisms of action: removal of profibrotic ECM and cells, and reorientation or elimination of tension. The most direct mechanism of eliminating excess ECM is to excise it and to allow the wound healing process to reoccur. In many cases, this healing is delayed until the factors that lead to HSc, bands, and contractures have resolved, thus promoting a more normal scar.[157] Scar revision can also make use of Z-plasties to reorient or eliminate tension, thus leading to improved healing.[158] The limitation is that scar excision can create an additional tissue deficit which must be filled, or risk an increase in mechanical tension, which promotes HSc.[158] Greater detail of these methods is discussed in the article on "Scar Management of the Burned Hand" by Drs Sorkin, Cholok, and Levi in this issue.

SUMMARY

HSc and contractures are a major source of morbidity and poor function in burned hands. The roots of these problems stem from burn injuries below a critical skin depth, which leads to a complex interplay of local and systemic cells, stimulated by various profibrotic factors that ultimately result in contractures and HSc. Numerous therapies have been developed that primarily target fibroblasts and myofibroblasts, profibrotic signaling molecules, or modulate the remodeling of collagen by decreasing production or increasing MMPs. Owing to this complexity, there is currently no silver bullet that can cure all pathologic scars, but hopefully with an increased understanding of the underlying pathophysiology, this will change, ultimately providing better outcomes for those with hand burns and other fibrotic diseases.

REFERENCES

1. Kwan P, Hori K, Ding J, et al. Scar and contracture: biological principles. Hand Clin 2009;25(4): 511–28.
2. Ewings EL, Pollack J. Pediatric upper extremity burns: outcomes of emergency department triage and outpatient management. J Burn Care Res 2008;29(1):77–81.
3. Fagenholz PJ, Sheridan RL, Harris NS, et al. National study of Emergency Department visits for burn injuries, 1993 to 2004. J Burn Care Res 2007;28(5):681–90.
4. Bayat A, McGrouther DA, Ferguson MW. Skin scarring. BMJ 2003;326(7380):88–92.
5. Robson MC, Smith DJ Jr, VanderZee AJ, et al. Making the burned hand functional. Clin Plast Surg 1992;19(3):663–71.
6. American Burn Association/American College of Surgeons. Guidelines for the operation of burn centers. J Burn Care Res 2007;28(1):134–41.
7. Monstrey S, Hoeksema H, Verbelen J, et al. Assessment of burn depth and burn wound healing potential. Burns 2008;34(6):761–9.
8. Cubison TC, Pape SA, Parkhouse N. Evidence for the link between healing time and the development of hypertrophic scars (HTS) in paediatric burns due to scald injury. Burns 2006;32(8):992–9.
9. Dunkin CS, Pleat JM, Gillespie PH, et al. Scarring occurs at a critical depth of skin injury: precise measurement in a graduated dermal scratch in human volunteers. Plast Reconstr Surg 2007;119(6): 1722–32 [discussion: 1733–4].
10. Ali-Bahar M, Bauer B, Tredget EE, et al. Dermal fibroblasts from different layers of human skin are heterogeneous in expression of collagenase and types I and III procollagen mRNA. Wound Repair Regen 2004;12(2):175–82.
11. Sorrell JM, Baber MA, Caplan AI. Site-matched papillary and reticular human dermal fibroblasts differ in their release of specific growth factors/cytokines and in their interaction with keratinocytes. J Cell Physiol 2004;200(1):134–45.
12. Wang J, Dodd C, Shankowsky HA, et al. Deep dermal fibroblasts contribute to hypertrophic scarring. Lab Invest 2008;88(12):1278–90.
13. Scott PG, Ghahary A, Tredget EE. Molecular and cellular aspects of fibrosis following thermal injury. Hand Clin 2000;16(2):271–87.
14. Niessen FB, Spauwen PH, Schalkwijk J, et al. On the nature of hypertrophic scars and keloids: a review. Plast Reconstr Surg 1999;104(5):1435–58.
15. Verhaegen PD, van Zuijlen PP, Pennings NM, et al. Differences in collagen architecture between keloid, hypertrophic scar, normotrophic scar, and normal skin: an objective histopathological analysis. Wound Repair Regen 2009;17(5):649–56.
16. Hayakawa T, Hashimoto Y, Myokei Y, et al. Changes in type of collagen during the development of human post-burn hypertrophic scars. Clin Chim Acta 1979;93(1):119–25.
17. Bailey AJ, Bazin S, Sims TJ, et al. Characterization of the collagen of human hypertrophic and normal scars. Biochim Biophys Acta 1975;405(2):412–21.
18. Lapiere CM, Nusgens B, Pierard GE. Interaction between collagen type I and type III in conditioning bundles organization. Connect Tissue Res 1977; 5(1):21–9.
19. Birk DE, Fitch JM, Babiarz JP, et al. Collagen fibrillogenesis in vitro: interaction of types I and V collagen regulates fibril diameter. J Cell Sci 1990; 95(Pt 4):649–57.

20. Scott PG, Dodd CM, Tredget EE, et al. Chemical characterization and quantification of proteoglycans in human post-burn hypertrophic and mature scars. Clin Sci (Lond) 1996;90(5):417–25.

21. Zhang G, Ezura Y, Chervoneva I, et al. Decorin regulates assembly of collagen fibrils and acquisition of biomechanical properties during tendon development. J Cell Biochem 2006;98(6):1436–49.

22. Yamaguchi Y, Mann DM, Ruoslahti E. Negative regulation of transforming growth factor-beta by the proteoglycan decorin. Nature 1990;346(6281):281–4.

23. Kolb M, Margetts PJ, Galt T, et al. Transient transgene expression of decorin in the lung reduces the fibrotic response to bleomycin. Am J Respir Crit Care Med 2001;163(3 Pt 1):770–7.

24. Bittner K, Liszio C, Blumberg P, et al. Modulation of collagen gel contraction by decorin. Biochem J 1996;314(Pt 1):159–66.

25. Gordon KJ, Blobe GC. Role of transforming growth factor-beta superfamily signaling pathways in human disease. Biochim Biophys Acta 2008;1782(4):197–228.

26. Prud'homme GJ. Pathobiology of transforming growth factor beta in cancer, fibrosis and immunologic disease, and therapeutic considerations. Lab Invest 2007;87(11):1077–91.

27. Roberts AB. Molecular and cell biology of TGF-beta. Miner Electrolyte Metab 1998;24(2–3):111–9.

28. Leask A, Abraham DJ. TGF-beta signaling and the fibrotic response. FASEB J 2004;18(7):816–27.

29. Wakefield LM, Smith DM, Masui T, et al. Distribution and modulation of the cellular receptor for transforming growth factor-beta. J Cell Biol 1987;105(2):965–75.

30. Ignotz RA, Massague J. Transforming growth factor-beta stimulates the expression of fibronectin and collagen and their incorporation into the extracellular matrix. J Biol Chem 1986;261(9):4337–45.

31. Cutroneo KR. TGF-beta-induced fibrosis and SMAD signaling: oligo decoys as natural therapeutics for inhibition of tissue fibrosis and scarring. Wound Repair Regen 2007;15(Suppl 1):S54–60.

32. Tredget EE, Shankowsky HA, Pannu R, et al. Transforming growth factor-beta in thermally injured patients with hypertrophic scars: effects of interferon alpha-2b. Plast Reconstr Surg 1998;102(5):1317–28 [discussion: 1329–30].

33. Occleston NL, Laverty HG, O'Kane S, et al. Prevention and reduction of scarring in the skin by Transforming growth factor beta 3 (TGFbeta3): from laboratory discovery to clinical pharmaceutical. J Biomater Sci Polym Ed 2008;19(8):1047–63.

34. Bock O, Yu H, Zitron S, et al. Studies of transforming growth factors beta 1-3 and their receptors I and II in fibroblast of keloids and hypertrophic scars. Acta Derm Venereol 2005;85(3):216–20.

35. Schultze-Mosgau S, Wehrhan F, Rodel F, et al. Anti-TGFbeta1 antibody for modulation of expression of endogenous transforming growth factor beta 1 to prevent fibrosis after plastic surgery in rats. Br J Oral Maxillofac Surg 2004;42(2):112–9.

36. Perbal B. CCN proteins: multifunctional signalling regulators. Lancet 2004;363(9402):62–4.

37. Leask A, Abraham DJ. The role of connective tissue growth factor, a multifunctional matricellular protein, in fibroblast biology. Biochem Cell Biol 2003;81(6):355–63.

38. Mori T, Kawara S, Shinozaki M, et al. Role and interaction of connective tissue growth factor with transforming growth factor-beta in persistent fibrosis: a mouse fibrosis model. J Cell Physiol 1999;181(1):153–9.

39. Colwell AS, Phan TT, Kong W, et al. Hypertrophic scar fibroblasts have increased connective tissue growth factor expression after transforming growth factor-beta stimulation. Plast Reconstr Surg 2005;116(5):1387–90 [discussion: 1391–82].

40. Stratton R, Shiwen X, Martini G, et al. Iloprost suppresses connective tissue growth factor production in fibroblasts and in the skin of scleroderma patients. J Clin Invest 2001;108(2):241–50.

41. Abraham D. Connective tissue growth factor: growth factor, matricellular organizer, fibrotic biomarker or molecular target for anti-fibrotic therapy in SSc? Rheumatology (Oxford) 2008;47(Suppl 5):v8–9.

42. Andrae J, Gallini R, Betsholtz C. Role of platelet-derived growth factors in physiology and medicine. Genes Dev 2008;22(10):1276–312.

43. Werner S, Grose R. Regulation of wound healing by growth factors and cytokines. Physiol Rev 2003;83(3):835–70.

44. Powell DW, Mifflin RC, Valentich JD, et al. Myofibroblasts. I. Paracrine cells important in health and disease. Am J Physiol 1999;277(1 Pt 1):C1–9.

45. Trojanowska M. Role of PDGF in fibrotic diseases and systemic sclerosis. Rheumatology (Oxford) 2008;47(Suppl 5):v2–4.

46. Younai S, Venters G, Vu S, et al. Role of growth factors in scar contraction: an in vitro analysis. Ann Plast Surg 1996;36(5):495–501.

47. Ghahary A, Shen YJ, Wang R, et al. Expression and localization of insulin-like growth factor-1 in normal and post-burn hypertrophic scar tissue in human. Mol Cell Biochem 1998;183(1–2):1–9.

48. Jones JI, Clemmons DR. Insulin-like growth factors and their binding proteins: biological actions. Endocr Rev 1995;16(1):3–34.

49. Ghahary A, Shen Q, Shen YJ, et al. Induction of transforming growth factor beta 1 by insulin-like growth factor-1 in dermal fibroblasts. J Cell Physiol 1998;174(3):301–9.

50. Ghahary A, Shen YJ, Nedelec B, et al. Collagenase production is lower in post-burn hypertrophic scar

fibroblasts than in normal fibroblasts and is reduced by insulin-like growth factor-1. J Invest Dermatol 1996;106(3):476–81.

51. Rolfe KJ, Cambrey AD, Richardson J, et al. Dermal fibroblasts derived from fetal and postnatal humans exhibit distinct responses to insulin like growth factors. BMC Dev Biol 2007;7:124.

52. Miele C, Rochford JJ, Filippa N, et al. Insulin and insulin-like growth factor-I induce vascular endothelial growth factor mRNA expression via different signaling pathways. J Biol Chem 2000;275(28): 21695–702.

53. Steenfos HH, Jansson JO. Gene expression of insulin-like growth factor-I and IGF-I receptor during wound healing in rats. Eur J Surg 1992; 158(6–7):327–31.

54. Tredget EE, Nedelec B, Scott PG, et al. Hypertrophic scars, keloids, and contractures. The cellular and molecular basis for therapy. Surg Clin North Am 1997;77(3):701–30.

55. Ghahary A, Shen YJ, Nedelec B, et al. Interferons gamma and alpha-2b differentially regulate the expression of collagenase and tissue inhibitor of metalloproteinase-1 messenger RNA in human hypertrophic and normal dermal fibroblasts. Wound Repair Regen 1995;3(2):176–84.

56. Castagnoli C, Stella M, Berthod C, et al. TNF production and hypertrophic scarring. Cell Immunol 1993;147(1):51–63.

57. Goldberg MT, Han YP, Yan C, et al. TNF-alpha suppresses alpha-smooth muscle actin expression in human dermal fibroblasts: an implication for abnormal wound healing. J Invest Dermatol 2007; 127(11):2645–55.

58. Verjee LS, Verhoekx JS, Chan JK, et al. Unraveling the signaling pathways promoting fibrosis in Dupuytren's disease reveals TNF as a therapeutic target. Proc Natl Acad Sci U S A 2013;110(10): E928–37.

59. Moscatello DK, Santra M, Mann DM, et al. Decorin suppresses tumor cell growth by activating the epidermal growth factor receptor. J Clin Invest 1998;101(2):406–12.

60. Schönherr E, Sunderkötter C, Iozzo RV, et al. Decorin, a novel player in the insulin-like growth factor system. J Biol Chem 2005;280(16):15767–72.

61. Goldoni S, Humphries A, Nyström A, et al. Decorin is a novel antagonistic ligand of the Met receptor. J Cell Biol 2009;185(4):743–54.

62. Vial C, Gutiérrez J, Santander C, et al. Decorin interacts with connective tissue growth factor (CTGF)/CCN2 by LRR12 inhibiting its biological activity. J Biol Chem 2011;286(27):24242–52.

63. Zhang Z, Garron TM, Li XJ, et al. Recombinant human decorin inhibits TGF-beta1-induced contraction of collagen lattice by hypertrophic scar fibroblasts. Burns 2009;35(4):527–37.

64. Davies JE, Tang X, Denning JW, et al. Decorin suppresses neurocan, brevican, phosphacan and NG2 expression and promotes axon growth across adult rat spinal cord injuries. Eur J Neurosci 2004; 19(5):1226–42.

65. Fabian MR, Sonenberg N, Filipowicz W. Regulation of mRNA translation and stability by microRNAs. Annu Rev Biochem 2010;79:351–79.

66. Kwan P, Ding J, Tredget EE. MicroRNA 181b regulates decorin production by dermal fibroblasts and may be a potential therapy for hypertrophic scar. PLoS One 2015;10(4):e0123054.

67. Chau BN, Xin C, Hartner J, et al. MicroRNA-21 promotes fibrosis of the kidney by silencing metabolic pathways. Sci Transl Med 2012;4(121):121ra118.

68. Duan LJ, Qi J, Kong XJ, et al. MiR-133 modulates TGF-beta1-induced bladder smooth muscle cell hypertrophic and fibrotic response: implication for a role of microRNA in bladder wall remodeling caused by bladder outlet obstruction. Cell Signal 2015;27(2):215–27.

69. Cushing L, Kuang P, Lu J. The role of miR-29 in pulmonary fibrosis. Biochem Cell Biol 2015;93(2):109–18.

70. Deitch EA, Wheelahan TM, Rose MP, et al. Hypertrophic burn scars: analysis of variables. J Trauma 1983;23(10):895–8.

71. Simon F, Bergeron D, Larochelle S, et al. Enhanced secretion of TIMP-1 by human hypertrophic scar keratinocytes could contribute to fibrosis. Burns 2012;38(3):421–7.

72. Werner S, Krieg T, Smola H. Keratinocyte-fibroblast interactions in wound healing. J Invest Dermatol 2007;127(5):998–1008.

73. Amjad SB, Carachi R, Edward M. Keratinocyte regulation of TGF-beta and connective tissue growth factor expression: a role in suppression of scar tissue formation. Wound Repair Regen 2007; 15(5):748–55.

74. Ghahary A, Marcoux Y, Karimi-Busheri F, et al. Differentiated keratinocyte-releasable stratifin (14-3-3 sigma) stimulates MMP-1 expression in dermal fibroblasts. J Invest Dermatol 2005;124(1):170–7.

75. Bellemare J, Roberge CJ, Bergeron D, et al. Epidermis promotes dermal fibrosis: role in the pathogenesis of hypertrophic scars. J Pathol 2005;206(1):1–8.

76. Singer AJ, Clark RA. Cutaneous wound healing. N Engl J Med 1999;341(10):738–46.

77. Schafer IA, Shapiro A, Kovach M, et al. The interaction of human papillary and reticular fibroblasts and human keratinocytes in the contraction of three-dimensional floating collagen lattices. Exp Cell Res 1989;183(1):112–25.

78. Feldman SR, Trojanowska M, Smith EA, et al. Differential responses of human papillary and reticular fibroblasts to growth factors. Am J Med Sci 1993; 305(4):203–7.

79. Sorrell JM, Baber MA, Caplan AI. Human dermal fibroblast subpopulations; differential interactions with vascular endothelial cells in coculture: non-soluble factors in the extracellular matrix influence interactions. Wound Repair Regen 2008; 16(2):300–9.

80. Rossio-Pasquier P, Casanova D, Jomard A, et al. Wound healing of human skin transplanted onto the nude mouse after a superficial excisional injury: human dermal reconstruction is achieved in several steps by two different fibroblast subpopulations. Arch Dermatol Res 1999;291(11):591–9.

81. Hinz B, Gabbiani G. Cell-matrix and cell-cell contacts of myofibroblasts: role in connective tissue remodeling. Thromb Haemost 2003;90(6): 993–1002.

82. Shin D, Minn KW. The effect of myofibroblast on contracture of hypertrophic scar. Plast Reconstr Surg 2004;113(2):633–40.

83. Junker JP, Kratz C, Tollback A, et al. Mechanical tension stimulates the transdifferentiation of fibroblasts into myofibroblasts in human burn scars. Burns 2008;34(7):942–6.

84. Moulin V, Larochelle S, Langlois C, et al. Normal skin wound and hypertrophic scar myofibroblasts have differential responses to apoptotic inductors. J Cell Physiol 2004;198(3):350–8.

85. Armour A, Scott PG, Tredget EE. Cellular and molecular pathology of HTS: basis for treatment. Wound Repair Regen 2007;15(Suppl 1):S6–17.

86. van der Veer WM, Bloemen MC, Ulrich MM, et al. Potential cellular and molecular causes of hypertrophic scar formation. Burns 2009;35(1):15–29.

87. Sunderkotter C, Steinbrink K, Goebeler M, et al. Macrophages and angiogenesis. J Leukoc Biol 1994;55(3):410–22.

88. Ishida Y, Gao JL, Murphy PM. Chemokine receptor CX3CR1 mediates skin wound healing by promoting macrophage and fibroblast accumulation and function. J Immunol 2008;180(1):569–79.

89. Zhu Z, Ding J, Ma Z, et al. The natural behavior of mononuclear phagocytes in HTS formation. Wound Repair Regen 2016;24(1):14–25.

90. Zhu Z, Ding J, Ma Z, et al. Systemic depletion of macrophages in the subacute phase of wound healing reduces hypertrophic scar formation. Wound Repair Regen 2016;24(4):644–56.

91. Wang JF, Jiao H, Stewart TL, et al. Fibrocytes from burn patients regulate the activities of fibroblasts. Wound Repair Regen 2007;15(1):113–21.

92. Ding J, Hori K, Zhang R, et al. Stromal cell-derived factor 1 (SDF-1) and its receptor CXCR4 in the formation of postburn hypertrophic scar (HTS). Wound Repair Regen 2011;19(5):568–78.

93. Abe R, Donnelly SC, Peng T, et al. Peripheral blood fibrocytes: differentiation pathway and migration to wound sites. J Immunol 2001;166(12):7556–62.

94. Yang L, Scott PG, Dodd C, et al. Identification of fibrocytes in postburn hypertrophic scar. Wound Repair Regen 2005;13(4):398–404.

95. Hong KM, Belperio JA, Keane MP, et al. Differentiation of human circulating fibrocytes as mediated by transforming growth factor-beta and peroxisome proliferator-activated receptor gamma. J Biol Chem 2007;282(31):22910–20.

96. Balmelli C, Alves MP, Steiner E, et al. Responsiveness of fibrocytes to toll-like receptor danger signals. Immunobiology 2007;212(9–10):693–9.

97. Chesney J, Bacher M, Bender A, et al. The peripheral blood fibrocyte is a potent antigen-presenting cell capable of priming naive T cells in situ. Proc Natl Acad Sci U S A 1997;94(12):6307–12.

98. Wynn TA. Cellular and molecular mechanisms of fibrosis. J Pathol 2008;214(2):199–210.

99. Goodman RE, Nestle F, Naidu YM, et al. Keratinocyte-derived T cell costimulation induces preferential production of IL-2 and IL-4 but not IFN-gamma. J Immunol 1994;152(11):5189–98.

100. Hauser C. The interaction between Langerhans cells and CD4+ T cells. J Dermatol 1992;19(11): 722–5.

101. Mosmann TR, Coffman RL. TH1 and TH2 cells: different patterns of lymphokine secretion lead to different functional properties. Annu Rev Immunol 1989;7:145–73.

102. Wang J, Jiao H, Stewart TL, et al. Increased TGF-beta-producing CD4+ T lymphocytes in postburn patients and their potential interaction with dermal fibroblasts in hypertrophic scarring. Wound Repair Regen 2007;15(4):530–9.

103. Wynn TA. Fibrotic disease and the T(H)1/T(H)2 paradigm. Nat Rev Immunol 2004;4(8):583–94.

104. Sandler NG, Mentink-Kane MM, Cheever AW, et al. Global gene expression profiles during acute pathogen-induced pulmonary inflammation reveal divergent roles for Th1 and Th2 responses in tissue repair. J Immunol 2003; 171(7):3655–67.

105. Kilani RT, Delehanty M, Shankowsky HA, et al. Fluorescent-activated cell-sorting analysis of intracellular interferon-gamma and interleukin-4 in fresh and frozen human peripheral blood T-helper cells. Wound Repair Regen 2005;13(4):441–9.

106. Tredget EE, Yang L, Delehanty M, et al. Polarized Th2 cytokine production in patients with hypertrophic scar following thermal injury. J Interferon Cytokine Res 2006;26(3):179–89.

107. Nedelec B, Ghahary A, Scott PG, et al. Control of wound contraction. Basic and clinical features. Hand Clin 2000;16(2):289–302.

108. Carlson MA, Longaker MT. The fibroblast-populated collagen matrix as a model of wound healing: a review of the evidence. Wound Repair Regen 2004;12(2):134–47.

109. Ramirez AT, Soroff HS, Schwartz MS, et al. Experimental wound healing in man. Surg Gynecol Obstet 1969;128(2):283–93.

110. Ramos ML, Gragnani A, Ferreira LM. Is there an ideal animal model to study hypertrophic scarring? J Burn Care Res 2008;29(2):363–8.

111. Ryan GB, Cliff WJ, Gabbiani G, et al. Myofibroblasts in human granulation tissue. Hum Pathol 1974;5(1):55–67.

112. Harris AK, Stopak D, Wild P. Fibroblast traction as a mechanism for collagen morphogenesis. Nature 1981;290(5803):249–51.

113. Ehrlich HP. Wound closure: evidence of cooperation between fibroblasts and collagen matrix. Eye (Lond) 1988;2(Pt 2):149–57.

114. Reed MJ, Vernon RB, Abrass IB, et al. TGF-beta 1 induces the expression of type I collagen and SPARC, and enhances contraction of collagen gels, by fibroblasts from young and aged donors. J Cell Physiol 1994;158(1):169–79.

115. Bell E, Ivarsson B, Merrill C. Production of a tissue-like structure by contraction of collagen lattices by human fibroblasts of different proliferative potential in vitro. Proc Natl Acad Sci U S A 1979;76(3):1274–8.

116. Nedelec B, Shen YJ, Ghahary A, et al. The effect of interferon alpha 2b on the expression of cytoskeletal proteins in an in vitro model of wound contraction. J Lab Clin Med 1995;126(5):474–84.

117. Stone PA, Madden JW. Effect of primary and delayed split skin grafting on wound contraction. Surg Forum 1974;25(0):41–4.

118. Ehrlich HP. The modulation of contraction of fibroblast populated collagen lattices by types I, II, and III collagen. Tissue Cell 1988;20(1):47–50.

119. Derderian CA, Bastidas N, Lerman OZ, et al. Mechanical strain alters gene expression in an in vitro model of hypertrophic scarring. Ann Plast Surg 2005;55(1):69–75 [discussion: 75].

120. Aarabi S, Bhatt KA, Shi Y, et al. Mechanical load initiates hypertrophic scar formation through decreased cellular apoptosis. FASEB J 2007;21(12):3250–61.

121. Wong VW, Rustad KC, Akaishi S, et al. Focal adhesion kinase links mechanical force to skin fibrosis via inflammatory signaling. Nat Med 2012;18(1):148–52.

122. Macintyre L, Baird M. Pressure garments for use in the treatment of hypertrophic scars–a review of the problems associated with their use. Burns 2006;32(1):10–5.

123. Anzarut A, Olson J, Singh P, et al. The effectiveness of pressure garment therapy for the prevention of abnormal scarring after burn injury: a meta-analysis. J Plast Reconstr Aesthet Surg 2009;62(1):77–84.

124. Engrav LH, Heimbach DM, Rivara FP, et al. 12-Year within-wound study of the effectiveness of custom pressure garment therapy. Burns 2010;36(7):975–83.

125. Perkins K, Davey RB, Wallis KA. Silicone gel: a new treatment for burn scars and contractures. Burns Incl Therm Inj 1983;9(3):201–4.

126. Momeni M, Hafezi F, Rahbar H, et al. Effects of silicone gel on burn scars. Burns 2009;35(1):70–4.

127. Cho YS, Jeon JH, Hong A, et al. The effect of burn rehabilitation massage therapy on hypertrophic scar after burn: a randomized controlled trial. Burns 2014;40(8):1513–20.

128. Ko WJ, Na YC, Suh BS, et al. The effects of topical agent (kelo-cote or contractubex) massage on the thickness of post-burn scar tissue formed in rats. Arch Plast Surg 2013;40(6):697–704.

129. Kanazawa Y, Nomura J, Yoshimoto S, et al. Cyclical cell stretching of skin-derived fibroblasts downregulates connective tissue growth factor (CTGF) production. Connect Tissue Res 2009;50(5):323–9.

130. Wang JH, Yang G, Li Z, et al. Fibroblast responses to cyclic mechanical stretching depend on cell orientation to the stretching direction. J Biomech 2004;37(4):573–6.

131. Kamolz LP, Kitzinger HB, Karle B, et al. The treatment of hand burns. Burns 2009;35(3):327–37.

132. Prasad JK, Bowden ML, Thomson PD. A review of the reconstructive surgery needs of 3167 survivors of burn injury. Burns 1991;17(4):302–5.

133. Atkinson JA, McKenna KT, Barnett AG, et al. A randomized, controlled trial to determine the efficacy of paper tape in preventing hypertrophic scar formation in surgical incisions that traverse Langer's skin tension lines. Plast Reconstr Surg 2005;116(6):1648–56 [discussion: 1657–48].

134. Longaker MT, Rohrich RJ, Greenberg L, et al. A randomized controlled trial of the embrace advanced scar therapy device to reduce incisional scar formation. Plast Reconstr Surg 2014;134(3):536–46.

135. Ketchum LD, Smith J, Robinson DW, et al. The treatment of hypertrophic scar, keloid and scar contracture by triamcinolone acetonide. Plast Reconstr Surg 1966;38(3):209–18.

136. Berman B, Viera MH, Amini S, et al. Prevention and management of hypertrophic scars and keloids after burns in children. J Craniofac Surg 2008;19(4):989–1006.

137. Atiyeh BS. Nonsurgical management of hypertrophic scars: evidence-based therapies, standard practices, and emerging methods. Aesthetic Plast Surg 2007;31(5):468–92 [discussion: 493–4].

138. Lama PJ, Fechtner RD. Antifibrotics and wound healing in glaucoma surgery. Surv Ophthalmol 2003;48(3):314–46.

139. Metterle L, Nelson C, Patel N. Intralesional 5-fluorouracil (FU) as a treatment for nonmelanoma skin

cancer (NMSC): a review. J Am Acad Dermatol 2016;74(3):552–7.

140. Goldan O, Weissman O, Regev E, et al. Treatment of postdermabrasion facial hypertrophic and keloid scars with intralesional 5-Fluorouracil injections. Aesthet Plast Surg 2008;32(2):389–92.

141. Fitzpatrick RE. Treatment of inflamed hypertrophic scars using intralesional 5-FU. Dermatol Surg 1999;25(3):224–32.

142. Chen MA, Davidson TM. Scar management: prevention and treatment strategies. Curr Opin Otolaryngol Head Neck Surg 2005;13(4):242–7.

143. Berman B, Villa AM, Ramirez CC. Novel opportunities in the treatment and prevention of scarring. J Cutan Med Surg 2004;8(Suppl 3):32–6.

144. Tredget EE, Wang R, Shen Q, et al. Transforming growth factor-beta mRNA and protein in hypertrophic scar tissues and fibroblasts: antagonism by IFN-alpha and IFN-gamma in vitro and in vivo. J Interferon Cytokine Res 2000;20(2):143–51.

145. Wang J, Chen H, Shankowsky HA, et al. Improved scar in postburn patients following interferon-alpha2b treatment is associated with decreased angiogenesis mediated by vascular endothelial cell growth factor. J Interferon Cytokine Res 2008; 28(7):423–34.

146. Wang J, Jiao H, Stewart TL, et al. Improvement in postburn hypertrophic scar after treatment with IFN-alpha2b is associated with decreased fibrocytes. J Interferon Cytokine Res 2007;27(11): 921–30.

147. Nedelec B, Shankowsky H, Scott PG, et al. Myofibroblasts and apoptosis in human hypertrophic scars: the effect of interferon-alpha2b. Surgery 2001;130(5):798–808.

148. Zhang J, Wong MG, Wong M, et al. A cationic-independent mannose 6-phosphate receptor inhibitor (PXS64) ameliorates kidney fibrosis by inhibiting activation of transforming growth factor-beta1. PLoS One 2015;10(2):e0116888.

149. Ferguson MW, Duncan J, Bond J, et al. Prophylactic administration of avotermin for improvement of skin scarring: three double-blind, placebo-controlled, phase I/II studies. Lancet 2009; 373(9671):1264–74.

150. Utley DS, Koch RJ, Egbert BM. Histologic analysis of the thermal effect on epidermal and dermal structures following treatment with the superpulsed CO2 laser and the erbium: YAG laser: an in vivo study. Lasers Surg Med 1999;24(2):93–102.

151. Taudorf EH, Danielsen PL, Paulsen IF, et al. Nonablative fractional laser provides long-term improvement of mature burn scars–a randomized controlled trial with histological assessment. Lasers Surg Med 2015;47(2):141–7.

152. Alster TS. Improvement of erythematous and hypertrophic scars by the 585-nm flashlamp-pumped pulsed dye laser. Ann Plast Surg 1994; 32(2):186–90.

153. Kuo YR, Wu WS, Jeng SF, et al. Suppressed TGF-beta1 expression is correlated with up-regulation of matrix metalloproteinase-13 in keloid regression after flashlamp pulsed-dye laser treatment. Lasers Surg Med 2005;36(1):38–42.

154. Kuo YR, Wu WS, Wang FS. Flashlamp pulsed-dye laser suppressed TGF-beta1 expression and proliferation in cultured keloid fibroblasts is mediated by MAPK pathway. Lasers Surg Med 2007;39(4):358–64.

155. Har-Shai Y, Amar M, Sabo E. Intralesional cryotherapy for enhancing the involution of hypertrophic scars and keloids. Plast Reconstr Surg 2003; 111(6):1841–52.

156. Wang XQ, Mill J, Kravchuk O, et al. Ultrasound assessed thickness of burn scars in association with laser Doppler imaging determined depth of burns in paediatric patients. Burns 2010;36(8):1254–62.

157. Mustoe TA, Cooter RD, Gold MH, et al. International clinical recommendations on scar management. Plast Reconstr Surg 2002;110(2):560–71.

158. Kwan PO, Cartotto R. Burn reconstruction basics. In: Greenhalgh DG, editor. Burn care for general surgeons and general practitioners. New York: Springer; 2016. p. 151–64.

Postburn Upper Extremity Occupational Therapy

Tiffany Williams, MS, OTR/L*, Tanya Berenz, MS, OTR/L

KEYWORDS

- Upper extremity • Burns • Occupational therapy • Splinting • Edema • Hand • Scar management

KEY POINTS

- The potential complications after an upper extremity burn injury can lead to loss of range of motion, joint contractures, and devastating functional limitations.
- A comprehensive occupational therapy program is essential in helping patients to regain optimal function after an upper extremity burn injury.
- Edema management, splinting, exercise, scar management, and activities of daily living are key elements of an occupational therapy treatment plan to achieve ideal postburn outcomes.
- Patient and family training is a vital component to successful carryover and recovery of function after an upper extremity burn.
- The pediatric burn patient population has additional considerations to be taken into account when treatment planning.

INTRODUCTION

An upper extremity burn injury can lead to life-long functional limitations due to the many potential challenges encountered throughout recovery.[1] The unique anatomy of the upper extremity leads to specific concerns and considerations throughout rehabilitation.[2] Early occupational therapy (OT) interventions are essential to achieve best functional outcomes, particularly because the hand is among the most common areas for scar contracture development after a burn.[3] The potential complications after an upper extremity burn injury can lead to loss of range of motion (ROM), joint contractures, and devastating functional limitations. A comprehensive OT program is essential to help patients regain optimal function.

INITIAL ASSESSMENT

A patient with an upper extremity burn should be assessed within 24 hours of a hospital admission by an occupational therapist with burn-specific training. This initial assessment includes evaluation of upper extremity edema, ROM, strength, sensation, burn depth, total burn surface area (TBSA), mechanism of injury, and functional status. This physical assessment is completed in conjunction with obtaining social history, previous medical history, prior functional status, and identification of patient goals. Current cognitive status, caregiver support, and surgical plans are equally important factors to consider upon initial assessment and will directly impact OT goals. This information is compiled to create a therapy treatment plan of care with the intent to return the patient to a preinjury level of functional independence.

TREATMENT
Edema Management

Edema is a common problem after a burn injury and should be one of the first areas assessed. Extra fluid accumulates in the affected upper

Disclosure Statement: The have nothing to disclose. The authors have no commercial or financial conflicts to report.
Occupational Therapy Division, Department of Physical Medicine and Rehabilitation, University of Michigan Health System, 1500 East Medical Center Drive, Ann Arbor, MI 48109, USA
* Corresponding author. 1693 Reserve Court, Ann Arbor, MI 48103.
E-mail address: tiffkw@med.umich.edu

Hand Clin 33 (2017) 293–304
http://dx.doi.org/10.1016/j.hcl.2016.12.015
0749-0712/17/© 2017 Elsevier Inc. All rights reserved.

hand.theclinics.com

extremity, causing discomfort, ROM limitations, and increased risk of infection.[1] Patients with partial-thickness and full-thickness burn injuries are especially at risk for the development of persistent edema.[4] Edema should be evaluated and treated in the acute phase and continually re-evaluated throughout all phases of burn recovery (**Fig. 1**).

Assessment of acute edema includes a description of the areas affected and a general description of edema severity. Generally, if edema remains after 48 to 72 hours, detailed measurements may be taken to monitor progress. Bilateral proximal upper extremity edema is measured with use of a soft measuring tape, with measurements taken circumferentially at specific intervals. More specifically, the hand can be measured using the figure-of-8 method to more accurately record hand edema[5] (**Fig. 2**). Measurements are reassessed periodically to track progress throughout recovery to assess the effectiveness of OT edema management interventions.

Treatment of edema in an affected upper extremity is acutely managed with supportive positioning and elevation to promote fluid reduction. The goal is to elevate the arm above heart level as tolerated. Elevation of the upper extremity can be achieved by a variety of supports. For example, a foam wedge arm support can be used to position the arm and hand in the appropriate position. Alternatively, an intravenous (IV) pole with a stockinette to suspend the upper extremity can be used to promote fluid reduction (**Fig. 3**).

After the acute phase of edema, after 72 hours, the use of compression may be initiated for edema

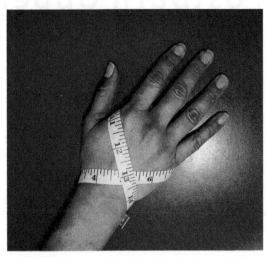

Fig. 2. The figure-of-8 method should be used to specifically record hand edema.[3] Measurements are reassessed periodically to monitor progress.

management.[2] Compression can be achieved with the use of edema gloves or self-adherent elastic wraps applied to edematous digits and/or hands (**Fig. 4**). Another option is the use of elasticized tubular bandages to provide even, continuous compression to affected upper extremities. After application of any type of compression, careful monitoring of the patient's tolerance must be observed to ensure patient's skin integrity is maintained. Compression should not limit a patient's participation in active use of the upper extremity.

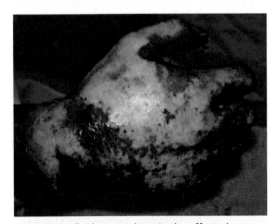

Fig. 1. Extra fluid accumulates in the affected extremity, causing discomfort, ROM limitations, and increased risk of infection. (*From* Moore ML, Dewey WS, Richard RL. Rehabilitation of the burned hand. Hand Clin 2009;25(4):530; with permission.)

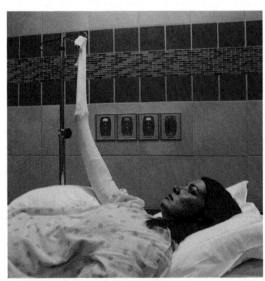

Fig. 3. An IV pole with a stockinette can be used to suspend the upper extremity to promote fluid reduction.

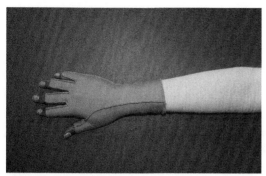

Fig. 4. Compression can be achieved to the affected areas with use of edema gloves or self-adherent elastic wraps applied to edematous digits and/or hands.

Active range of motion exercises (AROM) are a critical part of edema reduction. As soon as possible, patients should be instructed in an active upper extremity ROM exercise program. The goal is to promote circulation and to stimulate the lymphatic system.

Pediatric applications

Treatment of edema among pediatric patients should incorporate play activities as much as possible. Stuffed animals or colorful pillows can be used for positioning of the edematous arm. Compression gloves and bandages can be used in variety of colors or decorated to increase patient compliance. AROM exercises can be incorporated in play activities appropriate for the patient's age level.

Patient and caregiver education

Patients and caregivers should be instructed regarding the importance of edema reduction for overall recovery of upper extremity function. This education includes a strong emphasis on completion of edema management interventions beyond the patient's therapy sessions. Clear instructions should be provided to the patient and family members on edema reduction strategies, including home exercise programs, carryover of appropriate compression, and positioning recommendations. The goal is to provide patients and family members with the ability to actively participate in edema management throughout recovery.

ANTIDEFORMITY SPLINTING

After an upper extremity burn has been sustained, a patient is likely to assume a position of comfort, with the affected joints held in flexion. Splinting and positioning are essential components of OT treatment to prevent and correct joint limitations

that can occur from prolonged rest in this compromising position. The need for splinting intervention is assessed upon initial presentation and reassessed throughout a patient's recovery. Occupational therapists use splinting and positioning for upper extremity deformity prevention, achieved through tissue lengthening and proper joint alignment. Considerations for determining appropriate positioning include depth of the burn, current ROM, and the patient's participation in therapy. For example, patients who do not require surgical intervention, demonstrate full AROM, and participate in therapy would not require splinting.[1,6]

Despite skilled splinting interventions, upper extremity deformities can occur as a result of postburn edema, structural injury, and scarring.[1] Common upper extremity deformities include boutonniere deformity, mallet finger deformity, web space contractures, claw hand deformity, palmar arch contractures, elbow flexion contractures, and axillary scar bands. Splinting is a key treatment component to lessening the long-term effects of such deformities. Special attention is given to splint wear schedules and splint fit throughout burn recovery. In addition, patient and family education is a key component of upper extremity deformity prevention after a burn.

Boutonniere Deformity

Boutonniere deformity presents with the proximal interphalangeal (PIP) joint in flexion and the distal interphalangeal (DIP) joint in hyperextension. This position results from injury to the central slip, which can be damaged from a dorsal hand burn that exposes the PIP joint. It is best to keep the PIP and DIP joints immobilized in a finger extension splint until the tendon is no longer vulnerable (**Fig. 5**).[2]

Mallet Finger Deformity

Mallet finger deformity occurs when the burn injury has affected the distal portion of the extensor tendon. As a result, a DIP flexion contracture develops. A mallet finger splint or DIP extension splint can be fabricated to support the DIP joint in extension. This splint should be worn at all times of the day until the DIP joint is no longer susceptible to injury (**Fig. 6**).[1]

First Web Space Contractures

Burns that involve the digits of the upper extremity will often affect the web spaces of the hand. In particular, first web space contractures not only impact hand appearance but also largely impact hand function. Hand grasp, pinch, and opposition can all become impaired with such contractures,

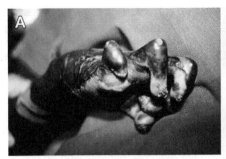
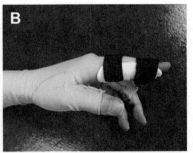

Fig. 5. (*A*, *B*) Boutonniere deformity presents with the PIP joint in flexion and the DIP joint in hyperextension. ([*A*] *From* Simpson RL. Management of burns of the upper extremity. In: Skiven TM, Osterman AL, Fedorczyk JM, editors. Rehabilitation of the hand and upper extremity. 6th edition. Philadelphia: Mosby, Inc; 2011:311; with permission.)

hindering independence with activities of daily living (ADL). Splinting for prevention includes use of a first web space or C-bar splint, which positions the thumb in abduction, promoting a position of function (**Fig. 7**).[6]

Claw Hand Deformity

Dorsal or circumferential deep partial and full-thickness burns of the hand can result in claw hand deformity. The presence of postburn edema and tendon injuries contributes to an increased likelihood of this deformity.[1] This position brings the metacarpophalangeal (MCP) joints into hyperextension and interphalangeal (IP) joints into flexion, potentially creating devastating functional deficits. Contracture in this position leads to difficulty with ADL, including self-feeding, grooming, and dressing. Splinting for prevention and correction of claw hand deformity places the hand in an intrinsic plus position. An intrinsic plus splint maintains the wrist in 20° to 30° of extension, MCP

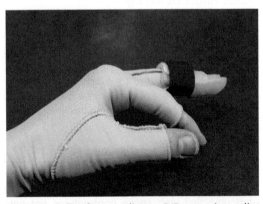

Fig. 6. A mallet finger splint or DIP extension splint supports the DIP joint, maintaining extension, and should be worn at all times of the day until the DIP joint is no longer susceptible to injury.

joints in 70° to 80° of flexion, and IP joints in extension (**Fig. 8**).

Palmar Arch Contractures

Impairment to the palmar arch of the hand can occur as a result of circumferential full-thickness hand or palmar surface burns. Despite the thick nature of the palmar skin, contractures can occur secondary to the resting position of the hand in flexion. A palmar extension splint provides antideformity positioning for this issue. The hand is positioned with the wrist in neutral, MCP and IP joints in extension, and thumb in abduction (**Fig. 9**).

Elbow Complications

Splinting of the elbow is typically limited to the days immediately following grafting. Such splints are used to immobilize the elbow joint for initial graft adherence. An anterior elbow extension splint with the elbow in 10° to 15° of flexion is fabricated for circumferential or antecubital space burns. Occasionally, when a burn involves the posterior portion of the elbow, a posterior elbow splint, also in 10° to 15° of flexion, can be created with the elbow portion floating in the splint. This posterior splint facilitates offloading of the olecranon whereby the skin grafts are quite fragile postoperatively.

OT treatment of elbow burns can be sidelined by the presence of heterotopic ossification (HO). HO occurs from bone growth in soft tissue, causing ROM limitations at nearby joints. Larger TBSA and full-thickness burns increase the likelihood of HO formation.[1] This presents additional challenges for the restoration of upper extremity function as it relates to ADL.

Axillary Complications

Axillary burns can lead to scar banding and shoulder ROM limitations that create challenging

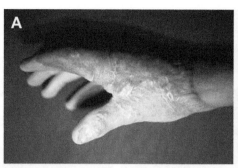
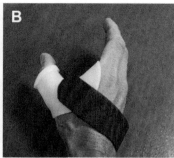

Fig. 7. (*A, B*) Thumb web space contractures not only impact hand appearance but also largely impact hand function. A thumb web space splint positions the thumb in abduction, promoting a functional position. ([*A*] *From* Simpson RL. Management of burns of the upper extremity. In: Skiven TM, Osterman AL, Fedorczyk JM, et al, editors. Rehabilitation of the hand and upper extremity. 6th edition. Philadelphia: Mosby, Inc; 2011:312; with permission.)

treatment complications for the occupational therapist. In the postgrafting phase, an airplane splint or foam wedge is used to position the patient in 90° of shoulder flexion and 70° of horizontal abduction with the forearm in neutral (**Fig. 10**). This can also be used after initial healing to provide an intermittent prolonged. Alternatively, if a patient only requires an axillary stretch while in supine position or while sedated, a bedside trough can be used (**Fig. 11**). This facilitates tissue lengthening at the axillary borders where scar bands frequently develop.

With each technique, care is taken to position and support the upper extremity without strain on the brachial plexus.

Advanced Stage Digit Complications

Upon later stages of wound healing, flexion of digits can become limited, affecting a patient's ability to form a composite fist. This position is often the result of full-thickness dorsal or circumferential hand burns. When this occurs, a dynamic flexion splint can be fashioned to facilitate active motion (**Fig. 12**). The dynamic flexion splint positions the thumb in abduction and permits the patient to actively extend the digits while providing assist for digit flexion. Conversely, digit extension may become limited by palmar surface burns. A low-profile dynamic extension splint can be fabricated to assist with finger extension (**Fig. 13**).

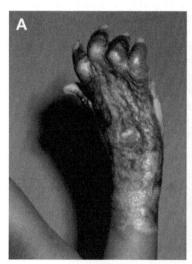
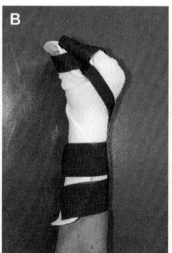
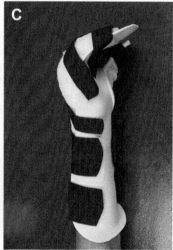

Fig. 8. (*A–C*) Claw hand position brings the MCP joints into hyperextension and IP joints into flexion, potentially creating devastating functional complications. An intrinsic plus splint maintains the wrist in 20° to 30° of extension, MCP joints in 70° to 80° of flexion, and IP joints in extension. ([*A*] *From* Wilhemi BJ, Burns MC, Cooney D. Orthoses for the burned hand. In: Hsu JD, Michael J, Fisk J, editors. AAOS atlas of orthoses and assistive devices. 4th edition. Philadelphia: Mosby, Inc; 2008:222; with permission.)

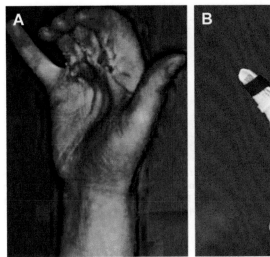
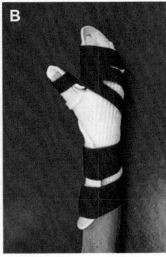
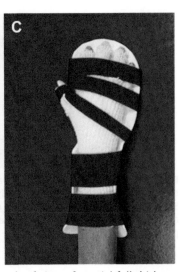

Fig. 9. (*A–C*) Impairment to the palmar arch of the hand can occur as a result of circumferential full-thickness hand or palmar surface burns. A palmar extension splint positions the wrist in neutral, MCP and IP joints in extension, and thumb in abduction. ([*A*] *From* Gulgonen A, Ozer K. The correction of postburn contractures of the second through fourth web spaces. J Hand Surg Am 2007;32(4):562; with permission.)

Dynamic splints are worn during the daytime when the patient can actively participate in ROM within the splint (**Table 1**).[2]

Splint Schedules

A patient's splint-wearing schedule depends on surgical interventions, level of alertness, and participation in therapy. Typically, initial grafting procedures require immobilization at the affected joints in splints for 3 to 5 days after surgery to facilitate graft adherence (**Fig. 14**). During this time, splints are donned with a gauze wrap to maintain splint position and to accommodate postoperative wound drainage. When a patient with deep partial or full-thickness hand burns is sedated, a hand splint is typically scheduled to be worn at all times, providing a prolonged antideformity posture while the patient is unable to actively engage in therapy sessions. A patient who is alert but not adequately participating in

therapy sessions or home exercise programs can benefit from intermittent daytime splint positioning. Intermittent daytime splint positioning may consist of wear for several daytime hours and at all hours of the night.

Pediatric Applications

Splints for pediatric patients are often successful when applied during naps and at nighttime. Daytime hours out of the splint permits active upper extremity use during play. The less participatory a child is with daytime active upper extremity use, the more wear time a splint will be recommended.[7] A stockinette or sock placed over the splint can deter a child from pulling at the straps of the splint and increase wear compliance.[1] Adequate splint wear time can be difficult for parents to achieve. It is especially imperative for the child's caregiver to understand the lifelong functional consequences of poor splint carryover.

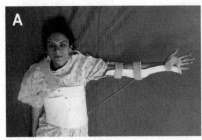
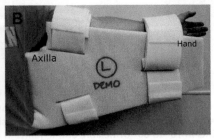

Fig. 10. (*A, B*) In the postgrafting phase, an airplane splint or foam wedge is used to position the patient in approximately 80° of scaption and the forearm in neutral.

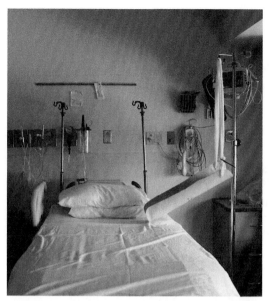

Fig. 11. If a patient only requires an axillary stretch while supine or if they are sedated, a bedside trough can be used for positioning.

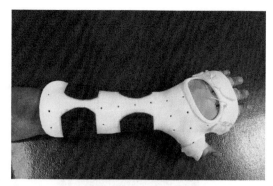

Fig. 13. A low-profile dynamic extension splint can be fabricated to assist with finger extension.

Patient and Caregiver Education

Successful upper extremity burn rehabilitation relies heavily on the participation of the patient and their support system. Education regarding the importance of adherence to splint wear schedules is initiated as soon as the need for a splint is determined. When appropriate, teaching the patient to apply their own splints can maximize his or her independence. Starting during hospitalization, family and caregiver training can assist with splint wear schedule carryover into discharge. Proper

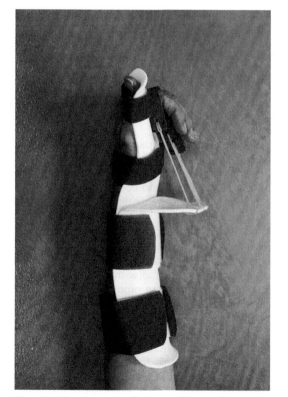

Fig. 12. The dynamic flexion splint positions the thumb in abduction and permits the patient to actively extend the digits and assists with digit flexion attempts.

Table 1
Splinting techniques for upper extremity deformities

Complication	Splint Recommendation
Boutonniere deformity	Finger extension splint—PIP and DIP joints in extension
Mallet finger deformity	Mallet finger splint or DIP extension splint—DIP joint in extension
Thumb web space contractures	Thumb web space splint—thumb in abduction
Claw hand deformity	Intrinsic plus splint—wrist in 20°–30° of extension, MCP joints in 70°–80° of flexion, PIP and DIP joints in extension
Palmar arch deformity	Palmar extension splint—wrist in neutral, MCPs, PIPs, and DIPs in extension, thumb in abduction
Axillary contractures	Airplane splint, foam wedge, or trough—shoulder in 80° of scaption, elbow in 10° of flexion, wrist in neutral

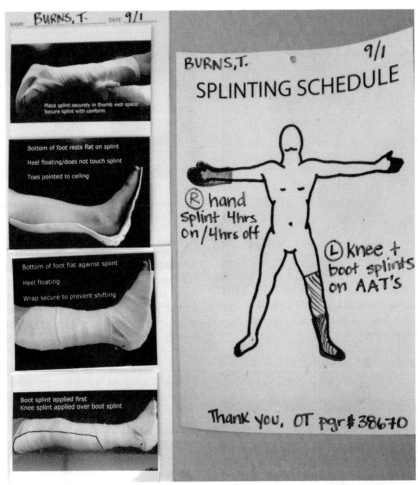

Fig. 14. Specific instructions for patients and families can assist with carryover of splint wear schedules starting during hospitalization through a patient's return to home.

splint care and skin checks must also be taught to decrease complications upon discharge.

RANGE OF MOTION AND STRENGTHENING

Full return of upper extremity function cannot rely on splinting alone. ROM and strengthening exercises assist with a patient's progress toward maximal functional recovery. ROM programs include AROM, active assistive ROM, and/or passive ROM exercises.

Opportunities to perform ROM and prolonged stretch when wound dressings are removed can be particularly helpful during the early healing phase postgrafting. This permits visibility of graft integrity and allows for maximal ROM without the restriction of bandages.[8] In addition, an occupational therapist may choose to perform ROM in the operating room when a patient is sedated preoperatively. This time affords the therapist an opportunity to determine a patient's maximal

available joint range, particularly if a patient is resistant with AROM treatment attempts.

Formal home programs that incorporate pictures, exercise logs, and concise instructions are helpful in patient carryover and compliance. Tendon glide AROM programs are particularly important after a hand burn has been sustained[6] (**Fig. 15**). Such programs need to become part of a patient's daily routine, because scars mature over 12 to 18 months after the burn. In addition, strengthening programs promote a well-rounded rehabilitation to facilitate a patient's return to previous level of function. Exercise programs should be completed at a minimum of 5 times a day. Utilization of hand exercisers and weighted therapy bars are useful tools for achieving AROM and strengthening of the upper extremity (**Fig. 16**).

Pediatric Applications

Formal ROM and strengthening programs can be difficult to implement with the pediatric burn

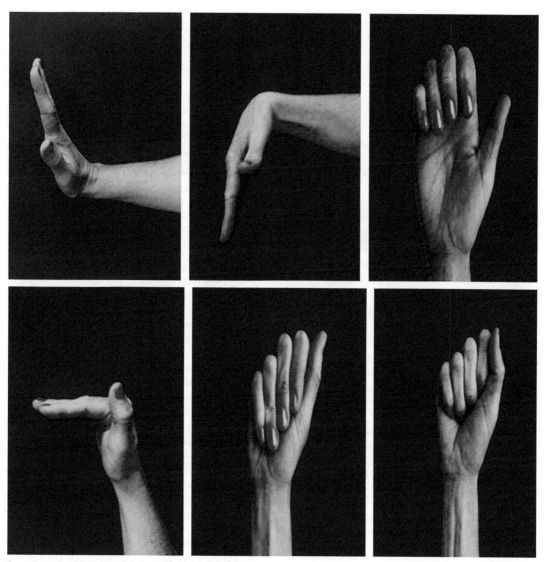

Fig. 15. Formal home programs that incorporate pictures, exercise logs, and concise instructions are helpful in patient carryover and compliance. Tendon glide AROM programs are particularly important after a hand burn has been sustained.

population. Caregivers are encouraged to incorporate AROM and stretching into age-appropriate play activities of interest to the child. Recently, use of virtual reality and video game systems has been found to be successful tools for incorporation of AROM with play, while providing a distraction from pain.[9] An alternative involves completing the stretching program while the child is sleeping, if tolerated.

Patient and Caregiver Education

Emphasis should be focused on the carryover of ROM, stretching, and strengthening home programs into daily routines. When the occupational therapist is not present, patients and family are responsible

for completion of exercise programs. Exercise checklists can allow caregivers to encourage home exercise program completion and follow through.

SCAR MANAGEMENT

After initial wound healing, the process of scar thickening and contraction begins. Scar development begins as the body replaces and reorganizes the structure of collagen fibers to the injured area. The new collagen fibers are aligned in a disorganized manner, creating the potential for raised and thickened scar tissue formation. Scar development typically begins 3 weeks after injury and continues for 12 to 18 months, and at times up to 24 months, after the initial burn injury.[6]

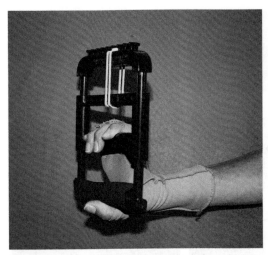

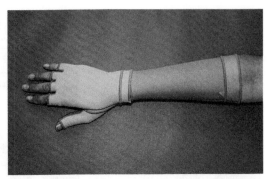

Fig. 17. Until custom compression garments can be provided for a patient, temporary compression can be achieved with use of edema gloves and elastic tubular bandages.

Fig. 16. Hand exercisers are useful tools for achieving AROM and strengthening of the digits.

Burn injuries that take longer than 2 weeks for wound healing and full-thickness burns are at an increased risk for developing hypertrophic scar tissue. Hypertrophic scars are initially characterized by a red, raised, and rigid appearance.

Scar formation can cause serious complications in the rehabilitation of an upper extremity burn. With increased scar development, there is the potential for loss of ROM, joint contracture, functional limitations, and decreased patient satisfaction in overall appearance.

Before the scar is fully matured, it is important to begin scar management strategies to positively affect scar healing. The goal is to assist the scar to become more pliable, less raised, and nonadhered to allow for optimal function:

- *Compression Garments:* when there is a risk for hypertrophic scar development, compression garments are recommended to assist with normalizing collagen fiber alignment. Patients should be measured for custom compression garments once the area is healed with no open areas larger than the size of a quarter. Compression garments for burn scar management provide 20 to 30 mm Hg of pressure and are worn 23 of 24 hours per day. The garments are typically replaced every 2 to 3 months in order to provide adequate compression for scar management.[10] Until custom compression garments can be provided for a patient, temporary compression can be achieved with use of edema gloves and elastic tubular bandages (**Fig. 17**).
  - *Inserts:* to provide appropriate compression to concave areas, such as palms, inserts fabricated from foam or an elastomer product

may be used under a compression garment. Digit web spaces at risk for developing scar tissue can be managed by molding web spacers out of foam or an elastomer product to be worn under a compression glove.[1]
- *Silicone:* silicone sheets are used to improve scar mobility and to assist in leveling rigid scar tissue. These silicone sheets may be worn under a custom or temporary compression garment. Initially, silicone is applied for several hours per day, progressing to 23 of 24 hours per day as tolerated[6] (**Fig. 18**).
- *Scar Massage:* scar massage is effective in softening scar tissue by reducing underlying tissue adhesions and desensitizing the newly healed skin.[11] Scar massage is applied only to healed areas with a lotion that is both alcohol and fragrance free. Initially, a gentle massage should be performed, progressing to a massage with moderate amount of pressure as the skin becomes more durable.[6] A typical home program consists of scar massage completed 3 to 5 times per day for approximately 10 minutes to each area.[11]

After the initiation of any scar-management intervention, it is important to evaluate treatment effectiveness. There are several scar scales available to closely monitor scar progression and development.[12]

Pediatric Applications

Scar massage instruction and hands-on practice should be provided to the patient's caregivers. Recommendations to incorporate scar massage with distracting activities such as singing, television shows, or video games can be helpful. Compression garments can be customized to incorporate specific colors, or appliqués of a

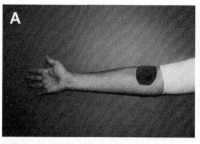
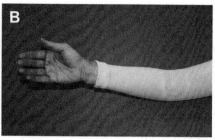

Fig. 18. (*A, B*) Silicone sheets are typically used under a custom or temporary compression garment.

favorite sports teams or character can be applied to increase compliance. Removable silicone gel sheeting should be carefully considered for patients younger than 5 years of age due to the potential concern for choking.

Patient and Caregiver Education

Patients and family members are provided with education on the potential for scar development and functional limitations associated with continued scar development. Instructions for the carryover of scar massage, compression, and silicone use for scar management are provided. For optimal functional recovery, emphasis is placed on the importance of patient and caregiver involvement in a scar management home program.

ACTIVITIES OF DAILY LIVING

Retraining for ADL is at the core of OT goals. As upper extremity ROM and strength improve, participation in ADL can further enhance a patient's recovery. Modifications such as adapted handles may be issued to maximize independence with feeding and grooming when hand ROM is limited (**Fig. 19**).[1] Engagement in ADL can promote a patient's sense of independence during the transition to previous life roles.

Postburn sun care should be taught to become a part of a patient's ADL routine. Proper education and compliance can prevent potential damage to grafted skin areas and improve long-term graft appearance. Patients are educated to apply sunscreen with a sun protection factor (SPF) of 30 or greater anytime they will be outdoors.[1] Reapplication is vital when outside for extended periods of time. Sweat-proof and waterproof lotion sunscreens that do not contain a fragrance or alcohol are recommended.

Pediatric Applications

Play and leisure-type activities are the basis for most OT treatments for pediatric patients. For infant and toddler burn patients, play is considered their ADL. Around the age of 5, they begin a greater participation in ADL, including dressing and grooming. In addition, utilization of child life specialists can assist with identifying and implementing the patient's interests in OT treatment sessions.

Adequate sun protection for children can be difficult to achieve. Appropriate reapplication of sunscreen after extended periods outdoors can be particularly challenging. Therefore, recommendations for swim shirts or clothing with an SPF protection can be an alternative.

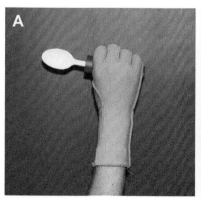
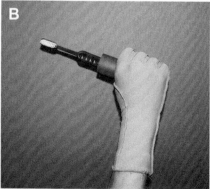

Fig. 19. (*A, B*) Adapted handles or tools may be issued for a patient to maximize independence during the healing phase or when contractures are limiting full ROM.

Patient and Caregiver Education

Often caregivers are eager to assist with the patient's ADL so they do not have to see their family member struggle. However, such assistance can lead to dependence on support and decreased opportunities for the patient to incorporate AROM into their daily routine. The occupational therapist should provide the family with instruction to allow the patient to attempt an ADL independently before initiating assistance.

Summary

Upper extremity burns can result in lifelong complications. A comprehensive OT program is imperative for the restoration of arm function. Edema management, splinting, exercise, scar management, and ADL are key treatment elements to achieve optimal postburn outcomes. Proper patient and caregiver education is essential for successful rehabilitation. Burn recovery requires the patient's commitment to the therapeutic process with the goal of achieving maximal independence. ROM, coordination, and strength show improvement with consistent participation in an OT burn rehabilitation program. Progress in these areas facilitate increased independence in ADL and improve overall quality of life.[13,14]

REFERENCES

1. Moore ML, Dewey WS, Richard RL. Rehabilitation of the burned hand. Hand Clin 2009;25(4):529–41.
2. Wilhemi BJ, Burns MC, Cooney D. Orthoses for the burned hand. In: Hsu JD, Michael J, Fisk J, editors. AAOS atlas of orthoses and assistive devices. 4th edition. Philadelphia: Mosby, Inc; 2008. p. 219–26.
3. Kraemer MD, Jones T, Deitch EA. Burn contractures: incidence, predisposing factors, and results of surgical therapy. J Burn Care Rehabil 1998;9:261–5.
4. Witte CL, Witte MH, Dumont AE. Significance of protein in edema fluid. Lymphology 1971;4:29–31.
5. Dewey WS, Hedman TL, Chapman TT, et al. The reliability and concurrent validity of the figure-of-eight method of measuring hand edema in patients with burns. J Burn Care Res 2007;28:157–62.
6. Tufaro PA, Bondoc SL. Therapist's management of the burned hand. In: Skirven TM, Osterman AL, Fedorczyk JM, et al, editors. Rehabilitation of the hand and upper extremity. 6th edition. Philadelphia: Mosby Inc; 2011. p. 317–41.
7. Daugherty MB, Carr-Collins JA. Splinting techniques for the burn patient. In: Richard RL, Staley MJ, editors. Burn care and rehabilitation principles and practice. Philadelphia: F.A. Davis; 1994. p. 242–321.
8. Richard RL, Staley MJ. Burn patient evaluation and treatment planning. In: Richard RL, Staley MJ, editors. Burn care and rehabilitation principles and practice. Philadelphia: F.A. Davis; 1994. p. 201–18.
9. Parry I, Painting L, Bagley A, et al. A pilot prospective randomized control trial comparing exercises using videogame therapy to standard physical therapy: 6 months follow-up. J Burn Care Res 2015; 36(5):534–44.
10. Sharp PA, Pan B, Yakuboff KP, et al. Development of a best evidence statement for the use of pressure therapy for management of hypertrophic scarring. J Burn Care Res 2016;37(4):255–64.
11. Serghiou MA, Ott S, Whitehead C, et al. Comprehensive rehabilitation of the burn patient. In: Herndon DN, editor. Total burn care. 4th edition. Edinburgh (Scotland): Saunders Elsevier; 2012. p. 517–49.
12. Tyack Z, Wasiak J, Spinks A, et al. A guide to choosing a burn scar rating scale for clinical or research use. Burns 2013;39:1341–50.
13. Cartotto R. The burned hand: optimizing long-term outcomes with a standardized approach to acute and subacute care. Clin Plast Surg 2005;32:515–27.
14. Tang D, Li-Tsang CW, Au RK, et al. Functional outcomes of burn patients with or without rehabilitation in mainland China. Hong Kong J Occup Ther 2015; 25:15–23.

Scar Management of the Burned Hand

Michael Sorkin, MD[a], David Cholok, BS[a], Benjamin Levi, MD[a,b],*

KEYWORDS

- Hand • Burn • Hypertrophic scar • Laser

KEY POINTS

- Early management of acute hand burns with debridement, grafting, and mobilization is critical to minimize development of hypertrophic scarring.
- Once hypertrophic scars have formed, surgical scar release can be achieved with a variety of procedures from local tissue rearrangement to free flaps to restore hand function.
- Many modalities including laser therapy have become the standard of care in the rehabilitation of hypertrophic scars and can ameliorate scar texture, thickness, color, and pruritus.

INTRODUCTION

According to the Burn Association Repository, approximately 500,000 burn victims seek medical treatment every year, with 39% of these injuries involving the upper extremity and hand as observed in previous studies.[1–3] Although the hand comprises only 3% to 5% of the body surface area, it is highly susceptible to injury, through its close proximity to the thermal source and because it is commonly used as a shield to protect other parts of the body.[4] The hand is therefore prone to absorb a high amount of energy, which may result in severe injury. Injury patterns can vary among different burn etiologies and can have significant impact on the expected severity and management. Although injuries from flame or fire are the predominant etiology during

recreational and work-related activities in adults, scald burns and contact burns account for most pediatric hand burn injuries.[5] Electrical injuries also pose a challenge in hand reconstruction, as these patients can require fasciotomies, which heal with hypertrophic scars.[6]

Acute management of hand burns should be performed at specialized burn centers that are equipped to provide a multidisciplinary team approach.

Aggressive early treatment of hand burns is critical and involves a combination of debridement, autografting, edema prophylaxis, early mobilization, splinting, and optimal hand rehabilitation.[7,8] A thorough initial assessment of the type of burn mechanism and burn depth should be accomplished to guide the need for surgical therapy. One should also be mindful that the acute burn

B. Levi Supported by funding from NIH/National Institute of General Medical Sciences Grant K08GM109105-0, Plastic Surgery Foundation, the Association for Academic Surgery Roslyn Award, American Association for the Surgery of Trauma Research & Education Foundation Scholarship, American Association of Plastic Surgery Academic Scholarship, American College of Surgeons Clowes Award, AAPS/PSF Pilot Award, International FOP Association.

[a] Section of Plastic and Reconstructive Surgery, Department of Surgery, University of Michigan, 1500 East Medical Center Drive, 2130 Taubman Center, SPC 5340, Ann Arbor, MI 48109, USA; [b] Burn/Wound and Regenerative Medicine Laboratory, Section of Plastic Surgery, Department of Surgery, University of Michigan Health System, 1500 East Medical Center Drive, 2130 Taubman Center, SPC 5340, Ann Arbor, MI 48109, USA
* Corresponding author: Burn/Wound and Regenerative Medicine Laboratory, Section of Plastic Surgery, Department of Surgery, University of Michigan Health System, Section of Plastic Surgery, 1500 E. Medical Center Dr., 2130 Taubman Center, SPC 5340, Ann Arbor, MI 48109.
E-mail address: blevi@med.umich.edu

Hand Clin 33 (2017) 305–315
http://dx.doi.org/10.1016/j.hcl.2016.12.009
0749-0712/17/© 2016 Elsevier Inc. All rights reserved.

wound is a dynamic environment and may be influenced by factors including edema, local and systemic inflammation, and bacterial contamination, which can contribute to conversion of the burn depth.[9] Although epidermal burns will likely go on to heal without scar formation, a delay in re-epithelialization of partial-thickness burns beyond 2 to 3 weeks will result in hypertrophic scarring. Deep partial thickness and full-thickness burns are therefore best treated with early excision to viable depth and skin grafting to preserve hand function.[10] In general, the palmar skin of the hand should be allowed more time to heal by secondary intention, as the properties of the glabrous skin are difficult to replace with a skin graft. Early grafting of the palm will place thin skin in an area that requires durability and can lead to severe contractures (**Fig. 1**). Although thin spilt-thickness grafts are sufficient to resurface other parts of the body, the hand is best treated with thick unmeshed autografts (0.012–0.018 inch thickness) or full-thickness grafts to prevent secondary contracture and to optimize the final appearance. In general, we use thick split-thickness grafts in the acute period and full-thickness grafts with subsequent contracture releases. Surgical management should be followed by hand splinting in anticontracture positioning, commonly intrinsic plus, and elevation followed by early range of motion when the skin graft has appropriately healed.[11]

Despite aggressive medical and surgical management in the acute phase of the burn injury, hypertrophic scar formation and contractures are complications resulting in substantial functional and aesthetic impairment. This impairment has the potential to not only limit quality of life but also impact the ability to perform a profession in which unimpaired hand function is required.[12,13] Therefore, adequate management of hand burn hypertrophic scars and contractures is paramount in the rehabilitation of the burned hand. This management will often present the surgeon with a challenging task.

This article reviews common approaches to the prevention and management of hypertrophic scars and contractures of the burned hand.

DEVELOPMENT OF HYPERTROPHIC SCARRING IN THE BURN WOUND

Several risk factors for hypertrophic scar formation have been identified and include young age, infection, skin stretch, and anatomic location (ie, axilla, neck).[14] Although superficial burn wounds tend to heal without complications, deeper partial and full-thickness burns have a significantly increased risk of resulting in hypertrophic scar formation.[1] In epidermal burns, the dermis remains entirely intact and re-epithelialization occurs from preserved keratinocytes within the superficial dermis. Similarly, superficial partial-thickness burns involve the epidermis and superficial dermis leading to blistering with complete regeneration occurring though migration of keratinocytes from preserved hair follicles and sweat glands. These superficial injuries may require careful monitoring alone. In contrast, in deep partial-thickness burns, the density of skin adnexa is significantly decreased, leading to prolonged time to re-epithelialization and

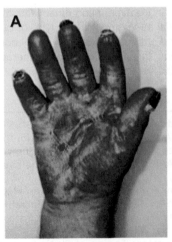 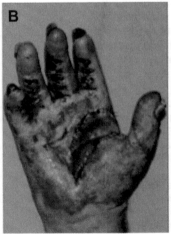 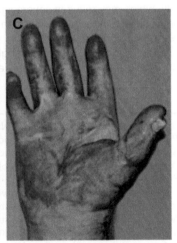

Fig. 1. A 58-year-old man with history of deep partial-thickness burns to the right hand from a natural gas explosion. (*A*) Initial presentation with scar band contractures involving the volar surfaces of the index, middle, ring, and small fingers and wide scar contracture over the ulnar border of thenar eminence. (*B*) Two weeks after z-plasty releases of digital contractures and full-thickness skin grafting from abdomen to palmar contracture. (*C*) Four months after surgery.

scarring.[10] Early assessment of burn depth is therefore critical to administer optimal treatment and prevent hypertrophic scar formation.

Normal wound healing proceeds through a complex balance of the 3 phases of inflammation, proliferation and remodeling. The principles underlying burn wound healing are unique secondary to a strong systemic immune response with increased production of proinflammatory cytokines (tumor necrosis factor-α, interleukin-1, and interleukin-6) and cell mobilization, which have a lasting impact on the local wound healing environment.[15,16] Furthermore, increased and persistent contractile forces across a large wound area trigger a cascade during which mechanical forces are translated into increased inflammation.[17] A recent study identified the focal adhesion kinase as a critical regulator of this process, which has been shown to sense mechanical forces and activate inflammatory downstream effectors that drive increased fibrosis through deposition of aberrant extracellular matrix.[18]

HYPERTROPHIC SCARRING IN THE HAND

Although measures to counteract hypertrophic scar formation in the acute phase of wound healing is critical, late complications cannot always be avoided.[19,20] The complex anatomy of the hand allows for an indispensable interaction with the environment through a balance of fine motor biomechanics and tactile sensation. Therefore, even small scar bands can result in significant functional impairment. The dorsum of the hand is especially susceptible to hypertrophic scar formation because of the thin and pliable nature of the skin in this area, which requires less thermal force to induce burn to the deeper dermal tissues and hypertrophic scarring. Dorsal scarring may not only inhibit passive flexion at the metacarpophalangeal joint but further result in hyperextension and subluxation of the joint in severe cases.[21] On the other hand, hypertrophic scar formation of the palm can ultimately result in a cupping deformity, which is characterized by convex warping of the longitudinal and horizontal palmar arches[19] (see **Fig. 1**).

Thermal injury involving opposing surfaces of border digits will often result in scar band or web formation, reducing the interdigital space and limiting abduction. Furthermore, if the first webspace is involved, thumb abduction is affected, causing adduction contractures and significantly reducing grip strength and function.

Flexion contracture of the small finger is one of the most difficult reconstructive challenges for surgeons, as this leads to contracture of the collateral ligaments, flexor tendons, and skin and results in shortening of the vessels and nerves (**Fig. 2**). Additionally, these scars can lead to significant functional and aesthetic deformities with its most severe form of burn syndactyly.[22] The best treatment for these patients is prevention. Thus, aggressive range of motion and splinting should be used in the acute period. If the flexion contracture continues to progress despite conservative

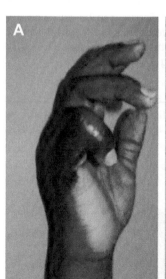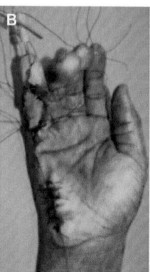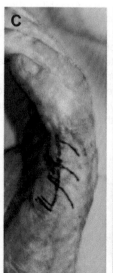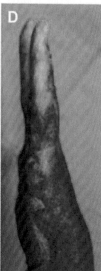

Fig. 2. A 6-year-old boy with small-finger contracture treated with hypothenar flap. (*A*) Preoperative photo of severe small-finger contracture. (*B*) Intraoperative photograph shows hypothenar flap inset and digit fixation in extension with K-wire. (*C*) Intraoperative placement of series of z-plasties along hypertrophic scar band. (*D*) One-month postoperative photograph shows good range of motion.

measures, then temporary K-wire placement should be performed to counteract the contracture forces.

Another common and stigmatic deformity of the burned hand includes the finger nail. Burn injury to the dorsum of the digit can result in retraction of the of the soft tissue proximal to the nail fold, leading to exposure of the germinal matrix and alterations in nail growth.[23]

TREATMENT OF HYPERTROPHIC SCARS
Early Scar Management

During the initial phase of thermal injury, the principles of acute management are directed toward reducing the extent of injury and minimizing or even preventing hypertrophic scar formation. Early surgical debridement and autografting when appropriate should be accomplished within the first 72 hours.[8] Debridement is performed with Goulian knife from 0.08- to 0.01-inch thickness to debride the necrotic tissue. Knowing the depth of debridement comes with experience and assessment of tissue moisture. Although pinpoint bleeding can be observed as an endpoint, the use of a tourniquet to minimize blood loss can require the surgeon to rely on tissue moisture. Grafts to the hand should be nonmeshed sheet grafts when possible and should be harvested at a thickness of 0.012 inches or thicker (**Fig. 3**). Meticulous hemostasis is needed, especially if sheet grafts are used. Dressings can be taken down after 48 to 72 hours, and any hematomas under the sheet graft can be aspirated with an 18G needle. If large area burns occur that prevent autograft coverage, debridement and homograft should be performed as a temporary coverage until autograft is available.

The initial weeks after a burn injury are characterized by consistent remodeling of the affected tissue, and several treatment modalities can be used to modulate hypertrophic scar formation in this critical period. In the early phase, the persistent presence of edema can prevent full range of motion in the finger joints and thus result in tightening of joint capsules and shortening of collateral ligaments leading to contractures. Hand elevation and elastic edema wraps can be used to promote absorption of the edema fluid. Furthermore, early range-of-motion exercises in a patient who is able to participate once surgically appropriate are imperative to prevent stiffening.[24] During the phase of operative recovery and in the unconscious patient, splinting of the hand in an antideformity position during which the ligamentous structures are taut is critical to counteract the forces of wound bed contraction. For the hand, this can be commonly accomplished with the intrinsic plus position, which is characterized by wrist extension, metacarpophalangeal joint flexion, and proximal interphalangeal/distal interphalangeal (DIP) joint flexion and thumb abduction.[25,26] Two to 3 weeks after the operative phase, scar massage can be initiated, which has been found to decrease pruritus and hypersensitivity associated with hypertrophic scarring in some studies,[27] although a lasting effect on the scar height is controversial. Although the scar continues to mature, pressure therapy can be an effective therapeutic adjunct in reducing hypertrophic scar formation. Although high-level evidence in the literature has been lacking, a recent meta-analysis concluded that pressure garments can result in a small decrease of hypertrophic scar height.[28] We typically begin compression therapy 4 weeks after grafting or once dressing changes are no longer necessary. In the recovering burn, hand pressure on the palm, dorsum and fingers can be achieved with custom-made gloves. Furthermore, special inserts are often used in the interdigital space to reduce webspace scarring.

Injectables

Intralesional injections of anti-inflammatory and antimitotic agents have been widely used to treat

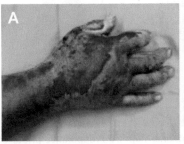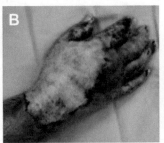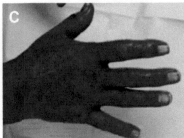

Fig. 3. Early debridement and sheet grafting to dorsal hand. (*A*) Preoperative photograph of burn injury. (*B*) Intraoperative placement of unmeshed thick STSG. (*C*) Two-month postoperative photograph shows good range of motion.

and prevent the formation of hypertrophic scarring. Intralesional corticosteroids, most commonly triamcinolone, are a prominent therapy for hypertrophic scars and have been effective in improving pigmentation and texture of formed scars.[29] Treatment regimens, including dose, frequency, and duration of triamcinolone injections are variable and range from 10 to 40 mg/mL every 2 to 4 weeks for a series of treatments until clinical improvement of the scar is observed. As a standalone treatment, triamcinolone injection has shown a response rate in 50% to 100% of patients; however, initial success is tempered by high rates of recurrence and side effects including hypopigmentation (more common in Fitzpatrick type III and higher), ulceration, and itching at the site of administration.[30] As such, intralesional corticosteroid injections are often used in conjunction with other treatment modalities including surgery and laser treatment to synergistically improve outcomes. Additionally, the surgeon must not inject too much corticosteroid at a single treatment (especially in children) to avoid adrenal insufficiency. Other injectable modalities include antineoplastic agents, such as 5-fluorouracil (5-FU) and bleomycin, and antibiotics such as mitomycin C and have been used to similar effect.[31] Similar to triamcinolone, these antimitotic agents have been found to reduce angiogenesis and diminish the proliferation of fibroblasts in the wound bed. 5-FU is a pyrimidine analogue antimetabolite and was initially found to reduce the proliferation of fibroblasts in culture.[32] Clinically, the drug has been used most often in combination with corticosteroids and other treatment modalities including pulsed-dye-laser therapy. Combination therapy shows significant resolution of hypertrophic scarring, and treatment with 5-FU mitigates the adverse effects induced by steroid injection alone.

Fat Grafting

Autologous fat grafting entails the harvest, enrichment, and injection of adipose tissue to improve scar resolution, fill contour deformity, and improve wound healing. The use of fat grafting has gained increasing favor in secondary burn reconstruction and has been used in multiple settings including relief of breast capsular contraction and treatment of postradiation skin changes to improve overlying skin quality.[33,34] The frequency of treatment required to achieve an optimal response remains uncertain, and many of the studies conducted to assess the utility of lipofilling remain limited by small sample sizes and subjective metrics. Nevertheless, several reports indicate improved scar outcomes after fat grafting. In hand reconstruction, Byrne

and colleagues[35] showed significant improvement of active motion, regression of scar tissue, and self-reported satisfaction of surgical outcome in patients who underwent a single fat grafting procedure. Fat grafting in burn regions can be challenging, as there is a constricted tissue envelope to allow for injection of the fat into multiple layers. Resolution of scar tissue after fat grafting remains incompletely understood, but the responsible mechanisms most likely include a multitude of biochemical and mechanical factors. Further studies are needed to validate the proposed mechanisms of improvement. Proponents claim that lipofilling replaces subdermal tissue, releasing the debilitating intrinsic and extrinsic tension caused by scar tissue. Caution not to inject excess adipose tissue must be taken to avoid a distorted appearance.

Laser Therapy

Recent advances in laser technology have paved the way for new techniques in hypertrophic scar management.[16,36] Besides functional disability, hypertrophic burn scars can result in significant discomfort because of the restrictive nature of the scar, erythematous discoloration, pruritus, pain, and abnormal appearance. Over the last decade, different modalities of laser therapy have become a versatile and integral part of scar management. Using selective photothermolysis and fractional ablation to target hypertrophic scar tissue provides a novel method to modulate the composition of the scar and may even result in reduction of scar restriction and contracture release.[37] Overall, laser therapy is associated with a low complication risk profile.[38] Laser therapy is usually initiated around 6 to 12 months.

Although the precise biologic mechanism accounting for the effect of scar improvement with laser treatment is a subject of ongoing investigation, its clinical effectiveness has been established in several clinical studies. A recently conducted prospective cohort study examining the effects of the pulse dye laser (PDL) and ablative carbon dioxide laser treatment on hypertrophic burn scars found significant improvement in scar texture, coloration, pain, and pruritus, whereas other clinical reports have successfully used laser therapy in the treatment of contractures in the adult and pediatric hand burn population.[39]

Pulse Dye Laser

The PDL has been found to be particularly effective in the treatment of erythematous and pruritic scars, although some reports suggest an additional positive effect on scar pliability and height.

PDL has a wavelength of 585 or 595 nm and has been widely used in the treatment of vascular malformations. The PDL laser demonstrates selective photothermolysis of microvessels within the hypertrophic scar and reduction of the inflammatory response. Thus, PDL is especially helpful in erythematous scars. Its use in nonerythematous scars, however, is minimal; therefore, its use in Fitzpatrick type V and higher is limited. The side-effect profile is limited and can include transient erythema and changes in pigmentation; therefore, it can be used cautiously in patients with darker skin tone. Serial treatments, which are commonly spaced 2 to 3 months apart, are often required to achieve a stable result (**Fig. 4**). Settings vary based on different systems; however, we usually begin treatment with a spot size of 7 mm and a fluence of 12 J/cm^2. If no blistering is seen, we often increase the fluence at the second treatment, whereas if blistering occurs, fluence will be decreased.

Fractional Carbon Dioxide Laser

The fractional carbon dioxide (CO_2) laser is particularly useful in the treatment of raised hypertrophic scars and uneven scars as commonly seen after meshed skin graft. Several reports also indicate substantial improvement with other associated symptoms including pruritus, erythema, and pain.[40] Mechanistically, because of its high wave length of 10,600 nm, the CO_2 laser targets water, which is stored in all layers of the skin, but specifically in collagen of the dermis. Although the exact mechanistic principles are yet to be established, the fractional CO_2 laser generates columns of microperforations that penetrate into the dermis and disrupt the disorganized collagen bundles of the hypertrophic scar and break up the disorganized collagen structure initially established after the burn. Each individual wound is separated from the next with a treatment density of less

than 10% of the skin. This generates an immediate mechanical release of tension in some restrictive scars and allows for adjacent, noninjured tissue to restore the ablated tissue.

Furthermore, this treatment breaks down the disorganized collagen organization and allows the microscopic wound to heal in a much more controlled low-inflammation state (several months after the inflammation from the burn injury). Histologic analysis found remodeling of the extracellular matrix with significant decrease in type I collagen and an increase in type III collagen with the dermal architecture closer resembling normal uninjured skin.[41] Similar to the PDL laser, fractional CO_2 photothermolysis requires multiple sessions to achieve a final result.

This treatment can be combined with corticosteroids, and laser-assisted triamcinolone delivery has recently been reported to be effective in the treatment of hypertrophic scars (**Fig. 5**). Settings again differ based on laser systems. We feel that deeper scar penetration with high energy (up to 150 mJ) is beneficial for thick burn scars. When using deep penetration settings, however, it is crucial to use a low density to avoid new thermal injuries. We typically use a density of 3% when using high energy (100–150 mJ). For less thick scars or when trying to improve the appearance of meshed grafts, we use lower settings, usually around 30 mJ, and increase the density to 5% to 10%. Additionally, for surface irregularities such as those used from previously meshed grafts, we use a superficial CO_2 handpiece or computerized pattern generator. With this laser, we use an energy of 80 to 100 mJ and 75 to 200 Hz. This handpiece, however, can cause hypopigmentation, so caution must be used in patients with Fitzpatrick type III or greater. If treating a scar that is thick and red, we only use the deep laser and superficial PDL (see **Fig. 5**). We do not use the PDL at the same time as the computerized pattern generator to avoid superficial skin injury.

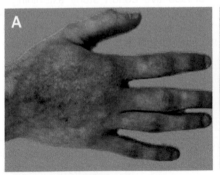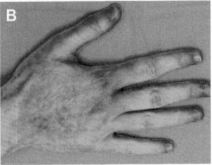

Fig. 4. A 23-year-old woman with history of right hand burn resulting in erythematous dorsal hand scar. (*A*) Initial appearance before treatment. (*B*) After 1 session of PDL treatment.

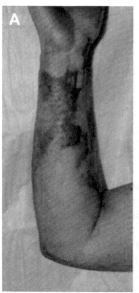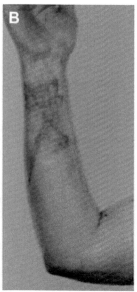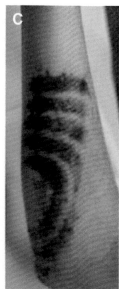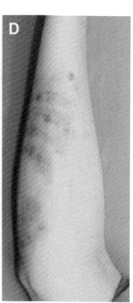

Fig. 5. A 43-year-old woman with history of deep partial-thickness grease burns to the right volar wrist resulting in a hypertrophic and erythematous scar. (*A*) Preoperative presentation before treatment. (*B*) After 2 sessions of fractional CO_2 laser photothermolysis with combined triamcinolone injection. (*C*) A 22-year-old woman after debridement and grafting of stove burn with thick, red, hypertrophic scars. (*C*) Preoperative presentation. (*D*) After 2 sessions of fractional CO_2 photothermolysis combined with PDL and triamcinolone injection.

Alexandrite Laser

This laser can be used for laser hair ablation. This laser is particularly useful in patients who had full-thickness grafts from hair-bearing regions grafted to regions in which hair is not desired (palm, face). When this arises, this laser modality can be used to ablate the hair by targeting the melanin in the hair follicles. Like PDL and CO_2, several treatments may be necessary to achieve an optimal result. Care must be taken not to use energy that is too high to avoid thermal injury. Additionally, this laser has improved efficacy in patients with dark hair and light skin (Fitzpatrick type I–II).

Operative Management

Scar management in the acute phase of the thermal injury and during initial scar maturation can significantly ameliorate hypertrophic scar formation and prevent sequelae leading to scar banding. However, after noninvasive treatment options are exhausted, operative techniques need to be considered for the treatment of persistent hand scars that cause functional or aesthetic impairment. Timing of the operative procedure should be carefully chosen, allowing enough time for complete scar maturation, as premature intervention can result in increased inflammation and additional scarring. We usually begin reconstructive procedures starting 6 months after injury. Although

a comprehensive review of operative techniques involved in burn hand reconstruction is beyond the scope of this report, several well-established techniques critical for scar management are discussed below.

Local skin flaps are commonly used to correct mild and moderate hypertrophic scar contractures thus avoiding the need for more complex procedures.[42] Simple linear scar bands, which can often occur across joints, are best addressed with a scar-lengthening z-plasty. The classic design of a z-plasty is oriented with its central limb along the hypertrophic scar band and with the lateral limbs at a 60° angle. Making the corner 90° before extending the z-plasty to 60° helps improve perfusion to the tip of the z-plasty[43] (**Fig. 6**). The flaps can safely be raised in scar tissue if maintained thick and incorporating underlying adipose tissue thus achieving active lengthening of 75%. Adjustments of the angle to 90° result in increased lengthening of 125%, however, involves larger limbs and thus increased sacrifice of adjacent width. This approach can be modified by including a series of smaller z-plasties along a scar thus effectively achieving similar lengthening but avoiding donor site morbidity with larger flaps (**Fig. 7**). We tend to use smaller flaps over the digits and palm, whereas we use larger flaps for axillary contractures.

Webspace contractures are commonly addressed with modifications of z-plasties, and a

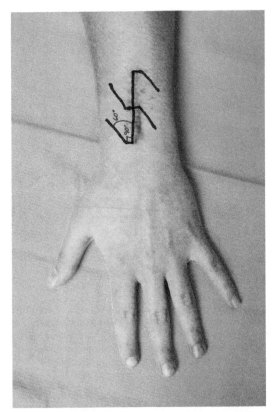

Fig. 6. Z-plasty design. Making the corner 90° before extending the z-plasty to 60° helps improve perfusion to the tip of the z-plasty.

variety of local flaps have been devised.[44,45] The 5-flap z-plasty is frequently used and is effective in creating a concavity and lengthening within the webspace because of its geometric design (**Fig. 8**). The Y to V region of this flap should be placed in the region of desired deepening. Other options include V-Y advancement flaps, which use the supple dorsal tissue that is advanced

into the webspace. These flaps can be further combined with forms of z-plasties.[46]

Axillary scar contractures are the second most common contractures behind neck contractures and are difficult to improve. Small linear bands can be released with z-plasties (see **Fig. 8**). Larger more restrictive contractures can be treated with release and thick split-thickness skin graft (STSG) or full-thickness skin graft (FTSG). Others describe treatment of severe contractures with pedicled flaps or with regional and free tissue transfer.[47]

Palmar burn scars commonly involve a large surface and can therefore result in tight contractures. Mild forms can be addressed with a sequence of z-plasties (see **Fig. 7**). If the contracture is severe, release of the scar may be required leaving a large defect. This defect can be filled with a full-thickness skin graft if no crucial structures are exposed.[48] Full-thickness skin grafts are preferred over split-thickness graft because of the decreased effect of secondary contraction to minimize scarring (see **Fig. 3**). If the contracture release leads to exposed tendon or bone, local or distant flaps may be required.[49] The extensor tendons dorsally often benefit from a fascia-only reverse radial forearm flap with a skin graft for coverage or a reverse dorsal interosseous flap. Alternatives include free fascia only or fasciocutaneous flaps, although bulky flaps should be avoided if possible.[50]

A common consequence of dorsal hand burns is contracture of the eponychial fold. This contracture is caused by excess tension across the dorsal digit, which often restricts DIP flexion. To address the contracture and eponychial fold deformity, we use a technique of release and full-thickness graft proximal to the DIP. This technique involves a distally based bipedicled flap, which is designed to release the proximal nail fold contracture. This is accompanied by an extensive release of the

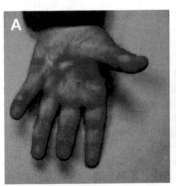
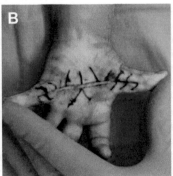
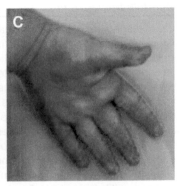

Fig. 7. A 4-year-old boy with history of left hand palm burn from a stove resulting in hypertrophic scar band extending from thumb, midpalm, and to small finger. (*A*) Preoperative presentation. (*B*) Intraoperative design of z-plasty releases. (*C*) Six-month follow-up after scar release.

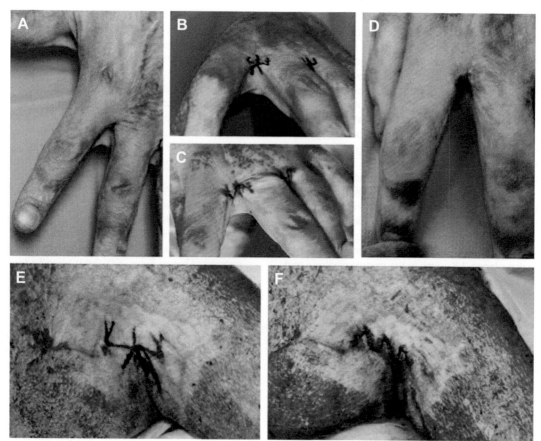

Fig. 8. Webspace contracture addressed with 5-flap jumping man z-plasty. (*A*) Preoperative webbing between index and middle fingers. (*B*) Intraoperative marking of 5-flap jumping man z-plasty. (*C*) Intraoperative release and rearrangement. (*D*) One-month postoperative appearance. (*E*) A 65-year-old man with deep partial-thickness burns to trunk and upper arms with resulting axillary scar contracture. Design of jumping man 5-flap z-plasty. (*F*) Immediate appearance after z-plasty transposition.

dorsal soft tissues and resurfacing of the resulting defect with a full-thickness skin graft. Restoration of normal anatomy can thus be achieved and results in normalized nail growth[23] (**Fig. 9**).

Another common and difficult reconstructive challenge as discussed above is small-finger scar contracture. For these patients, preoperative radiograph and analysis of the level of contracture of the

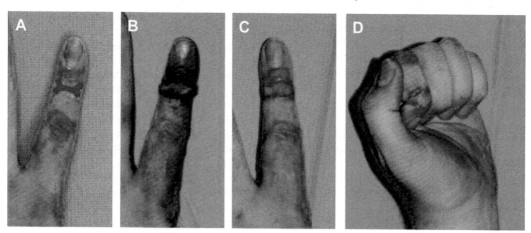

Fig. 9. A 25-year-old man with left index finger nail bed deformity from flame burn injury. (*A*) Presentation before treatment. (*B*) Two weeks after nail bed release and full-thickness skin grafting. (*C*) Six-week postoperative follow-up with improved DIP flexion. (*D*) Postoperative range of motion of the DIP joint.

joint is crucial to a successful outcome. If severe joint contracture is present or the patient has a boutonnière deformity from previous debridement or injury to the extensor tendon, the condition will not be improved by an operation addressing the skin contracture alone. The surgeon should also avoid the urge to straighten the small finger in one operation, as this often leads to venous congestion or ischemia caused by the shortening of the vessels from the contracture. If the skin is the only area causing the contracture then a z-plasty or series of z-plasties can be used. In more severe contractures, a release and full-thickness hypothenar flap can be used (see **Fig. 2**). Finally, in those cases of joint and skin contracture, a Joint Jack can be used for slow distraction and stretching of the contracture. This device places 2 K-wires in the middle phalanx and has a series of bands that connect to the wrist slowly stretching the contracture.[51]

SUMMARY

Hypertrophic scarring after burn injury of the hand can result in detrimental functional deficits and impaired appearance. Although early management of the acute burn injury is critical to minimize the sequelae of scar formation, hypertrophic scarring cannot always be avoided. A variety of noninvasive and invasive therapeutic modalities are available to the reconstructive hand surgeon to treat and modulate a formed scar with the goal to restore hand function. Local tissue rearrangement techniques form a central pillar to address deforming scar tissue, whereas adjunct therapies including laser treatment, and injectables have shown excellent results in scar rehabilitation.

ACKNOWLEDGMENTS

Collaborate with Boehringer Ingleheim on project not discussed here. We have filed a patent application for the new use of Rapamycin in heterotopic ossification. IP has not yet been licensed.

REFERENCES

1. McKee DM. Acute management of burn injuries to the hand and upper extremity. J Hand Surg Am 2010;35(9):1542–4.
2. Ng D, Anastakis D, Douglas LG, et al. Work-related burns: a 6-year retrospective study. Burns 1991; 17(2):151–4.
3. Sheridan RL, Hurley J, Smith MA, et al. The acutely burned hand: management and outcome based on a ten-year experience with 1047 acute hand burns. J Trauma 1995;38(3):406–11.
4. Richards WT, Vergara E, Dalaly DG, et al. Acute surgical management of hand burns. J Hand Surg Am 2014;39(10):2075–85.e2.
5. McCauley RL. Reconstruction of the pediatric burned hand. Hand Clin 2009;25(4):543–50.
6. Arnoldo BD, Purdue GF. The diagnosis and management of electrical injuries. Hand Clin 2009; 25(4):469–79.
7. Pan BS, Vu AT, Yakuboff KP. Management of the acutely burned hand. J Hand Surg Am 2015;40(7): 1477–84 [quiz: 1485].
8. Mohammadi AA, Bakhshaeekia AR, Marzban S, et al. Early excision and skin grafting versus delayed skin grafting in deep hand burns (a randomised clinical controlled trial). Burns 2011;37(1):36–41.
9. Ong YS, Samuel M, Song C. Meta-analysis of early excision of burns. Burns 2006;32(2):145–50.
10. Monstrey S, Hoeksema H, Verbelen J, et al. Assessment of burn depth and burn wound healing potential. Burns 2008;34(6):761–9.
11. Dewey WS, Richard RL, Parry IS. Positioning, splinting, and contracture management. Phys Med Rehabil Clin N Am 2011;22(2):229–47, v.
12. Fufa DT, Chuang SS, Yang JY. Postburn contractures of the hand. J Hand Surg Am 2014;39(9): 1869–76.
13. Hegge T, Henderson M, Amalfi A, et al. Scar contractures of the hand. Clin Plast Surg 2011;38(4):591–606.
14. Butzelaar L, Ulrich MM, Mink van der Molen AB, et al. Currently known risk factors for hypertrophic skin scarring: A review. J Plast Reconstr Aesthet Surg 2016;69(2):163–9.
15. Kwan P, Hori K, Ding J, et al. Scar and contracture: biological principles. Hand Clin 2009;25(4):511–28.
16. Tredget EE, Levi B, Donelan MB. Biology and principles of scar management and burn reconstruction. Surg Clin North Am 2014;94(4):793–815.
17. Wong VW, Paterno J, Sorkin M, et al. Mechanical force prolongs acute inflammation via T-cell-dependent pathways during scar formation. FASEB J 2011;25(12):4498–510.
18. Wong VW, Rustad KC, Akaishi S, et al. Focal adhesion kinase links mechanical force to skin fibrosis via inflammatory signaling. Nat Med 2012;18(1):148–52.
19. Cartotto R, Cicuto BJ, Kiwanuka HN, et al. Common postburn deformities and their management. Surg Clin North Am 2014;94(4):817–37.
20. Kreymerman PA, Andres LA, Lucas HD, et al. Reconstruction of the burned hand. Plast Reconstr Surg 2011;127(2):752–9.
21. Graham TJ, Stern PJ, True MS. Classification and treatment of postburn metacarpophalangeal joint extension contractures in children. J Hand Surg Am 1990;15(3):450–6.
22. Grishkevich VM. Flexion contractures of fingers: contracture elimination with trapeze-flap plasty. Burns 2011;37(1):126–33.

23. Donelan MB, Garcia JA. Nailfold reconstruction for correction of burn fingernail deformity. Plast Reconstr Surg 2006;117(7):2303–8 [discussion: 2309].

24. Moore ML, Dewey WS, Richard RL. Rehabilitation of the burned hand. Hand Clin 2009;25(4):529–41.

25. Rrecaj S, Hysenaj H, Martinaj M, et al. Outcome of physical therapy and splinting in hand burns injury. Our last four years' experience. Mater Sociomed 2015;27(6):380–2.

26. Schouten HJ, Nieuwenhuis MK, van Zuijlen PP. A review on static splinting therapy to prevent burn scar contracture: do clinical and experimental data warrant its clinical application? Burns 2012;38(1):19–25.

27. Richard R, Baryza MJ, Carr JA, et al. Burn rehabilitation and research: proceedings of a consensus summit. J Burn Care Res 2009;30(4):543–73.

28. Anzarut A, Olson J, Singh P, et al. The effectiveness of pressure garment therapy for the prevention of abnormal scarring after burn injury: a meta-analysis. J Plast Reconstr Aesthet Surg 2009;62(1):77–84.

29. Maguire HC Jr. Treatment of keloids with triamcinolone acetonide injected Intralesionally. JAMA 1965; 192:325–6.

30. Tang YW. Intra- and postoperative steroid injections for keloids and hypertrophic scars. Br J Plast Surg 1992;45(5):371–3.

31. Wang XQ, Liu YK, Qing C, et al. A review of the effectiveness of antimitotic drug injections for hypertrophic scars and keloids. Ann Plast Surg 2009; 63(6):688–92.

32. Jemec B, Linge C, Grobbelaar AO, et al. The effect of 5-fluorouracil on Dupuytren fibroblast proliferation and differentiation. Chir Main 2000;19(1):15–22.

33. Klinger M, Caviggioli F, Klinger FM, et al. Autologous fat graft in scar treatment. J Craniofac Surg 2013; 24(5):1610–5.

34. Brongo S, Nicoletti GF, La Padula S, et al. Use of lipofilling for the treatment of severe burn outcomes. Plast Reconstr Surg 2012;130(2):374e–6e.

35. Byrne M, O'Donnell M, Fitzgerald L, et al. Early experience with fat grafting as an adjunct for secondary burn reconstruction in the hand: Technique, hand function assessment and aesthetic outcomes. Burns 2016;42(2):356–65.

36. Hultman CS, Friedstat JS, Edkins RE, et al. Laser resurfacing and remodeling of hypertrophic burn scars: the results of a large, prospective, before-after cohort study, with long-term follow-up. Ann Surg 2014;260(3):519–29 [discussion: 529–32].

37. Taudorf EH, Danielsen PL, Paulsen IF, et al. Non-ablative fractional laser provides long-term improvement of mature burn scars–a randomized controlled trial with histological assessment. Lasers Surg Med 2015;47(2):141–7.

38. Clayton JL, Edkins R, Cairns BA, et al. Incidence and management of adverse events after the use of laser therapies for the treatment of hypertrophic burn scars. Ann Plast Surg 2013;70(5):500–5.

39. Krakowski AC, Goldenberg A, Eichenfield LF, et al. Ablative fractional laser resurfacing helps treat restrictive pediatric scar contractures. Pediatrics 2014;134(6):e1700–5.

40. Levi B, Ibrahim A, Mathews K, et al. The Use of CO2 Fractional Photothermolysis for the Treatment of Burn Scars. J Burn Care Res 2016; 37(2):106–14.

41. Ozog DM, Liu A, Chaffins ML, et al. Evaluation of clinical results, histological architecture, and collagen expression following treatment of mature burn scars with a fractional carbon dioxide laser. JAMA Dermatol 2013;149(1):50–7.

42. Hop MJ, Langenberg LC, Hiddingh J, et al. Reconstructive surgery after burns: a 10-year follow-up study. Burns 2014;40(8):1544–51.

43. Rohrich RJ, Zbar RI. A simplified algorithm for the use of Z-plasty. Plast Reconstr Surg 1999;103(5): 1513–7 [quiz: 1518].

44. Sari E, Tellioglu AT, Altuntas N, et al. Combination of rhomboid flap and double Z-plasty technique for reconstruction of palmar and dorsal web space burn contractures. Burns 2015;41(2):408–12.

45. Grishkevich VM. First web space post-burn contracture types: contracture elimination methods. Burns 2011;37(2):338–47.

46. Peker F, Celebiler O. Y-V advancement with Z-plasty: an effective combined model for the release of post-burn flexion contractures of the fingers. Burns 2003; 29(5):479–82.

47. Ogawa R, Hyakusoku H, Murakami M, et al. Reconstruction of axillary scar contractures–retrospective study of 124 cases over 25 years. Br J Plast Surg 2003;56(2):100–5.

48. Yotsuyanagi T, Yamashita K, Gonda A, et al. Double combined Z-plasty for wide-scar contracture release. J Plast Reconstr Aesthet Surg 2013;66(5): 629–33.

49. Karanas YL, Buntic RF. Microsurgical reconstruction of the burned hand. Hand Clin 2009;25(4): 551–6.

50. Jones NF, Jarrahy R, Kaufman MR. Pedicled and free radial forearm flaps for reconstruction of the elbow, wrist, and hand. Plast Reconstr Surg 2008; 121(3):887–98.

51. Houshian S, Gynning B, Schroder HA. Chronic flexion contracture of proximal interphalangeal joint treated with the compass hinge external fixator. A consecutive series of 27 cases. J Hand Surg Br 2002;27(4):356–8.

Postburn Contractures of the Hand

Matthew Brown, MD*, Kevin C. Chung, MD, MS

KEYWORDS

- Postburn • Contracture • Hand • Finger • Flexion • Claw • Boutonniere

KEY POINTS

- Burn contractures present as a spectrum of deformities that significantly limit hand function.
- Appropriate care during the acute burn phase can help limit the incidence or severity of postburn contracture.
- Surgical release with graft or flap coverage is the primary treatment modality.
- Postoperative splinting, hand therapy, and scar care are vital to a successful outcome.

INTRODUCTION

Burns are among the most common causes of hand contractures. Failure to seek timely medical attention, inadequate treatment, and healing by secondary intention are common causes of burn contractures. Postburn deformities of the hand are functionally limiting and serve as constant visual stigma to the patient and will occur at a certain rate regardless of the initial treatment method. Sheridan and colleagues[1] reported their experience with 698 hand burns in children. Children treated with dressing changes during the initial burn went on to develop contractures that required operative correction in 4.4% of cases. Of patients requiring grafting during their initial burn care, 32% developed contractures requiring subsequent surgery. The severity of a burn contracture depends on several factors: the location of the burn, the depth of the burn, the timing of surgical or nonsurgical treatment, postinjury splinting, hand therapy and scar care during the maturation process.[2] McCauley[3,4] provided a severity rating for burn contractures of the hand, grading them I to IV (**Table 1**). Grade 1 and 2 contractures can typically be managed with therapy. Grade III and IV contractures are subcategorized as flexion, extension, or mixed deformities. More severe contractures require more complex reconstruction; however, even good functional outcomes have been achieved in grade IV contractures.[4]

Care of these deformities is more appropriately termed postburn hand reconstruction rather than treatment of burn scar contracture. In addition to release of the contracted skin and coverage of the soft-tissue defect, the surgeon must address the secondary changes to the musculotendinous unit, ligaments, and joints.[5,6] The appropriate procedures must be selected to provide a patient with the best functional outcome. For example, arthrodesis of a finger proximal interphalangeal (PIP) joint may provide a better functional outcome than complex soft tissue repair of a boutonniere deformity for some patients because of the unpredictable outcomes in boutonniere deformity, especially in the setting of postburn scar contracture,

M. Brown has no commercial or financial conflicts of interest or any funding sources to disclose. K. Chung has no commercial or financial conflicts of interest and is funded in part by Midcareer Investigator Award (2K24 AR053120-06). The content is solely the responsibility of the authors and does not necessarily represent the official views of the National Institutes of Health.
Division of Plastic Surgery, Department of Surgery, University of Michigan, 2130 Taubman Center, 1500 East Medical Center Drive, Ann Arbor, MI 48109-0340, USA
* Corresponding author.
E-mail address: matbro@med.umich.edu

Hand Clin 33 (2017) 317–331
http://dx.doi.org/10.1016/j.hcl.2016.12.005
0749-0712/17/© 2016 Elsevier Inc. All rights reserved.

hand.theclinics.com

Table 1
Severity ratings for burn contractures of the hand

Grade	Description
I	Reports symptomatic tightness, no visible changes
II	Mild decrease in range of motion
III	Functional deficit with mild changes to hand architecture
IV	Severe functional deficit with dramatic changes to hand architecture

Adapted from McCauley RL. Reconstruction of the pediatric burned hand. Hand Clin 2009;25(4):545; with permission.

which often overpowers soft tissue reconstructions. In severely burned hands, creating stable key pinch or tripod grasp may provide the functional improvement necessary for performance of daily activities. Finally, postoperative hand therapy must be tailored to the individual contracture and surgery. For example, patients with joint release need earlier mobilization in comparison with those undergoing skin contracture release and grafting. Surgical treatment presents unique challenges but functional improvement and patient satisfaction remain high after these operations.

CONDITIONS AND PRESENTATION OF BURN CONTRACTURES IN THE HAND

The acute treatment of a burn depends on the depth of the injury. Surgery is indicated for deep or full-thickness burns that are not expected to heal within 3 weeks. Healing potential cannot always be determined at the time of injury and often requires serial assessment. Early excision and grafting is the mainstay of surgical treatment.[1,7] If the surgeon believes the burn will progress or if the burn is too large cover

the hands immediately, allograft can be used for temporary coverage. Burns with deep dermal or full-thickness injury that are left to heal by secondary intention have fibroblast deposition and scar formation resulting in contracture. The distinct anatomic differences between the dorsal and volar skin also change the outcome after burn injury. The thinner more pliable dorsal skin is more easily destroyed by contracture and the relatively superficial extensor tendons are at increased risk of exposure or injury. Burns of the thicker glabrous skin of the palm and volar fingers are less commonly full-thickness dermal injuries. The palmar fascia and fibrous septae provide additional layers that protect flexor tendons and digital neurovascular bundles. Deep palmar burns take more than 3 weeks to epithelize but still have comparatively mild scarring and contracture.[8,9] Soft tissue reconstruction either with skin grafting or flaps are commonly done for dorsal hand burns but are not commonly performed for palmar burns that often can heal completely.

Untreated or severe burns of the hand result in a characteristic appearance of wrist extension, metacarpophalangeal (MCP) joint hyperextension, and interphalangeal (IP) joint flexion commonly referred to as the burn claw deformity (**Fig. 1**A, B). This is primarily a result of direct thermal injury to the dorsal skin and extensor apparatus but is potentiated by immobility, edema, and joint distension. In a patient with a large surface area burn, aggressive fluid management is initiated to fight against evaporative losses and maintain intravascular volume. Burn injuries result in third spacing with severe edema of extracellular spaces of the body. Edema and swelling of the joints encourage extension at the MCP because more joint space exists in this position versus flexion. The collateral ligaments of the MCP are lax in extension but with prolonged periods of extension they will shorten, which prevents passive MCP flexion. Extension at the MCP increases the relative flexion forces at the IP joints, leading to a

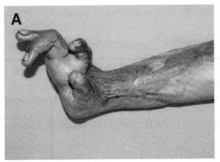
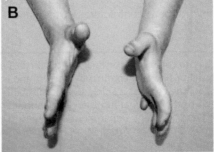

Fig. 1. Burn claw deformity. (*A*) Severe burn claw deformity with wrist and MCP extension and PIP flexion. (*B*) Mild claw deformity with MCP hypertension and slight PIP flexion.

flexion deformity and intrinsic minus positioning. Additionally, the wrist is extended from dorsal skin contracture and the thumb is often flexed at the IP and adducted toward the palm. Preoperative and postoperative splinting and aggressive hand therapy is aimed to combat these forces by maintaining ligament length and joint mobility.[10]

In children, volar contact burns are more common because children usually injure themselves while grasping something hot. In a study of 953 pediatric burns, Brown and colleagues[11] found that contact burns of the palm and volar fingers were most frequent injuries to the hand. Burned or grafted skin does not expand and grow with the same plasticity as normal skin. It is not uncommon for a child who is initially asymptomatic to develop a function-limiting contracture over time. Furthermore, a child with an early age burn injury may require multiple procedures over their lifetime. Prolonged skin contracture can also cause deformities to developing bones and joints, leading to a more complicated surgical correction. In a study of 61 children with burn contractures, Gupta and colleagues[2] demonstrated that patients with more than 10 years of neglect of a burn contracture had worse outcomes than those with 5 to 10 years of neglect. Although postburn reconstruction is not a surgical emergency, timely intervention is beneficial and essential.

PREVENTION OF CONTRACTURE

The ideal outcome after burn injury is to avoid contracture. Following skin grafting, the burned extremity and hand are elevated and splinted to prevent ligament and joint contracture. The wrist is placed in 30° of extension, the MPs are flexed to 90°, the IP joints fully extended, and the thumb is maximally abducted. Buchan[12] reported his experience with thermoplastic splints as early as 1975. Although no objective outcome data were reported, they advocated early treatment of patients for the prevention of contracture. Most physicians use splinting at the earliest possible stage in hand burns.[13–15] It is imperative that patients are kept to a strict regimen of splinting and therapy. Delayed or missed splinting periods will increase the likelihood of contractures developing. Also, a bulky wound dressing may make the thermoplast splints less effective and maintenance of joint position is better secured with Kirschner (K) wires. The K-wires are at risk of infection but if good pin care is maintained these can mean the difference between functional and nonfunctional outcomes. Early supervised range of motion is started immediately in nonoperative cases and within 1 to 2 weeks of operative cases. Once the epithelium is healed,

silicone sheeting and compression garments are worn for 23 hours a day for the first 6 months. Despite these preventative measures, burn contracture may still develop, which is explained to patient and family when highlighting the importance of therapy and close follow-up.

PREOPERATIVE EVALUATION, TIMING, AND PRINCIPLES

Preoperative evaluation helps determine what structures may be involved in the contracture and if surgical intervention is safe to proceed. Patients with isolated burns to the hand and minor health problems can be treated electively with minimal concern. A patient recovering from a burn with total body surface area involvement greater than 20% may have additional medical issues, including a compromised immune system, acute renal or hepatic injury, and depleted nutrition. For these patients, a thorough medical work-up should be completed before operative intervention. Patients with compromised immune systems or poor kidney function may be at increased anesthetic risk. Patients with poor nutrition have a lower capacity to heal additional skin graft or flap procedures. Loss of grafts after contracture release may lead to recurrence or worsening of the contracture.

Physical examination helps isolate involved structures in a burn contracture. The skin is examined for the texture and laxity. Skin that has healed secondarily or with skin grafts does not have the same viscoelastic properties as normal skin. Local or adjacent tissue transfer is only an option if the surrounding skin or scar tissue is of reasonable quality. Areas of prior skin graft are less reliable because the associated blood supply is compromised and aggressive elevation or rotation of these areas may result in flap necrosis. The involvement of the tendons and joints in the contracture is determined next. The resting posture, active motion, and passive motion of each joint are assessed. Distal joints are tested with off-loading at the proximal joint. For example, an extension contracture of the MCP joint should be evaluated with the wrist extended and flexed. Wrist extension helps offload the restricting forces that contracted extrinsic extensor tendons or dorsal skin may have on MCP flexion. Inability to flex the MCP with wrist extended indicates possible MCP joint involvement. The same principle can be used to evaluate a volar burn contracture. With the MCP in neutral, the patient may be unable to fully extend the PIP of the finger because of volar skin contracture (**Fig. 2**). With the MCP flexed, the patient illustrates complete PIP

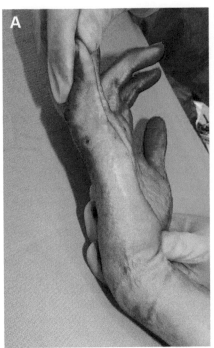
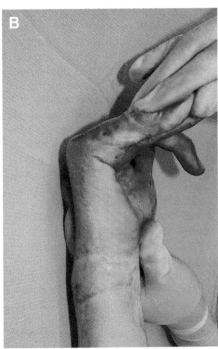

Fig. 2. Physical examination of flexion contracture. (*A*) With MCP in extension, the PIP joint cannot be fully extended. (*B*) With MCP in flexion, PIP is able to be fully extended, illustrating that contracture does not involve the PIP joint capsule.

extension, which indicates that there is no direct PIP joint contracture. These maneuvers may aid in determining tendon or joint involvement but sometimes it is still not clear until operative release. The surgeon should be prepared to release skin, scar, and muscle, lengthen tendons, release joints, and provide the appropriate soft tissue coverage.

Patients with a burn contracture can present from months to years after their injury. Patients with thickened scars a few months after injury with minimal change in their range of motion are more appropriately treated with compression garments, splinting, and scar massage. These interventions may eliminate the need for surgery or lessen the degree of the deformity requiring correction. If a significant limitation in range of motion exists, then an earlier operative intervention may be more appropriate to prevent long-term joint contracture or changes to the developing bones of a child. Scar contracture release is usually delayed until 6 to 12 months after injury to allow for scar maturity.

Adjacent tissue transfer is a powerful method to address linear scar contractures and web spaces. There are several common flap designs and techniques that the hand surgeon should be familiar with, including the standard z-plasty, 4-flap plasty,[16] and the jumping man 5-flap plasty[17]

(**Fig. 3**). These flaps use the same principle of rotating skin lateral to the scar to increase length. Increasing the angle of the flap or increasing the number of flaps (where the angles are additive), increases the gain in length (**Table 2**).

This article highlights specific strategies to address burn contractures of the wrist and hand but contracture of the elbow or shoulder often accompanies these burns. In most instances the shoulder and elbow are addressed before the wrist and hand. If a hand cannot be appropriately positioned in space, then any type of hand reconstruction is unlikely to improve a patient's quality of life. Additionally, reconstruction of a hand that is flexed at the elbow and adducted at the shoulder is inherently more difficult to position in the operating room.

FLEXION CONTRACTURES

Flexion contractures of the palm and fingers are usually the result of direct injury to the volar skin from contact burns and most often occur in children. Linear contractures can create a volar web of skin that attaches from the midpalm to the distal finger causing flexion deformities of both the PIP and MCP joints (**Fig. 4**). Stern and colleagues[18] classified flexion deformities of the PIP joint based on correction of the deformity with MCP flexion

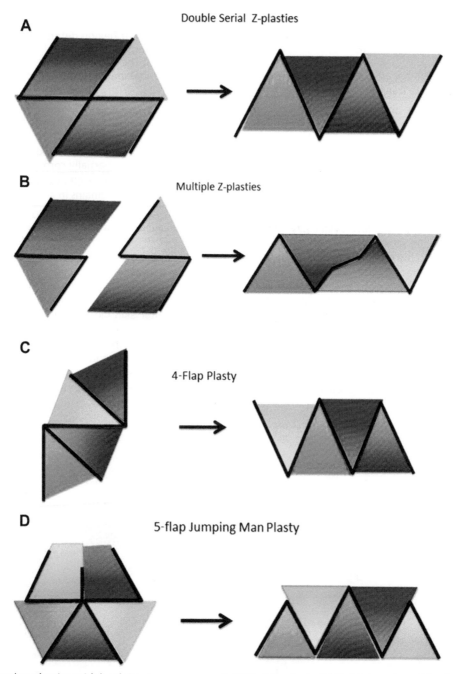

Fig. 3. Scar lengthening with local tissue rearrangement. (*A*) Serial z-plasty. (*B*) Multiple z-plasty. (*C*) 4-flap plasty. (*D*) 5-flap plasty.

(**Table 3**). Local tissue rearrangement using z-plasties is usually sufficient in most cases with a linear scar band (**Fig. 5**). A longitudinal midline incision is made down to the level of the tendon sheath and full-thickness flaps are raised. The oblique cuts of the z-plasties are then incised to release the contracted skin and underlying scar. Scissors are used to gently release any scar around the neurovascular bundles. If the skin contracture is significant, the flaps are rotated by prioritizing coverage of exposed joint or tendon, and skin grafting is used to fill in remaining defects (**Fig. 6**). PIP contractures of the joint with volar burns are uncommon except in the most severe or delayed cases. PIP contracture also present in the setting of a dorsal burn and associated

Table 2
Flap designs and techniques that can be rotated to increase length

Adjacent Tissue Transfer	Estimated Increase in Length (%)
Z-plasty with 60° angles	75
4-Flap plasty or 90° z-plasty	100
Jumping man 5-flap plasty	125

Table 3
Classifications of flexion deformities of the proximal interphalangeal joint based on correction of the deformity with metacarpophalangeal flexion

Class	Physical Examination Finding
Type I	With MCP flexed the PIP fully extends
Type II	With MCP flexed the PIP only partially corrects
Type III	With MCP flexed the PIP remains in a fixed deformity

Data from Stern PJ, Neale HW, Graham TJ, et al. Classification and treatment of postburn proximal interphalangeal joint flexion contractures in children. J Hand Surg Am 1987;12(3):450–7.

boutonniere deformity (see later discussion). If joint contracture exists with a volar injury, the volar plate is released after raising the skin flaps. The lateral aspect of the A-3 pulley is incised, the flexor tendons are retracted, and curvilinear incision is made along the volar plate separating it from the accessory collateral ligaments. The volar plate is elevated with a freer and the joint is released until the finger is fully extended. Care is taken to ensure the neurovascular bundles are not placed on excessive traction and the vascularity of the finger is inspected before leaving the operating room. If the finger is pale with full extension, the amount of extension can be relaxed to see if the finger

becomes pink. If the finger is still pale, the arteries must be explored under the microscope and repaired. After skin closure, the hand is splinted in extension and therapy is initiated after 1 week. Stern[18] reported that 88% of surgically treated flexion contractures had less than 20° of residual contracture. They found that older patients and those with more severe contractures had poorer outcomes.

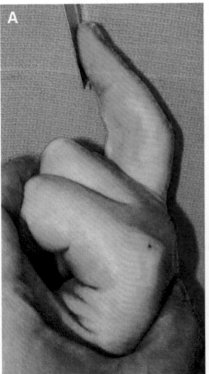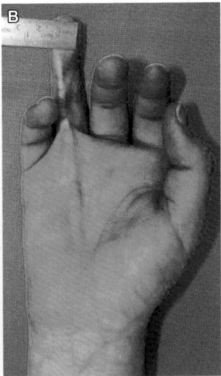

Fig. 4. Volar flexion contraction. (*A*) Side view of finger illustrating volar web of skin. (*B*) Volar view of hand illustrating linear scar contracture from distal phalanx to the midpalm.

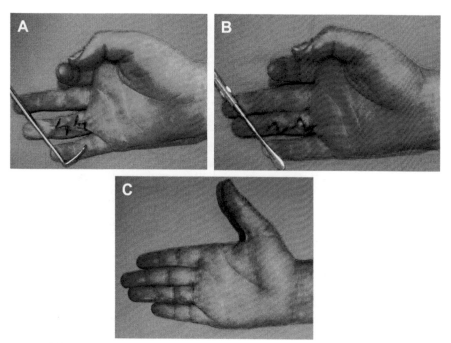

Fig. 5. Treatment of flexion contracture with multiple z-plasties. (*A*) Preoperative marking. (*B*) Incision at end of surgery. (*C*) Final function result showing complete extension.

THUMB

Burn contractures of the thumb can severely limit function because of inability to open the hand for grasping larger objects. Thumb contractures were formally classified by Stern and colleagues[19] into 4 groups: adduction, opposition, extension, and flexion contractures. Adduction contractures draw the thumb metacarpal toward the index metacarpal in the plane of the palm. Opposition contractures cause pronation and rotation of the thumb metacarpal anterior to the plane of the palm. Extension contractures cause the thumb metacarpal to be radially abducted in the plane of the palm. Flexion contractures have a contracture band running parallel to the metacarpal

producing a flexion deformity of the MP and IP joint. Stern and colleagues[19] reported the distribution of these contractures to be 66% adduction, 24% opposition, 5% extension, and 5% flexion.

Similar to finger flexion contractures, local tissue rearrangement, and skin grafting are the mainstay of treatment of thumb contractures. In unilateral injuries, measurement of the maximal abduction of the opposite thumb may be helpful in determining the functional deficit. For opposition contractures, a tight band is usually felt over the palmar skin of the thumb and a z-plasty is designed appropriately to release it (**Fig. 7**). With adduction contractures, the flap design is made along the edge of the web space skin (**Fig. 8**). The rotation of the flaps will increase the skin available for thumb abduction and

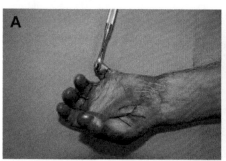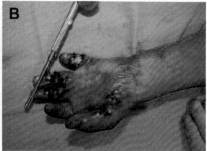

Fig. 6. Treatment of flexion contractures with z-plasty and skin grafts. (*A*) Surgical flap design. (*B*) Incisions and grafts at the end of surgery.

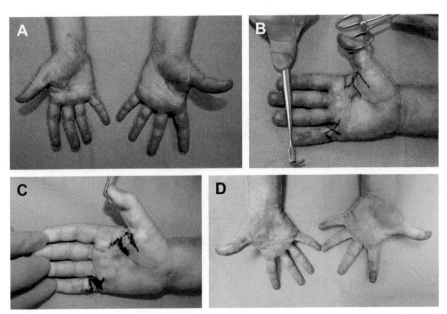

Fig. 7. Treatment of palmar thumb contracture. (*A*) Preoperative photo showing restriction of thumb abduction and extension. (*B*) Intraoperative flap markings. (*C*) Postsurgical closure. (*D*) Final surgical result illustrating symmetric thumb abduction.

simultaneously deepen the web space. After flap elevation, the apices of the flaps cuts are released based on the ability to advance the tips of the rotated flaps. This assessment is critical to maximizing the use of the flap skin and gaining additional web space. A 5-flap jumping man can also be used placing the V-Y over the region of the web space that you want to deepen. In cases with extremely poor skin quality, the thumb is released with an incision perpendicular to the line of contracture and the resulting defect is covered with a graft or regional flap.[20] It is rare and not advantageous to excise skin. Deeper burns may require release of the palmar fascia or the adductor aponeurosis. Fraulin and Thompson[21] looked specifically at 4-flap versus 5-flap plasties using a pig model designed to replicate the first web space. They concluded that 4-flap plasty

was more effective in deepening the web space than the 5-flap plasty. Grishkevich[22] reported his experience with over 500 first web space contractures, classifying them as edge, medial, or total web space contractures. He advocated his trapeze flap of opposing trapezoid flaps that are advanced and transposed as an effective method of reconstruction. Regardless of the method of reconstruction, postoperatively, patients are splinted in maximal thumb abduction and are transitioned to a removable splint once therapy is started.

BOUTONNIERE DEFORMITY

A boutonniere deformity can form in conjunction with the burned claw hand or separately as a result of distal burns of the dorsal fingers. The primary

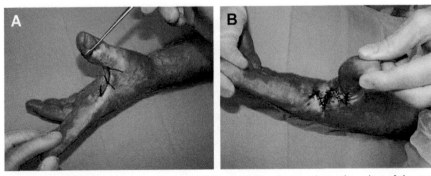

Fig. 8. Treatment of thumb adduction contracture. (*A*) Surgical flap design along the edge of the web space. (*B*) Closure after serial z-plasty.

mechanism is denaturation of the central slip from direct thermal injury or secondary desiccation from prolonged exposure. The central slip has been postulated to undergo further ischemic changes when it is isolated between overlying eschar and the head of the proximal phalanx.[23] Loss of the central extensor attachment leads to volar translocation of the lateral bands. The function of the lateral bands changes from extension of the PIP joint to flexion as they pass palmar to the central axis of the PIP joint. Reconstruction of this deformity is extremely challenging and the prevention with PIP extension splinting is imperative. Early stable wound coverage of the exposed areas avoids delayed rupture of the central slip. Therapy can be initiated with isolation of 1 joint at time during flexion exercises. Composite flexion of all joints simultaneously places maximal tension on an attenuated extensor attachment. Development of an early boutonniere deformity is treated with splinting and soft tissue coverage of any exposed tendon or joint.

Long-standing burn boutonniere deformities have 3 treatment options:

1. Reconstruction
2. Arthrodesis of the PIP joint
3. Amputation of the finger.

Any patient with signs of joint destruction and poor skin quality is better treated with either amputation or arthrodesis. Reconstruction should be attempted in highly motivated patients, with reasonable dorsal skin and no articular damage to the PIP joint. The first step in reconstruction is to release pathologic structures to correct the deformity. To release the lateral bands from their volar malposition, the distal volar attachments to the oblique and transverse retinacular ligaments are incised.[24,25] If the finger still cannot be passively extended, the volar plate is released as described previously under flexion contractures. After passive correction, if a there is enough substance to the central slip, it is mobilized, advanced, and reattached to the middle phalanx. Practically, a postburn injury rarely has any central slip to advance. Other options for reconstruction include centralizing the lateral bands to each other, or dividing 1 lateral band proximally and attaching it to the central extensor tendon and opposite lateral band, although there is concern that these procedures limit the excursion.[24,25] Tendon graft reconstructive procedures of the central slip have also been described.[24–29] A tendon graft is attached the middle phalanx with sutures or a drill hole. The tendon is then wrapped around the lateral bands to prevent their volar migration and then secured to central extensor

tendon dorsally. A tenotomy of the terminal tendon, proximal to the attachment of the oblique retinacular ligament is performed to correct the distal interphalangeal (DIP) hyperextension deformity. The finger PIP and DIP joint are pinned in 0° of extension for 3 to 4 weeks. Unfortunately, a purely soft tissue reconstruction for the treatment of chronic postburn boutonniere deformities will most likely fail because the deforming forces that led to the original contracture will likely overcome the soft tissue reconstruction over time. Additionally, the vessels of the fingers have often contracted and large changes in finger extension can lead to congestion or ischemia. Groenevelt and Schoorl reported a series of 54 long-standing boutonniere deformities, 26 of which were treated with arthrodesis and 4 that were amputated.[24] The remaining 24 were reconstructed and the investigators rated their outcomes on improvement active range of motion. Active range of motion was improved greater than 60° in 1 subject, 30° to 60° in 5 subjects, 15° to 30° in 15 subjects, and less than 15° in 2 subjects. Based on these results, the investigators advocated fusion in a more functional position as the procedure of choice over reconstruction. Rico and colleagues[25] reported their experience in 22 fingers of 12 subjects, all of which had previous skin grafting to the dorsal fingers. They rated 32% of their results as excellent with total active motion (TAM) greater than 70° and 36% as good, indicated by TAM between 50 to 70°. The investigators reported that the poorest outcomes occurred in the small finger, which has been corroborated by other investigators. Reconstruction of a burn boutonniere is possible; however, patients are advised of the possible outcomes and the possibility of need for salvage arthrodesis.

BURN SYNDACTYLY

In a normal hand, the skin between the fingers is rectangular in shape and slopes 45° in a distal palmar direction from the metacarpal head to the midproximal phalanx.[30] A burn of the web space can alter the anatomy by contracting the web space transversely, lengthening the distance of the web space skin attachment, and changing the normal slope of the skin. The main concern of patients with burn syndactyly is limited finger abduction.

Interdigital burn deformities were categorized into 3 types by Gulgonen and Ozer[31] (**Table 4**). Based on these categorizations, the investigators advocated deformity-specific release and, in most cases, reconstruction with a skin graft. For dorsal contractures, a rectangular flap based on

Table 4
Categories of interdigital burn deformities

Category	Web Slope (N = 45°)	Palm to Finger-Length Ratio (N = 5/4)	Additional Complications
Dorsal web contraction	Increased	Normal	Can lead to MCP hyperextension
Palmar web contraction	Decreased	Increased	Associated with various MCP, PIP, or DIP contractures
Interdigital Contraction	Increased	Increased	Can result in almost complete fusion

Modified from Gulgonen A, Ozer K. The correction of postburn contractures of the second through fourth web spaces. J Hand Surg Am 2007;32(4):557; with permission.

the side of the finger was designed with the width of the flap determining the width of the web space and the length of the flap determining the slope (**Fig. 9**). For palmar web contraction, the correct location of the palmar web space was established by comparing the ratio of the length of the palm to the middle finger, which may be helpful in a hand completely distorted after burn.

Surgical correction releases any abnormal interdigital connection and moves new skin to the web space with either flaps or grafts. Local tissue flaps can work extremely well for lengthening the web space. The authors prefer 4-flap or 5-flap plasty options (**Fig. 10**). The 5-flap jumping man plasty uses a combination of multiple z-plasties with a central Y to V advancement. It is important not to draw the flaps too small or the angles too acute, which may limit the flap base and vascular supply.

The central stem of the Y can be back cut further if the skin is supple enough to further advance the central V-flap. The underlying scar, which may be near the bifurcation of common digital artery, is released with scissors after flap elevation. When the interdigital contracture or webbing extends more than 75% of the proximal phalanx, it may be more prudent to design a dorsal flap for resurfacing of the web space with skin grafting to the sides of the fingers, as would be done for congenital syndactyly.[30] Postoperatively, finger abduction exercises and massage to the web space helps maintain the added length.

METACARPOPHALANGEAL JOINT CONTRACTURES

MCP joint extension contracture results from deep burns to the dorsum of the hand. Contractures of the MCP joint in children were classified by Graham and colleagues[32] (**Table 5**). Surgical correction starts with release of the contracted skin proximal to MP joint. If this fails to correct the deformity, the joint capsules and collateral ligaments are released. The capsulotomy is performed with a dorsal approach. The sagittal bands are partially incised to mobilize the overlying extensor tendon. After elevating the extensor tendon, the dorsal capsule is then transversely released and the dorsal aspect of the collateral ligaments is partially released from the distal metacarpal. If there is a long-term contracture, the volar plate is mobilized off the metacarpal head with a Freer elevator or knife. The proximal phalanx is then reduced and flexed. For patients with dorsally subluxated proximal phalanges, the MCP joints are temporarily fixated in position with K-wires for 10 days. Improvement was reported as 95% successful of type I fingers, 73% of type II fingers, and 47% of type III fingers, with the ring and small fingers representing 68% of the failures.[32]

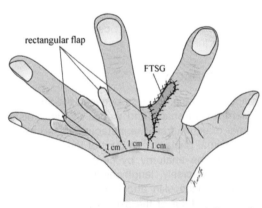

Fig. 9. Drawing of flap from the lateral finger for filling the web space after release of dorsal web space contracture. The most proximal aspect of the web space for insetting the flap is 1 cm distal to the metacarpal head. The width of the flap determines the width of the web space and the length will determine the slope of the web space. The donor site is treated with a full-thickness skin graft (FTSG). (*Courtesy of* N. Fujihara, MD, Ann Arbor, MI.)

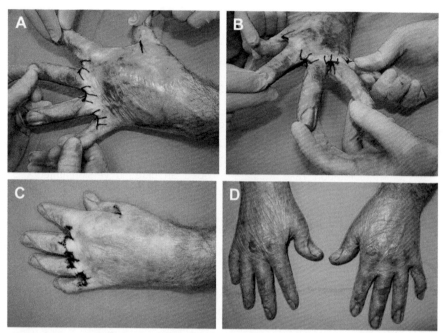

Fig. 10. Treatment of burn syndactyly. (*A*) Dorsal view of jumping man 5-flap plasty. (*B*) Axial view of 5-flap plasty. (*C*) Closure after surgical release and flap rearrangement. (*D*) 3-month postoperative result.

WRIST CONTRACTURES

Wrist contractures are usually dorsal or volar and rarely circumferential. As with many burns cases, preoperative assessment may not delineate the depth of involvement of the contracture, which could involve the skin, tendons, or wrist capsule. The burn scar or contracted skin is released with a z-plasty or transverse incision. After skin release, passive wrist movement is assessed (**Fig. 11**). For a dorsal contracture, the wrist extensors, including the extensor carpi radialis longus, extensor carpi radialis brevis, and extensor carpi ulnaris, are individually palpated for tightness. If the tendons are tight, a step-cut lengthening is performed. If the wrist is still held in extension, the extensor tendons are mobilized between the third and fourth extensor compartments. Through this exposure, the dorsal capsule is incised transversely over any areas of tension. A complete dorsal capsulotomy is rarely necessary.

Flexion contractures are approached similarly with release of the skin, appropriate tendon lengthening, and a limited capsulotomy. After release of the wrist, finger extension is tested. If the fingers can be fully extended with the wrist flexed but not with the wrist in neutral, then fractional lengthening of finger flexors tendons at the musculotendinous junction may be appropriate. If the fingers cannot be passively moved with the wrist flexed, then the MCP and PIP joint are addressed as previously described.

Coverage of wrist defects has more options than the fingers or the hand. If there is an underlying vascular tissue bed with no exposed tendon or nerve, full-thickness or split-thickness skin grafting is favored. Perforator flaps of the ulnar or radial artery are readily available in the forearm and usually reach the wrist without tension. Additional flaps

Table 5		
Classifications of contractures of the metacarpophalangeal joint in children		
Class	**Physical Examination Finding**	**Pathology**
Type I	MCP flexes past 30° with wrist maximally extended	Usually limited to skin
Type II	Cannot flex MCP past 30° with wrist extended	Contracture of the MCP joint that will require release
Type III	Fixed deformity despite wrist position	Often boney or articular change

From Graham TJ, Stern PJ, True MS. Classification and treatment of postburn metacarpophalangeal joint extension contractures in children. J Hand Surg Am 1990;15(3): 450–6; with permission.

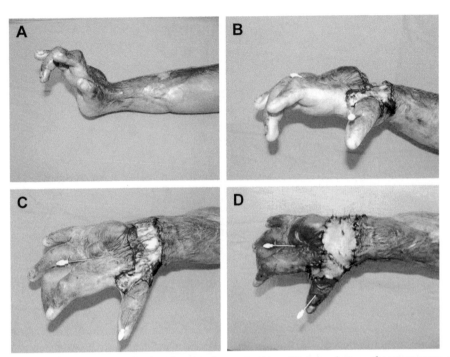

Fig. 11. Wrist contracture. (*A*) Preoperative dorsal wrist contracture. (*B*) Lateral view after transverse release of scar contracture. (*C*) Dorsal view illustrating defect created by contracture release. A K-wire was used to maintain the wrist in neutral position. (*D*) Closure of defect with full-thickness skin graft.

include the distally based posterior interosseous flap (PIA) flap, dorsal ulnar artery flap, or reverse radial artery forearm flap.

BURN CLAW HAND DEFORMITY

These injuries represent some of the most challenging problems to correct after development and represent a culmination of the previously discussed contractures. Surgery is aimed at correcting the deformity to place the wrist and fingers in a more useful position so the patient can perform rudimentary grasp. In most cases of a burn claw hand, there is MCP joint contracture or subluxation in addition to a skin deficit. The skin is released first with transverse incision and the wrist and metacarpal joints are addressed as previously presented. In cases of severely hypertrophic scar, the scarred tissue is removed (**Fig. 12**). Coverage of the soft tissue defect may be suitable with skin grafting but if there are small areas of tendon exposure or joint then a dermal substitute is used. For significant exposure of tendon, nerve, or bone, regional or free tissue transfer is performed. Davami and Pourkhameneh[33] reported their experience with 53 burn claw deformities. They reported 6 cases of superficial necrosis and 5 cases of K-wire migration but in the end all patients had stable correction of the deformity. Their choice of flap was a groin flap that required

subsequent division and inset. Any K-wires that are placed are removed after 10 to 14 days and therapy is begun. A full composite grasp or finger flexion is not always realistic for these patients but a functional key and tripod pinch can is a primary priority (**Fig. 13**).

POSTOPERATIVE CARE

The treatment of burn scar contracture does not stop at the end of the operation. Early mobilization is critical to an optimal outcome. In cases of joint subluxation or instability, K-wire fixation for 10 days is used to ensure congruity of the joint. Patients with joint release and no instability start therapy within the first week of the operation. Patients with skin graft are seen back in clinic at 1 week for removal of dressings. Those with good take of the graft will then begin therapy. In combination with therapy, most patients are splinted at night and during periods of rest. Nonadherence to splinting, especially those with skin grafting, has been attributed to recurrence of contracture.[34] Incisional wounds or areas of skin graft loss are treated with local wound care. Prophylactic antibiotics are not routinely prescribed during the postoperative period. After sutures are removed and grafts have healed, patients begin aggressive scar massage, which they are asked to maintain for at least 1 year postoperatively. Patients are followed

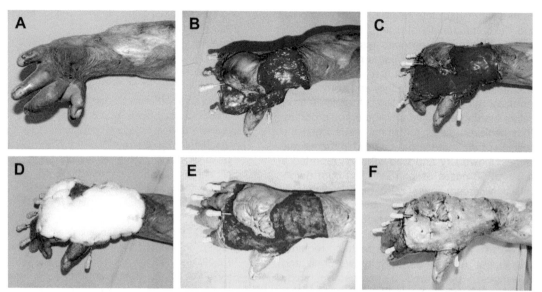

Fig. 12. Burn claw deformity. (*A*) Preoperative view of deformity. (*B*) Dorsal view after wrist and MCP joint release with pinning of reduced joint. (*C*) Placement of dermal substitute over defect. (*D*) Placement of bolster to secure dermal substitute. (*E*) Revascularization of dermal substitute. (*F*) Placement of split-thickness skin graft.

annually for recurrence, especially during years of active growth.

OUTCOMES

Most the literature surrounding burn contracture is reported as the retrospective experience of surgeons demonstrating their techniques, functional outcomes, and complications. Guven and colleagues[35] reported their experience with 38 patients with burn contractures of the hand. One patient with a PIA flap had partial necrosis; 63 of 71 phalangeal contractures achieved full motion. In 8 cases, recurrence was seen and

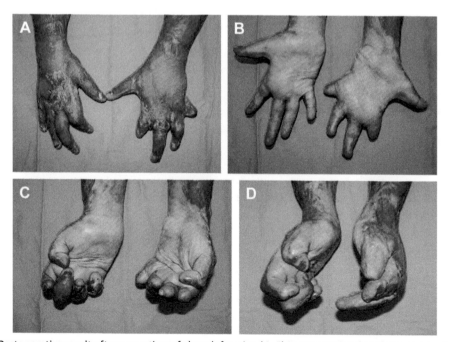

Fig. 13. Postoperative result after correction of claw deformity. (*A, B*) Postoperative dorsal view and palmar view of the hands in extension. (*C, D*) Postoperative view with active flexion and thumb pinch.

treated with volar plate release, flexor tenotomy, and flexor tendon lengthening. Saleh and colleagues[36] reported described results in 40 subjects with a variety of postburn contractures, including dorsal, volar, and first web space contractures, as well as syndactyly and complex deformities. Subjects were splinted for 8 to 10 days before starting an active physiotherapy program. They achieved better functional result when the position of the metacarpal was within the normal range. Chowdhury and Chowdhury[34] reported a series of 50 cases of long-standing burn deformities. Nineteen cases were treated with skin grafting and 31 were treated with local or regional flaps. They found that contractures treated at an earlier date from injury had better functional recovery. Three children treated required subsequent release as they grew. Sunil and colleagues[37] performed a prospective study following 50 subjects treated for burn contracture deformities of the hand. They reported good outcomes (TAM >75% of normal) in 66% of their cases. They experienced the greatest amount of contracture recurrence in subjects treated with split-thickness skin grafting. In summary, the literature indicates that release of burn scar contracture is a useful procedure with minor complications, including wound healing and flap loss, which may require secondary surgery in a low percentage of cases.

SUMMARY

Postburn contractures can present in with a variety of deformities, and surgery remains the standard for treatment of grade III and grade IV contractures. Simple or linear burn contractures can be treated to restore near normal function. Reconstruction of boutonniere deformities and claw hand remains a challenging problem although surgery can still offer marked improvement in hand function. A variety of surgical techniques exist with investigators demonstrating and reporting their specific techniques with variable success. Long-term prospective studies with patient-reported measures might provide better guidance on the ideal surgical interventions.

REFERENCES

1. Sheridan RL, Hurley J, Smith MA, et al. The acutely burned hand: management and outcome based on a ten-year experience with 1047 acute hand burns. J Trauma 1995;38(3):406–11.
2. Gupta RK, Jindal N, Kamboj K. Neglected post burns contracture of hand in children: analysis of contributory socio-cultural factors and the impact of neglect on outcome. J Clin Orthop Trauma 2014;5(4):215–20.
3. McCauley RL. Reconstruction of the pediatric burned hand. Hand Clin 2009;25(4):543–50.
4. McCauley RL. Reconstruction of the pediatric burned hand. Hand Clin 2000;16(2):249–59.
5. Bhattacharya V, Purwar S, Joshi D, et al. Electrophysiological and histological changes in extrinsic muscles proximal to post burn contractures of hand. Burns 2011;37(4):692–7.
6. Saraiya H. Is 20 years of immobilization, not sufficient to render metacarpophalangeal joints completely useless?–Correction of a 20-year old post-burn palmar contracture: a case report. Burns 2001;27(2):192–5.
7. Mahler D, Hirshowitz B. Tangential excision and grafting for burns of the hand. Br J Plast Surg 1975;28(3):189–92.
8. Baryza MJ, Hinson M, Conway J, et al. Five-year experience with burns from glass fireplace doors in the pediatric population. J Burn Care Res 2013;34(6):607–11.
9. Scott JR, Costa BA, Gibran NS, et al. Pediatric palm contact burns: a ten-year review. J Burn Care Res 2008;29(4):614–8.
10. Bhattacharya S. Avoiding unfavorable results in postburn contracture hand. Indian J Plast Surg 2013;46(2):434–44.
11. Brown M, Coffee T, Adenuga P, et al. Outcomes of outpatient management of pediatric burns. J Burn Care Res 2014;35(5):388–94.
12. Buchan NG. Experience with thermoplastic splints in the post-burn hand. Br J Plast Surg 1975;28(3):8193–7.
13. Saleh Y, El-Shazly M, Adly S, et al. Different surgical reconstruction modalities of the post-burn mutilated hand based on a prospective review of a cohort of patients. Ann Burns Fire Disasters 2008;21(3):141–9.
14. Woo SH, Seul JH. Optimizing the correction of severe postburn hand deformities by using aggressive contracture releases and fasciocutaneous free-tissue transfers. Plast Reconstr Surg 2001;107(1):1–8.
15. Fufa DT, Chuang SS, Yang JY. Prevention and surgical management of postburn contractures of the hand. Curr Rev Musculoskelet Med 2014;7(1):53–9.
16. Woolf RM, Broadbent TR. The four-flap Z-plasty. Plast Reconstr Surg 1972;49(1):48–51.
17. Peker F, Celebiler O. Y-V advancement with Z-plasty: an effective combined model for the release of postburn flexion contractures of the fingers. Burns 2003;29(5):479–82.
18. Stern PJ, Neale HW, Graham TJ, et al. Classification and treatment of postburn proximal interphalangeal joint flexion contractures in children. J Hand Surg Am 1987;12(3):450–7.

19. Stern PJ, Neale HW, Carter W, et al. Classification and management of burned thumb contractures in children. Burns Incl Therm Inj 1985;11(3):168–74.

20. Moody L, Galvez MG, Chang J. Reconstruction of first web space contractures. J Hand Surg Am 2015;40(9):1892–5 [quiz: 1896].

21. Fraulin FO, Thomson HG. First webspace deepening: comparing the four-flap and five-flap Z-plasty. Which gives the most gain? Plast Reconstr Surg 1999;104(1):120–8.

22. Grishkevich VM. First web space post-burn contracture types: contracture elimination methods. Burns 2011;37(2):338–47.

23. Maisels DO. The middle slip or boutonniere deformity in burned hands. Br J Plast Surg 1965;18: 117–29.

24. Groenevelt F, Schoorl R. Reconstructive surgery of the post-burn boutonniere deformity. J Hand Surg Br 1986;11(1):23–30.

25. Rico AA, Holguin PH, Vecilla LR, et al. Tendon reconstruction for postburn boutonniere deformity. J Hand Surg Am 1992;17(5):862–7.

26. Fowler SB. The management of tendon injuries. J Bone Joint Surg Am 1959;41-A(4):579–80.

27. Nichols HM. Repair of extensor-tendon insertions in the fingers. J Bone Joint Surg Am 1951;33-A(4): 836–41.

28. Grishkevich VM. Surgical treatment of postburn boutonniere deformity. Plast Reconstr Surg 1996; 97(1):126–32.

29. Groenevelt F. Some aspects of the burned little finger. Br J Plast Surg 1986;39(2):225–8.

30. Krizek TJ, Robson MC, Flagg SV. Management of burn syndactyly. J Trauma 1974;14(7):587–93.

31. Gulgonen A, Ozer K. The correction of postburn contractures of the second through fourth web spaces. J Hand Surg Am 2007;32(4):556–64.

32. Graham TJ, Stern PJ, True MS. Classification and treatment of postburn metacarpophalangeal joint extension contractures in children. J Hand Surg Am 1990;15(3):450–6.

33. Davami B, Pourkhameneh G. Correction of severe postburn claw hand. Tech Hand Up Extrem Surg 2011;15(4):260–4.

34. Chowdhury SR, Chowdhury AK. Management of long standing post burn deformities of hand. J Indian Med Assoc 1989;87(11):251–3.

35. Guven E, Ugurlu AM, Hocaoglu E, et al. Treatment of post-burn upper extremity, neck and facial contractures: report of 77 cases. Ulus Travma Acil Cerrahi Derg 2010;16(5):401–6.

36. Saleh Y, El-Shazly M, Adly S, et al. Different surgical reconstruction modalities of the post-burn mutilated hand based on a prospective review of a cohort of patients. Ann Burns Fire Disasters 2008; 21(2):81–9.

37. Sunil NP, Ahmed F, Jash PK, et al. Study on surgical management of post burn hand deformities. J Clin Diagn Res 2015;9(8):PC06–10.

Reconstruction of the Adult and Pediatric Burned Hand

Ryan P. Cauley, MD, MPH[a], Lydia A. Helliwell, MD[a],
Matthias B. Donelan, MD[a,b], Kyle R. Eberlin, MD[b,c],*

KEYWORDS

- Burns • Reconstruction • Hand surgery • Skin grafting • Locoregional flaps

KEY POINTS

- Thermal injuries to the hand can greatly affect long-term function.
- Initial treatment should focus on contracture prevention.
- Surgical intervention should follow the standard reconstructive ladder and can involve several techniques from simple to complex including laser and steroid injection, contracture release and skin grafting, regional flaps and local tissue rearrangement, and pedicled and free flaps.
- Appropriately planned and well executed reconstructive interventions can help promote meaningful functional recovery.

INTRODUCTION

The hands represent 3% to 5% of the body's surface area; however, they are involved in 80% to 90% of large burns.[1] The dorsal aspect of the hand has thin cutaneous coverage over critical structures, such as extensor tendons, nerves, and veins, making this area highly vulnerable to thermal injury.[2–4] Although the thick glabrous skin of the palm is protective and less frequently injured, its important functional role in tactile sensation and grasping can make palmar burn injuries particularly disabling.[5]

Hands are important for the ability to manipulate the surrounding world. Therefore, hand burns can have a great impact on both quality of life and long-term functional outcomes.[3,6] Burns to the hand are often associated with significant motor and sensory deficits, tissue loss, and functionally limiting contracture.[4] The presence and severity of functional deficits of the hand may be associated with several factors, including the mechanism, location, and depth of the burn injury.[2,7] Given the complexity and importance of optimal treatment, all hand burns should be referred to a specialized burn center.[8,9]

The surgical treatment of contracture after burn injury should follow standard reconstructive principles and is determined by

1. The type, location, and severity of the deficit
2. The location and quality of uninjured tissue to be used in the reconstruction

Conflicts of Interest and Source of Funding: None of the authors has a financial interest in any of the products, devices, or drugs mentioned in this article. This study has not been presented in any form prior to submission of this article.
[a] Division of Plastic and Reconstructive Surgery, Massachusetts General Hospital, Harvard Medical School, 55 Fruit Street, Boston, MA 02114, USA; [b] Plastic and Reconstructive Surgery, Shriner's Hospital for Children, 51 Blossom Street, Boston, MA 02114, USA; [c] MGH Hand Surgery Fellowship, Division of Plastic and Reconstructive Surgery, Massachusetts General Hospital, Harvard Medical School, 55 Fruit Street, Boston, MA 02114, USA
* Corresponding author. MGH Hand Surgery Fellowship, Division of Plastic and Reconstructive Surgery, 55 Fruit Street, Boston, MA 02114.
E-mail address: keberlin@mgh.harvard.edu

3. The patient's functional requirements and goals for reconstruction

Reconstructive options to treat functional deficits in the burned hand range from the simple (contracture release with skin grafting or local tissue rearrangement) to the complex (pollicization and free tissue transfer). This review focuses on contracture prevention, defining the functional deficits of the burned hand, and the myriad reconstructive options.

CONTRACTURE PREVENTION

The first aim in the treatment of hand burns is to minimize a patient's long-term functional impairment. The seeds for functionally significant contractures are planted early in the course of a burn patient's care; techniques for the prevention of contractures should begin in the acute phase. The authors strongly believe that one of the most important aspects of contracture prevention is a strong focus on tissue sparing, not only through the use of judicious tangential excision but also through the support of any potentially viable tissue through the optimization of resuscitation, hemodynamics, and infection control.

Occupational and physical therapy should be closely involved in a burn patient's care. Positioning is an important aspect of both acute and long-term treatment. Hands at risk of edema should be elevated and compression dressings may be needed. For awake patients, active range-of-motion exercises are often important.[6] The most common burn deformity is the intrinsic-minus position, in which the wrist is flexed, the metacarpophalangeal (MCP) joint is extended, and the interphalangeal (IP) joints are flexed (Fig. 1). Early splinting should be used to maintain

a stable intrinsic-plus position, in which the wrist is extended, the MCP joint is flexed, the proximal interphalangeal joint (PIP) and distal interphalangeal joint (DIP) are maximally extended, and the thumb abducted.[1,6]

FUNCTIONAL DEFORMITIES AND REQUIREMENTS OF RECONSTRUCTION OF THE BURNED HAND

Burn scar contractures of the hand have been classified by McCauley[10] to include 4 grades (Table 1). Burn deformities occur because of thermal injury to the skin, but secondary changes occur in the tendons, ligaments, and joints of the hand that may also have an impact on function and require correction. Surgeons should primarily focus their reconstructive efforts on restoring the function of the hand, rather than improving the range of motion of individual digits.[11]

The typical burned hand deformity comprises several anatomic and functional impairments (Table 2). The classic deformity includes hyperextension of the MCP joints of the fingers, with flexion of the PIP and DIP joints resulting in a clawed posture of the digits. There can be syndactyly and/or nail bed deformity, with contracture of the first web space and adduction of the thumb.

Despite the complexity of the burned hand deformity, the reconstructive needs can often be simplified. Like other challenging reconstructive problems in the hand, there is a need for palmar breadth and a convex metacarpal arch. Additionally, there is a need for a palmarly abducted and

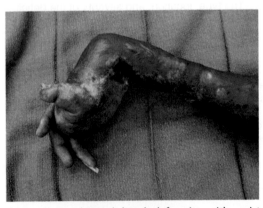

Fig. 1. Severe burned hand deformity with wrist flexion contracture, MCP joint hyperextension, IP joint flexion, and thumb adduction.

Table 1
McCauley grades of burn scar contracture

Grade I	Symptomatic tightness but no limitations in range of motion, normal architecture
Grade II	Mild decrease in range of motion without significant impact on activities of daily living, no distortion of normal architecture
Grade III	Functional deficit noted, with early changes in normal architecture of the hand
Grade IV	Loss of hand function with significant distortion of normal architecture of the hand

Subset classification for grade III and grade IV contractures: A, flexion contractures; B, extension contractures; and C, combination of flexion and extension contractures.

Adapted from McCauley RL. Reconstruction of the pediatric burned hand. Hand Clin 2009;25(4):545; with permission.

Table 2
Surgical intervention should follow the standard reconstructive ladder and can involve several techniques

Defect/Contracture	Treatment (s)
Dorsal hand	Mild • Laser therapy or steroid injections Moderate • Release and skin graft • Random local flaps: Z-plasty, square flap, rhomboid flap • Anatomic local flaps: reverse DMCA Flap Severe/tendon exposure • Release and dermal substitute with subsequent autograft • Regional flap: radial forearm flap, PIA flap • Distal pedicled flap: groin flap, abdominal flap • Free flap
Palmar hand	Primary: local tissue rearrangement, STSG/FTSG (STSG from the plantar aspect of the foot) Secondary: local/regional flap coverage Tertiary: abdominal flap, groin flap, free flap
Dorsal digit	Primary: local tissue rearrangement, release and STSG/FTSG Secondary: local/regional flap coverage (reverse cross-finger flap, homodigital flap, DMCA flap) Tertiary: abdominal flap/groin flap, free flap
Volar digit	Primary: local tissue rearrangement, release and STSG/FTSG Secondary: Local/regional flap coverage (cross-finger flap, homodigital flap, DMCA flap if proximal to DIP) Tertiary: abdominal flap/groin flap, free flap
Web space	Single fold affected (dorsal or palmar): release and STSG/FTSG, z-plasty, starplasty Both folds affected (dorsal and palmar): release and STSG/FTSG, pedicled rhomboid flap Severe (no identifiable fold): release and STSG/FTSG, pedicled rhomboid flap, DMCA flap, bilobed flap, radial forearm flap, abdominal/groin flap, free flap
Boutonneire/swan neck	Release and STSG ± tendon rebalancing Arthrodesis if deformity is functionally limiting
Nail bed	Primary: distally based bipedicled flap and FTSG Secondary: homodigital flaps Tertiary: ablation, composite grafts, transplantation of nail bed from toe
Loss of thumb/digit	Partial loss: web space deepening, distraction lengthening Total loss: pollicization, toe transfer

opposable thumb, with sufficient length and sensibility to interact with the other digits. These critical functions are often affected during thermal injury and should be corrected.

Dorsal Hand Burns

The dorsal skin of the hand is thin and susceptible to thermal injury. After a dorsal burn, the extensor tendons may shorten, and the MCP joint capsule may become stiff and adherent, preventing the ability to flex at the MCP joint. The goals for treatment of dorsal hand contractures are to completely release the contracture and allow for MCP joint flexion and IP joint extension, in addition to restoring palmar abduction of the thumb outside the plane of the second to fifth metacarpals (recreating the transverse metacarpal arch).

Reconstruction of dorsal hand burns in the proximal-distal plane typically involves a transverse release of the contracted dorsal hand skin; the release is performed proximal to or at the level of the MCP joint (**Fig. 2**). Soft tissue release is meticulously performed in the subcutaneous plane, carefully preserving the dorsal veins (if possible) as well as the extensor tendons and paratenon. In addition, release of the burn scar in the radial/ulnar dimension is often required to restore the width and breadth of the hand, along with the convexity of the metacarpal arch. MCP joint capsulotomy and/or release of the

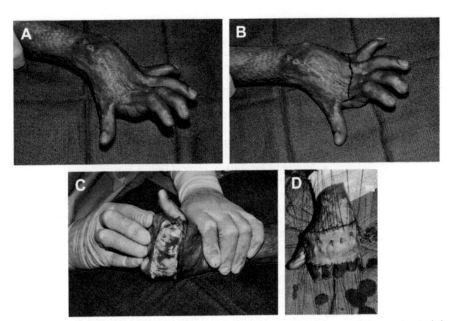

Fig. 2. Reconstruction of dorsal hand burns typically involves a transverse release of the contracted dorsal hand skin; the release is performed proximal to or at the level of the MCP joint. (*A*) Dorsal hand contracture. (*B*) Markings for and (*C*) Transverse incision for contracture release with pinning of MCP joints. (*D*) STSG used to cover the resulting defect.

collateral ligaments may be necessary to optimize flexion at the MCP joint.

Once adequate contracture release is performed to allow for flexion at the MCP joint, percutaneous Kirschner wires are used to maintain flexion of the MCP joints and stretch of the collateral ligaments. The authors typically use 1.143-mm (0.045-in) wires in adults and 0.889-mm (0.035-in) wires in children. These are usually maintained for 3 weeks to 5 weeks depending on the clinical scenario. Soft tissue coverage after dorsal burn scar contracture release can take the form of thick skin grafting (0.014-in or greater), local/regional flaps, or free flap coverage. In practice, a vast majority of dorsal burns involve the skin only, and as such thick skin grafts may be the ideal soft tissue coverage unless there are exposed tendons, joints, or severe injury to underlying structures.

Palmar Hand Burns

Palmar burns are less common than dorsal hand burns; the volar surface of the hand contains thick, glabrous skin that is highly resistant to thermal injury. These are most common in the pediatric population, where the curiosity of young children results in a higher incidence of contact burns to the palm compared with adults.[12] Most palmar hand burns do not require surgical intervention. When full thickness, however, these injuries can result in significant contracture, limiting the breadth of the palm and the ability to grasp objects. The

reconstructive needs of the palmar surface of the hand include sensate, thin cutaneous coverage without significant bulk or shearing and a durable surface to withstand the contact forces of daily use.

Palmar hand burns are often sufficiently treated with local tissue rearrangement, such as Z-plasty, and skin grafts are commonly reserved for more severe or recurrent contractures. When skin grafts are used, one consideration is the use of split-thickness grafts from the plantar surface of the foot (**Fig. 3**). This replaces like with like and may be a better color and texture match. It is the authors' practice to first inject tumescent fluid (with dilute epinephrine) into the subcutaneous space to allow for ease of graft harvest; the dermatome is usually set to 22/1000-in to 24/1000-in and the graft is obtained from the non–weight-bearing plantar instep of the foot. Some investigators have suggested harvesting 2 sequential grafts from the same location on the plantar aspect of the foot (each taken at 8–10/1000 of an inch); the inner (dermal) layer is used to graft the palmar defect of the hand and the outer layer is used to regraft the donor site.[13]

First Web Space Contractures

First web space contractures resulting in thumb adduction are extremely common in thermal injuries to the hand and can be especially debilitating. These contractures have an impact on thumb circumduction at the carpometacarpal

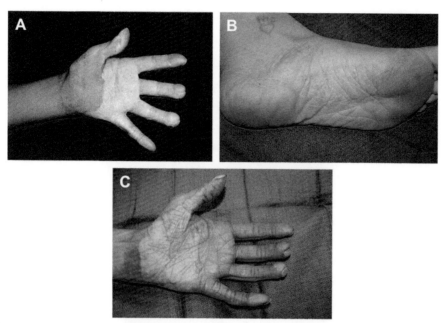

Fig. 3. (*A*) Nonglabrous skin grafts are often a poor color match when treating the burned palm. The plantar surface of the foot can be used as a donor site for palmar hand coverage and typically heals with minimal visible scarring. (*B*) This patient underwent skin graft harvest on 4 occasions without significant untoward effect on the donor site. (*C*) The use of glabrous plantar skin to treat palmar defects can result in both improved aesthetics and a good functional outcome.

(CMC) joint as well as opposition and palmar abduction of the thumb. In addition, the MCP joint of the thumb may become contracted in the hyperextended or hyperflexed position, which can also secondarily affect the IP joint. The goals of first web space reconstruction in the burned hand are to allow for adequate palmar abduction, opposition, and pronation of the thumb and to ensure stability at the MCP joint.

Given the importance of the thumb, concerted effort must be undertaken to restore function. There are many critical elements of first web space contracture release, including complete release of the first CMC joint, restoration of the full breadth of the palm and the convexity of the metacarpal arch, release of the leading edge of the web space, and restoration of palmar skin to the volar surface of the hand. In the authors' experience, surgeons often focus exclusively on release of the leading edge of the contracture and thus may perform an incomplete release of the base of the thumb near the CMC joint.

Many techniques have been described for reconstruction of the first web space after contracture release, including skin grafts as well as regional and free flaps (**Fig. 4**).

Swan Neck and Boutonniere Deformities

Swan neck deformities commonly arise from dorsal cutaneous burn contractures at the level of the proximal phalanx, which cause a compensatory hyperextension at the PIP joint and secondary flexion at the DIP joint. Swan neck deformities may also be caused by rupture of the terminal extensor tendon at its distal insertion or alternatively by intrinsic scarring and fibrosis. The treatment of swan neck deformities depends on their etiology: if the result of dorsal soft tissue deficiency, contracture release and skin grafting may remedy the problem; if a chronic, severe, or fixed deformity, arthrodesis may be the best option.

Boutonniere deformities can result from dorsal burn injuries and resultant rupture of the central slip tendon resulting in flexion at the PIP joint, volar translation of the lateral bands, and a secondary hyperextension at the DIP joint. Patients with boutonniere deformities may remain quite functional secondary to the position of flexion at the PIP joint; the authors typically reserve operative intervention for patients with hyperextension at the DIP joint or the MCP joint.

In the authors' experience, tendon rebalancing and transfers are extremely challenging in burn patients, because the soft tissue envelope is poor, and arthrodesis or amputation may be a better option.

Burn Syndactyly

Burn syndactyly is common after burn injury. This can be functionally incapacitating and the goal of

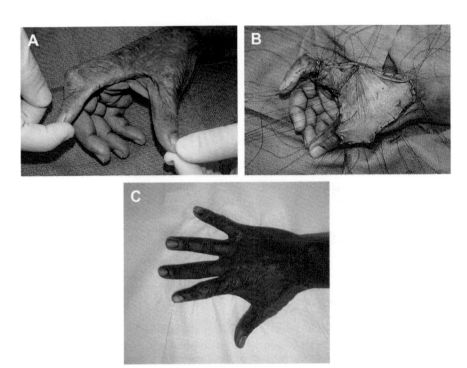

Fig. 4. (*A*) First web space contractures resulting in thumb adduction are common. (*B*) The contracture is released to the level of the CMC joint and then soft tissue coverage is provided. (*C*) Reconstruction of the web space can lead to an improved functional result.

treatment is to recreate normal anatomic relationships of the web space and to adequately separate the digits. Full-thickness skin flaps are often not available as a result of the burn, but when they are, the authors' preferred technique involves either an hourglass-shaped dorsally based flap or triangular flaps. Existing scars should be considered during flap design. If the existing skin is insufficient, the authors perform a longitudinal division of the syndactyly and skin grafts are used for correction. Splinting and conforming dressings are extremely important after burn syndactyly release and critical to success.

Nail bed deformities

Nail deformities include poor appearance or absence of the nail plate. Dorsal burn injuries to the finger can result in proximal migration of the eponychial fold, which results in an elongated, contracted appearance of the nail (**Fig. 5**). If the nail plate is absent or severely injured, ablation or composite graft may be indicated.

Digital necrosis

Acute digital necrosis resulting from thermal injury can be a challenge for the reconstructive surgeon. Depending on the level of digital loss, patients may

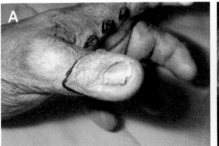
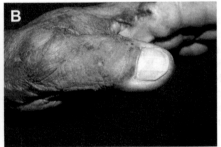

Fig. 5. (*A*) Dorsal burn injuries to the finger can result in proximal migration of the eponychial fold causing an elongated, contracted appearance of the nail. Dorsal contracture release and full-thickness skin grafts can allow for restoration of normal nail growth over time. (*B*) Image at 8-year follow-up.

be candidates for various reconstructive options, including pedicled metacarpal transfers, distraction lengthening, or toe transfer. The type and complexity of reconstructive procedures offered depends on many factors, including the remaining digits and their function, the status of the contralateral hand, and functional needs of the patient.

DIFFERENCES IN RECONSTRUCTION OF THE PEDIATRIC AND THE ADULT BURNED HAND

Although many principles of hand reconstruction are similar in adults and children, there are a few salient differences. Although flame burns are common in both adults and children, scald and contact burns are significantly more common in the pediatric population.[14] Repeated, large, bilateral, or circumferential scald burns of the wrist and hand, or those with concomitant trauma, should raise suspicion for nonaccidental injury.[15]

Children are more susceptible to palmar contact burns given their intellectual and digital curiosity.[12] As in adults, however, these injuries seldom require treatment given the thickness of palmar skin. In 1 series of approximately 700 burned hands in children, palmar burns occurred in 68% of cases but required skin resurfacing in only 15% of cases.[16] Although palmar burns often heal without surgical intervention, given that pediatric dermis is significantly thinner than in adults, full-thickness injury and surgical intervention are more likely in dorsal, digital, and web space injuries.[17] Sheridan and colleagues[16] found that reconstructive surgery was necessary in just 4.4% of patients with partial-thickness burns but in 32% of patients with full-thickness injuries and in 65% of patients with bone or tendon injury. Compared with adults, children recover more quickly from joint stiffness and immobilization; they are more adaptable and have greater cortical plasticity.[18] With good occupational therapy and timely reconstructive surgery, pediatric patients often have good long-term functional outcomes.

SPECIFIC TECHNIQUES FOR RECONSTRUCTION

This section reviews the specific techniques available to the reconstructive hand surgeon. The authors' suggestions for reconstructive techniques for various common deformities of the burned hand are described in **Table 2**.

Minimally Invasive Techniques

Hypertrophic scarring is most likely to occur in areas that require more than 2 weeks to heal primarily.[6] Nonsurgical techniques to treat hypertrophic scarring include compression with or without silicone, laser therapy, and steroid injection. Acutely, elastic bandage wraps can be used to reduce edema and apply pressure to hypertrophic scars. Over the longer term, however, custom-fit elastic pressure garments and specialized pressure inserts may be more efficacious.[19]

Burns that are deep, infected, or heavily colonized may have a higher risk of forming hypertrophic scars.[20,21] These scars can form early, especially in higher tension areas, and may take years to mature. Symptoms of hypertrophic scarring can include contracture as well as pruritus, pain, abnormal pigmentation, and a poor aesthetic outcome. Recently, both fractional carbon dioxide and pulsed dye lasers have been successfully used to ameliorate hypertrophic scarring.[21] Studies have demonstrated that laser treatment is both safe and efficacious for this purpose.[20,22]

Intralesional corticosteroid injection has been used for treatment of hypertrophic scar and may also be useful in the treatment of mild superficial contractures of the hand.[23] The use of fractional CO_2 laser prior to steroid injection has been suggested as an adjunctive way to optimize drug delivery.[24]

Skin Grafting

Contracture release followed by split-thickness skin grafting (STSG) is perhaps the most common method of burn reconstruction. It is a reliable, first-line option for most patients with burn contractures of the hand as long as donor sites for skin autograft are available and the recipient bed is sufficiently vascularized to receive a skin graft.

Using this technique, the contracture is carefully released, carrying the incision through the scarred dermis into the underlying soft tissue.[7] Y-shaped extensions, or darts, can be used to extend the bipedicled flaps diagonally and optimize the contracture release (see **Fig. 2**). The authors recommend that the skin graft be placed into the wound without any tenting or tension to reduce the chance of graft loss and secondary contracture. It is optimal to use sheet grafts on the hand to improve the aesthetic outcome. If meshed grafts are necessary, it is the authors' practice to limit the size of the interstices as much as possible.[25] Silk tie-over bolster and vacuum dressings are the most common methods to secure the graft, and these are often kept in place until postoperative days 5 to 7. In children, it is the authors' practice to maintain these dressings for 2 weeks to 3 weeks depending on the age of the child and the area of burn.

Dermal substitutes

Dermal substitutes can be used in combination with an STSG and may reduce the risk of secondary contracture while providing additional coverage over sensitive structures, such as tendon sheaths and bone, when a flap is not possible. Integra (Integra LifeSciences Corporation, Plainsboro, NJ), a dermal regeneration template made of bovine collagen and glycosaminoglycans covered with a silicon epidermal substitute, is often used for this purpose. STSG can be used once the vascularity of the bed is sufficient.[26] When using this technique, it is important that the wound bed is clean with a low bacterial load because Integra provides no antimicrobial properties.[26,27] It is the authors' practice to wait 3 weeks to 4 weeks after placement of Integra prior to autografting, depending on the patient and the functional needs for rehabilitation.

Full-thickness autograft versus split-thickness autograft

Compared with STSGs, full-thickness autografts may be associated with a higher risk of early graft failure given greater nutrient requirements.[17] Nevertheless, full-thickness grafts may have a lower risk of secondary contracture given their greater dermal thickness and may result in a superior functional and aesthetic outcome.[28]

In the authors' practice, the hands of most severely burned patients tend to be grafted using split-thickness grafts given donor site limitations.[29] Sheet grafts may be less likely to contract than meshed grafts, although some investigators have demonstrated that as long as the meshed grafts remain unexpanded, there is no significant difference in wound contraction.[30]

Release and autograft for nail bed deformities

Even mild digital burns can cause abnormalities of the perionychium, or nail apparatus. The most common cause of nail bed deformity is contracture of the dorsal matrix, which displaces the tissue proximally and prevents the creation of a normal nail.

Treatment of this deformity typically involves the release of the distal dorsal contracture to allow for a return of normal nail growth.[31] Donelan and Garcia[32] reported the largest series of nail bed reconstructions using a distally based bipedicled flap. Full-thickness grafts are used to fill the resulting defect and are held in place using tie-over bolsters (see Fig. 5). Other investigators have reported the use of local flaps to facilitate a similar release of dorsal nail bed contractures.[31]

If an injury to the matrix is complete, signified by segmental or complete loss of nail growth, normal nail growth cannot be restored by simple contracture release. In these cases, nail ablation can be performed.[31] For highly motivated patients, composite grafts or toe transfers may be appropriate.

Local Flaps

Local flaps continue to be one of the mainstays of treatment when reconstructing the burned hand.[33] Compared with simple contracture release and skin grafting, the benefits of using local/regional flaps include a shorter period of immobilization, a minimal donor site, lower risk of contracture recurrence, and potentially greater functional and aesthetic improvement.[34]

Local digital flaps

Digital flexion contractures on the volar aspect of the digit can be challenging when providing local tissue coverage. For smaller defects, cross-finger flaps can be effective, providing soft tissue coverage and an improved neurosensory outcome.[35] The traditional cross-finger flap is used to cover defects on the volar aspect of the digit, but a reverse cross-finger flap or a dorsal adipofascial cross finger flap may be used to repair dorsal defects. For larger defects, homodigital island flaps may be useful in combination with cross-finger flaps.[36]

Anatomic local flaps

Dorsal metacarpal artery flaps Flaps based on the dorsal metacarpal artery (DMCA) can be used to relocate uninjured tissue from the dorsum of the hand or proximal phalanx to either the web space or to other more proximal dorsal hand defects.[37] Although the first and second DMCAs are the most commonly used for local anatomic flaps, the third and fourth DMCAs can also be used.[38,39] Flaps based on the DMCAs have been shown effective for both dorsal and volar defects up to the level of the middle phalanx.[37,38,40] Many investigators have used extended reverse DMCA flaps based on the retrograde flow from the points of extensive palmar-dorsal vascular anastomosis at the base of the phalanges. These reverse DMCA flaps can be used to transpose uninjured tissue from the dorsal hand as far distal as the middle phalanx or DIP joint.[37]

Pollicization For partial loss of the thumb, locoregional flaps can be used to improve thumb circumduction and abduction.[41] Although more commonly used for hypoplasia of the thumb, index finger pollicization may also be used when most or all of the thumb metacarpal is injured or missing secondary to trauma or burn.[42] Over the past 30 years, pollicization has been refined, allowing for improved aesthetic outcomes, greater strength and mobility from optimizing extrinsic and intrinsic tendon repositioning, and incisional modifications that improve the web space contour.[18]

Local flaps for treatment of web space contracture/neosyndactyly

Grishkevich[43] divided web space contractures into 3 types: contractures that involve either the dorsal or palmar aspect of the fold, contractures that involve both the dorsal and palmar aspects of the fold, and more severe contractures in which there is total adduction without a fold. For contractures that involve only one side of the fold,

techniques, such as the trapezoid flap or starplasty, may allow for advancement of the more pliable uninjured edge.[44,45] In cases of web space contractures that involve both aspects of the fold, bilateral advancement is needed through multiple trapezoid flaps, multiple Z-plasties, or a subcutaneously pedicled rhomboid flap.[33,43,46]

Z-plasty is a simple and flexible way to provide additional scar length. Z-plasties work best when there is adjacent tissue laxity on both sides of a linear contracture (**Fig. 6**).[45] More complicated tissue arrangements, such as the jumping man, may

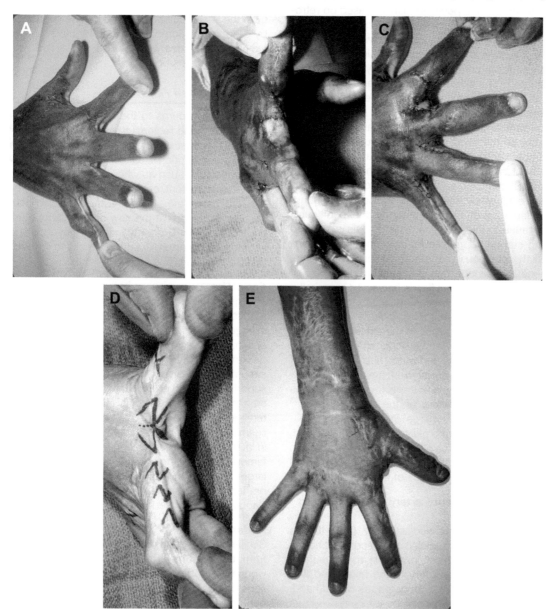

Fig. 6. (*A*) For milder webspace contractures that involve the dorsal or palmar fold. (*B–C*) Single or double Z-plasties can adequately release the contracture. (*D, E*) For more severe contractures, greater tissue advancement may be needed through trapezoid flaps, a rhomboid flap, multiple Z-plasties, or a jumping man flap.

provide more tissue advancement than a single Z-plasty.[47]

Regional Flaps

Several regional flaps can be used to reconstruct postburn defects of the hand when local flaps are insufficient.

Reverse radial forearm flap

The reverse radial forearm fasciocutaneous flap was first described in 1982.[48] This flap uses the same fasciocutaneous paddle as a free radial forearm flap but in a pedicled fashion based on retrograde flow through the palmar arch.[49]

The radial artery is located between the flexor carpi radialis and the brachioradialis, and venous drainage is primarily provided by venae comitantes.[50] The skin paddle is thin and pliable and can be harvested on a long pedicle, allowing it to reach distal wounds on the hand. It can be used for defects involving the palmar and dorsal surfaces of the hand and digits, including first web space contractures.[51] A preoperative Allen test should be performed to verify that the palmar arch is intact and sacrificing the radial artery does not result in any issues with perfusion of the hand.

Flap harvest can be performed expeditiously because no microsurgical anastomosis is required and can be neurotized by including the antebrachial cutaneous nerves. Additionally, muscle, bone and tendon can be transferred as part of the flap.[52] The fascial flap is harvested in a similar fashion and has a similarly reliable blood supply. Disadvantages of this flap include sacrifice of one of the major arteries in the extremity and the conspicuous nature of the donor site.[51]

The radial artery perforator flap is based off perforating vessels arising from the distal radial artery, which supply a complex vascular plexus within the deep fascia of the volar forearm.[53] These perforators emerge in an area approximately 2 cm to 4 cm proximal to the radial styloid, which acts as the pivot point for the flap.[54] This flap shares many of the same benefits of the radial artery flap without sacrifice of the radial artery.

Posterior interosseous artery fasciocutaneous flap

The posterior interosseous artery (PIA) flap is another option for pedicled flap reconstruction in the hand. It provides thin, pliable tissue without sacrifice of a major artery to the hand, and it is used for coverage of wounds on the dorsal hand, first web space, and wrist.[55]

The PIA fasciocutaneous flap is based off perforators from the PIA, which can be found in the septum between the extensor carpi ulnaris and the extensor digiti minimi. When used as a pedicled flap for hand coverage, arterial inflow is provided via retrograde perfusion through a distal communication between the anterior and posterior interosseous arteries.[56]

The cutaneous paddle supported by the PIA can be as large as 12 cm to 15 cm in length and 8 cm to 10 cm in width.[57] Small flaps up to 3 cm to 4 cm in width can allow for primary closure of the donor site. The PIA is found along a line joining the distal radioulnar joint and the lateral epicondyle. A large perforator from the PIA is usually found at the midpoint of this line (approximately 7.5–9.5 cm from the lateral epicondyle) and can be confirmed by Doppler.[55] Some investigators have shown excellent outcomes with the use of this flap with few complications or flap loss.[55]

Remote Pedicled Flaps

With extensive burns to the hand and upper extremity, local and regional flaps may not be available for reconstruction. Distant pedicled flaps can be a good option in cases where microsurgery is not possible, such as when there are no recipient vessels present, or the patient is a poor microsurgical candidate. Because the pedicled flap must revascularize at the new site, patients must undergo at least 2 operations and they must be immobilized for approximately 3 weeks to 4 weeks prior to division of the flap.

Groin Flap

The groin flap can be especially useful in burn reconstruction because the groin is often spared in large burns (**Fig. 7**). It can supply a large amount of thin, supple skin and is often hairless if the flap is designed laterally.[58] It is supplied by the superficial circumflex iliac artery, which originates from the superficial femoral artery either alone or as a common trunk with the superficial inferior epigastric artery approximately 3 cm below the inguinal ligament.[59] The flap is centered over the vessel in a line drawn from its origin at the superficial femoral artery to the anterior iliac spine. A flap as large as 10 cm in width and 15 cm in length can be harvested based off the superficial circumflex iliac artery and closed primarily.[60]

Abdominal Flap

Similar to the groin flap, fasciocutaneous flaps from the abdomen can be designed to cover wounds of both the hand and the forearm. These flaps can be random or can be based off discrete periumbilical perforators, allowing large skin flaps to be raised for coverage of the entire hand or large portions of the forearm with primary closure of the donor site.

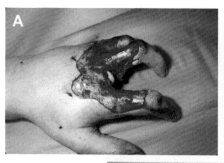
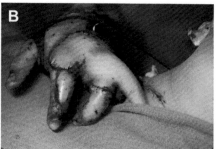
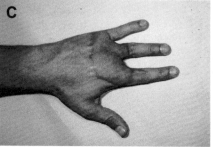

Fig. 7. (*A*) The groin flap can be useful for reconstructing complex 3-D defects of the hand. (*B*) The flap is tubularized if possible and typically divided at 3 weeks to 4 weeks, (*C*) ultimately yielding a satisfactory outcome.

The paraumbilical perforator flap, first described by Taylor and colleagues[61] in 1983, is based off periumbilical perforators from the deep inferior epigastric artery. The size of the potential flap can be up to 8 cm × 30 cm. The flap is raised in the suprafascial plane above the external oblique until the lateral border of the rectus abdominus muscle is reached. It is inset and subsequently divided at approximately 3 weeks to 4 weeks, although division can be staged or delayed if a wound is large or the patient's wound healing is compromised.[62]

If coverage of an entire hand is required, the use of large random abdominal flaps in a pocket or glove configuration can be used. These flap designs leave a large, aesthetically undesirable donor site, however, and may require STSG for closure. These flaps also often require revision procedures to remove syndactyly between the digits.[63]

Free Tissue Transfer

Free tissue transfer has become the reconstructive option of choice for large wounds because they allow for a significant amount of tissue to be used for wound coverage without additional operations required for pedicle division. Free tissue transfer also allows for remote tissue to be transferred to a wound that may be a better match. This requires microsurgical expertise and resources but can result in excellent cosmetic and functional outcomes.[64]

Hand transplantation

Vascularized composite allotransplantation has been developed as an alternative method of reconstruction in severe deformities or total hand loss. Hand transplantation has been performed successfully more than 70 times since the first hand transplantation by Dubernard and colleagues[65] in 1998. There are specific considerations involved with hand transplantation in patients with significant burns, including a paucity of cutaneous veins for drainage of the allograft.[66]

SUMMARY

Although thermal injuries of the hand do not typically affect mortality, they can have a great impact on both quality of life and long-term functional outcome. The optimal treatment of functionally significant hand burns should initially focus on the prevention of contracture through the use of tissue-sparing techniques and good occupational therapy. Surgical intervention should follow the standard reconstructive ladder and includes minimally invasive techniques, such as laser and steroid injection, contracture release and skin grafting, local/regional tissue rearrangements, pedicled flaps, and/or complex microsurgical techniques. Reconstructive hand surgery after thermal injury can be a complex and time intensive process; however, with optimal planning and good surgical technique, there is hope for functional improvement for even severe burn injuries.

REFERENCES

1. Schneider JC, Holavanahalli R, Helm P, et al. Contractures in burn injury part II: investigating joints of the hand. J Burn Care Res 2008;29(4):606–13.

2. Sunil NP, Ahmed F, Jash PK, et al. Study on surgical management of post burn hand deformities. J Clin Diagn Res 2015;9(8):PC06–10.

3. Hop MJ, Langenberg LC, Hiddingh J, et al. Reconstructive surgery after burns: a 10-year follow-up study. Burns 2014;40(8):1544–51.

4. Kamolz LP, Kitzinger HB, Karle B, et al. The treatment of hand burns. Burns 2009;35(3):327–37.

5. Pensler JM, Steward R, Lewis SR, et al. Reconstruction of the burned palm: full-thickness versus split-thickness skin grafts–long-term follow-up. Plast Reconstr Surg 1988;81(1):46–9.

6. Moore ML, Dewey WS, Richard RL. Rehabilitation of the burned hand. Hand Clin 2009;25(4):529–41.

7. Kreymerman PA, Andres LA, Lucas HD, et al. Reconstruction of the burned hand. Plast Reconstr Surg 2011;127(2):752–9.

8. Richards WT, Vergara E, Dalaly DG, et al. Acute surgical management of hand burns. J Hand Surg 2014;39(10):2075–85.e2.

9. Pan BS, Vu AT, Yakuboff KP. Management of the acutely burned hand. J Hand Surg 2015;40(7):1477–84 [quiz: 1485].

10. McCauley RL. Reconstruction of the pediatric burned hand. Hand Clin 2000;16(2):249–59.

11. Sabapathy SR, Bajantri B, Bharathi RR. Management of post burn hand deformities. Indian J Plast Surg 2010;43(Suppl):S72–9.

12. Chan QE, Barzi F, Harvey JG, et al. Functional and cosmetic outcome of full- versus split-thickness skin grafts in pediatric palmar surface burns: a prospective, independent evaluation. J Burn Care Res 2013;34(2):232–6.

13. Friel MT, Duquette SP, Ranganath B, et al. The use of glabrous skins grafts in the treatment of pediatric palmar hand burns. Ann Plast Surg 2015;75(2):153–7.

14. Clarke HM, Wittpenn GP, McLeod AM, et al. Acute management of pediatric hand burns. Hand Clin 1990;6(2):221–32.

15. Pawlik MC, Kemp A, Maguire S, et al. Children with burns referred for child abuse evaluation: burn characteristics and co-existent injuries. Child Abuse Negl 2016;55:52–61.

16. Sheridan RL, Baryza MJ, Pessina MA, et al. Acute hand burns in children: management and long-term outcome based on a 10-year experience with 698 injured hands. Ann Surg 1999;229(4):558–64.

17. Feldmann ME, Evans J, O SJ. Early management of the burned pediatric hand. J Craniofac Surg 2008;19(4):942–50.

18. Taghinia AH, Littler JW, Upton J. Refinements in pollicization: a 30-year experience. Plast Reconstr Surg 2012;130(3):423e–33e.

19. Cowan AC, Stegink-Jansen CW. Rehabilitation of hand burn injuries: current updates. Injury 2013;44(3):391–6.

20. Levi B, Ibrahim A, Mathews K, et al. The Use of CO2 Fractional Photothermolysis for the treatment of burn scars. J Burn Care Res 2016;37(2):106–14.

21. Friedstat JS, Hultman CS. Hypertrophic burn scar management: what does the evidence show? A systematic review of randomized controlled trials. Ann Plast Surg 2014;72(6):S198–201.

22. Clayton JL, Edkins R, Cairns BA, et al. Incidence and management of adverse events after the use of laser therapies for the treatment of hypertrophic burn scars. Ann Plast Surg 2013;70(5):500–5.

23. Ledon JA, Savas J, Franca K, et al. Intralesional treatment for keloids and hypertrophic scars: a review. Dermatol Surg 2013;39(12):1745–57.

24. Waibel JS, Wulkan AJ, Shumaker PR. Treatment of hypertrophic scars using laser and laser assisted corticosteroid delivery. Lasers Surg Med 2013;45(3):135–40.

25. Kowalske KJ. Hand burns. Phys Med Rehabil Clin N Am 2011;22(2):249–59, vi.

26. Lohana P, Hassan S, Watson SB. Integra in burns reconstruction: our experience and report of an unusual immunological reaction. Ann Burns Fire Disasters 2014;27(1):17–21.

27. Watt AJ, Friedrich JB, Huang JI. Advances in treating skin defects of the hand: skin substitutes and negative-pressure wound therapy. Hand Clin 2012;28(4):519–28.

28. Pham TN, Hanley C, Palmieri T, et al. Results of early excision and full-thickness grafting of deep palm burns in children. J Burn Care Rehabil 2001;22(1):54–7.

29. Chandrasegaram MD, Harvey J. Full-thickness vs split-skin grafting in pediatric hand burns–a 10-year review of 174 cases. J Burn Care Res 2009;30(5):867–71.

30. Fifer TD, Pieper D, Hawtof D. Contraction rates of meshed, nonexpanded split-thickness skin grafts versus split-thickness sheet grafts. Ann Plast Surg 1993;31(2):162–3.

31. Goutos I, Jennings CL, Pandya A. Reconstruction of the burnt perionychium: literature review and treatment algorithm. J Burn Care Res 2011;32(4):451–7.

32. Donelan MB, Garcia JA. Nailfold reconstruction for correction of burn fingernail deformity. Plast Reconstr Surg 2006;117(7):2303–8 [discussion: 2309].

33. Ulkur E, Uygur F, Karagoz H, et al. Flap choices to treat complex severe postburn hand contracture. Ann Plast Surg 2007;58(5):479–83.

34. Emsen IM. The cross incision plasty for reconstruction of the burned web space: introduction of an

alternative technique for the correction of dorsal and volar neosyndactyly. J Burn Care Res 2008;29(2): 378–85.

35. Kappel DA, Burech JG. The cross-finger flap. An established reconstructive procedure. Hand Clin 1985; 1(4):677–83.

36. Ulkur E, Acikel C, Karagoz H, et al. Treatment of severely contracted fingers with combined use of cross-finger and side finger transposition flaps. Plast Reconstr Surg 2005;116(6):1709–14.

37. Gregory H, Heitmann C, Germann G. The evolution and refinements of the distally based dorsal metacarpal artery (DMCA) flaps. J Plast Reconstr Aesthet Surg 2007;60(7):731–9.

38. Wang H, Chen C, Li J, et al. Modified first dorsal metacarpal artery island flap for sensory reconstruction of thumb pulp defects. J Hand Surg Eur Vol 2016;41(2):177–84.

39. Zhang X, He Y, Shao X, et al. Second dorsal metacarpal artery flap from the dorsum of the middle finger for coverage of volar thumb defect. J Hand Surg 2009;34(8):1467–73.

40. Chang LY, Yang JY, Wei FC. Reverse dorsometacarpal flap in digits and web-space reconstruction. Ann Plast Surg 1994;33(3):281–9.

41. Kurtzman LC, Stern PJ, Yakuboff KP. Reconstruction of the burned thumb. Hand Clin 1992;8(1):107–19.

42. Taghinia AH, Upton J. Index finger pollicization. J Hand Surg 2011;36(2):333–9.

43. Grishkevich VM. First web space post-burn contracture types: contracture elimination methods. Burns 2011;37(2):338–47.

44. Grishkevich VM. The post-burn elbow medial flexion scar contracture treatment with trapeze-flap plasty. Burns 2009;35(2):280–7.

45. Hultman CS, Teotia S, Calvert C, et al. STARplasty for reconstruction of the burned web space: introduction of an alternative technique for the correction of dorsal neosyndactyly. Ann Plast Surg 2005;54(3): 281–7.

46. Ertas NM, Kucukcelebi A, Bozdogan N, et al. Treatment of recontracture with the subcutaneous pedicle rhomboid flap. Plast Reconstr Surg 2006; 117(5):1590–8.

47. Peker F, Celebiler O. Y-V advancement with Z-plasty: an effective combined model for the release of post-burn flexion contractures of the fingers. Burns 2003; 29(5):479–82.

48. Lu KH. The forearm radial arterial turnover flap and its clinical applications. Zhonghua Wai Ke Za Zhi 1982;20(11):695–7, 704. [in Chinese].

49. Lin SD, Lai CS, Chiu CC. Venous drainage in the reverse forearm flap. Plast Reconstr Surg 1984; 74(4):508–12.

50. Piza-Katzer H, Weinstabl R, Firbas W. The venous blood-flow of the flexor aspect of the human

forearm. Clinical relevance to the distally-pedicled forearm flap. Surg Radiol Anat 1988;10(3):229–32.

51. Megerle K, Sauerbier M, Germann G. The evolution of the pedicled radial forearm flap. Hand (NY) 2010; 5(1):37–42.

52. Soucacos PN, Zoubos AB, Korompilias AV, et al. Versatility of the island forearm flap in the management of extensive skin defects of the hand. Injury 2008;39(Suppl 3):S49–56.

53. Zhang YT. The use of reversed forearm pedicled fascio-cutaneous flap in the treatment of hand trauma and deformity (report of 10 cases). Zhonghua Zheng Xing Shao Shang Wai Ke Za Zhi 1988; 4(1):41–2 [in Chinese].

54. Ho AM, Chang J. Radial artery perforator flap. J Hand Surg 2010;35(2):308–11.

55. Agir H, Sen C, Alagoz S, et al. Distally based posterior interosseous flap: primary role in soft-tissue reconstruction of the hand. Ann Plast Surg 2007; 59(3):291–6.

56. Lu LJ, Gong X, Lu XM, et al. The reverse posterior interosseous flap and its composite flap: experience with 201 flaps. J Plast Reconstr Aesthet Surg 2007; 60(8):876–82.

57. Page R, Chang J. Reconstruction of hand soft-tissue defects: alternatives to the radial forearm fasciocutaneous flap. J Hand Surg 2006;31(5):847–56.

58. McGregor IA, Jackson IT. The groin flap. Br J Plast Surg 1972;25(1):3–16.

59. Knutson GH. 7. The groin flap: a new technique to repair traumatic tissue defects. Can Med Assoc J 1977;116(6):623–5.

60. Schlenker JD. Important considerations in the design and construction of groin flaps. Ann Plast Surg 1980;5(5):353–7.

61. Taylor GI, Corlett R, Boyd JB. The extended deep inferior epigastric flap: a clinical technique. Plast Reconstr Surg 1983;72(6):751–65.

62. Gutwein LG, Merrell GA, Knox KR. Paraumbilical perforator flap for soft tissue reconstruction of the forearm. J Hand Surg 2015;40(3):586–92.

63. Pradier JP, Oberlin C, Bey E. Acute deep hand burns covered by a pocket flap-graft: long-term outcome based on nine cases. J Burns Wounds 2007;6:e1.

64. Abramson DL, Pribaz JJ, Orgill DP. The use of free tissue transfer in burn reconstruction. J Burn Care Rehabil 1996;17(5):402–8.

65. Dubernard JM, Owen E, Herzberg G, et al. Human hand allograft: report on first 6 months. Lancet 1999;353(9161):1315–20.

66. Eberlin KR, Leonard DA, Austen WG Jr, et al. The volar forearm fasciocutaneous extension: a strategy to maximize vascular outflow in post-burn injury hand transplantation. Plast Reconstr Surg 2014; 134(4):731–5.

Microsurgical Reconstruction of the Burned Hand and Upper Extremity

Mauricio De la Garza, MD[a],*,
Michael Sauerbier, MD, PhD[b,c], Germann Günter, MD, PhD[c],
Curtis L. Cetrulo Jr, MD[d], Reuben A. Bueno Jr, MD[e],
Robert C. Russell, MD[f], Michael W. Neumeister, MD[a]

KEYWORDS

• Microsurgery • Hand • Burn • Reconstruction • Free flap • Contracture

KEY POINTS

- Although the majority of burned hand wounds can be covered with skin grafts, many of these wounds require complex microsurgical reconstruction.
- Special considerations must be taken when planning for microsurgical reconstruction of the burned hand and upper extremity.
- Early excision has been shown to improve outcomes, and one must ensure that the recipient site is free of any remaining burned tissues prior to reconstruction.
- Timing of the microsurgical reconstruction of the burned hand requires careful planning.
- With adequate early management, careful planning, and selection of the reconstructive technique, microsurgical reconstruction of the burned hand is safely performed with good functional and aesthetic outcomes.

INTRODUCTION

The improvements in critical care and burn victim resuscitation have led to increased survival of severely burned patients. Initial resuscitation, early excision of burned tissues, prevention of burn wound sepsis, and wound coverage remain mainstays of care. Although the majority of burn wounds can be covered with skin grafts, many of these wounds require complex reconstruction.[1] This is particularly important in the hand, where a small cross-sectional area contains multiple specialized structures that when burned lead to devastating injuries, resulting in loss of hand

Disclosure Statement: The authors have nothing to disclose.
[a] The Institute for Plastic Surgery, Southern Illinois University, 747 North Rutledge Street, Springfield, IL 62702-6700, USA; [b] Department for Plastic, Hand and Reconstructive Surgery, BG Trauma Center, Friedberger Landstrasse 430, Frankfurt am Main 60389, Germany; [c] Department for Plastic, Hand and Reconstructive Surgery, Burn Center, BG Trauma Center Ludwigshafen, University of Heidelberg, Ludwig Guttman Street 13, Ludwigshafen 67071, Germany; [d] Department of Surgery, Division of Plastic Surgery, Massachusetts General Hospital, 55 Fruit Street, Boston, MA 02114-2621, USA; [e] Department of Plastic Surgery, Monroe Carell, Jr Children's Hospital, Vanderbilt University Medical Center, D-4207 Medical Center North, Nashville, TN 37232-2345, USA; [f] Heartland Plastic Surgery Center, 320 East Carpenter, Spfingfield, IL 62702-5185
* Corresponding author.
E-mail address: mdelagarza@siumed.edu

Hand Clin 33 (2017) 347–361
http://dx.doi.org/10.1016/j.hcl.2016.12.007
0749-0712/17/Published by Elsevier Inc.

function and permanent disability. Coverage of tendons, ligaments, joints, vessels, nerves, and bones of the hand requires healthy vascularized tissue to maintain viability and function. Local flaps or regional flaps, such as reverse radial forearm flaps or posterior interosseous artery flaps, may be within the burn zone of injury and therefore not available for pedicled transfer. Refined microvascular free tissue transfer techniques along with the growing availability of microsurgical instrumentation and increased experience in microsurgery of the burned patient offer free tissue transfer as a procedure that can be safely performed with good functional and aesthetic outcomes.

PREPARING FOR MICROSURGERY

Special considerations must be taken when planning for microsurgical reconstruction of the burned hand and upper extremity (**Table 1**). Particular attention is placed on hemodynamic stability of

Table 1
Special considerations prior to free tissue transfer in the acutely burned patient

Resuscitation	Acutely burned patients lose an enormous amount of fluid through insensible losses. Adequate fluid resuscitation means the patient is hemodynamically stable with appropriate urine output, normal vital signs, and homeostatic in pH, lactate, and electrolyte status.
Escharotomies and Fasciotomies	All decompressive procedures are complete before the free tissue transfer. Late releases may lead to flap loss, muscle necrosis, lack of functional recovery of the limb, increased chance of infection, and the need for further free tissue transfer to cover newly exposed vital structures.
Debridement	All devitalized tissue must be excised. An adequate debridement treats the wound like a pseudo-tumor. Take a second or third look after 24 or 48 hours to further debride the wound. Electrical and friction burns are notorious for progressive tissue necrosis. Large vessels may be patent; therefore the tissues bleed, but capillary beds have coagulated, resulting in tissue death.
Temporary Dressings	The patient's condition must be optimized before the free tissue transfer surgery. The wounds can be temporized with opsite, allograft, xenograft, negative pressure wound therapy, or moist dressings. The goal is to keep tissues and vital structures from desiccation.
Donor Sites	Larger TBSA burns require ample skin graft donor sites. The same donor sits may be the site of flap harvest. Wait for the skin graft donor site to heal to minimize the infection rates.
Bone Stabilization	It is preferable to have the skeletal foundation stable prior to performing the free tissue transfer. Internal fixation is usually preferable to minimize infection rates and improve logistics of the free tissue transfer. The acutely burned patient is at higher risk for many insults including hemodynamic instability, hypothermia, coagulopathy, infection, malnutrition, electrolyte disturbances, blood product reactions, and organ failure. Minimizing surgery duration and complexity will minimize risk to the patient.
Multidisciplinary Team Participation	The acutely burned patient may be very ill or in critical condition. All services looking after the patient should be aware of any pending free tissue transfer surgery. The team may include burn surgeons, critical care intensivists, nurses, anesthesiologists, infectious disease specialists, nephrologists, cardiologists, pulmonologists, nutritionists, and other health professionals. Optimization by all specialists includes resolving organ failure, being off pressors, hemodynamically stable, and an informed consent. The informed consent is particularly important when patients are sedated, medicated, or on the ventilator. The power of attorney (POA) must be fully aware of all risks of the free tissue transfer in these patients.
Vascular Status	Vessel compromise may be present despite a well-vascularized limb in the acutely burned patient. Angiograms remain a gold standard for vessel visualization, but computed tomography angiography (CTA) is often acceptable

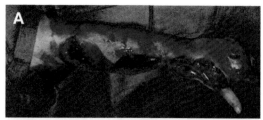

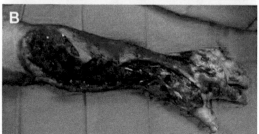

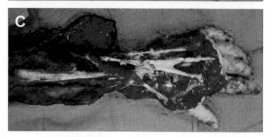

Fig. 1. Photos of a burned hand demonstrating the need for a second look as zones of stasis progress after (A) initial debridement to (B) necrosis, ultimately leading to (C) large defects with exposed vital structures that may require microsurgical reconstruction for salvage.

the patient, where the net body fluid and hemoglobin levels must be optimized in preparation for a microvascular procedure. Diet supplementation, nutritional support via enteric tube feeds or even parenteral feeding, if necessary, should be established with a goal of maximizing protein levels to assist with wound healing. Early management of the severely burned hand will often include early decompression of all 10 fascial compartments, via escharotomies and/or fasciotomies if needed. Release of the carpal tunnel and Guyon canal should also be an early consideration to avoid median and ulnar compressive neuropathy, respectively. The pathophysiologic differences between thermal, chemical, and electrical burns must be considered when planning on preparing the wound for microsurgical reconstruction. Early excision has been shown to improve outcomes, and one must ensure that the recipient site is free of any remaining burned tissues prior to reconstruction.[2] Necrotic tissues provide a medium for bacterial and fungal colonization and produce leucotoxins and systemic immunosuppressants, jeopardizing any vascular anastomosis. Adequate debridement consists of excision of necrotic and ischemic tissues until a viable and healthy bleeding wound bed is reached. It is not unusual to require a second-look procedure to excise zones of stasis that have progressed to necrosis (**Fig. 1**). This is particularly common in electrical burns, where not only the direct thermal injury causes damage, but tissues also undergo electroporation and electroconformational changes in addition to the Joule heat effect on the bones (**Table 2**). Because bone has the highest resistance, the greatest heat is generated in the deep tissues. This means that during debridement, muscle attached to the bones may require excision because of nonviability. This often results in exposure of vital structures such as tendons, nerves, vessels, joints, and bone. Adequate

Table 2 Special considerations of electrical burns	
Direct Thermal Injury	Direct cutaneous burn from the entrance site or the arc across joint as the current skips
Joule Heat Effect	The effect is defined as the passage of current through a solid conductor, resulting in a conversion of electrical energy to heat Joule's law states, $J = 0.24 \times I^2 \times R \times T$, where J is the heat production, I is the current, R is the resistance, and T is the time of exposure Each of these factors has an effect on the ultimate outcome of tissue damage in electrical burns
Electroconformation	Changes in functional reductions in membrane proteins and Na and K channels, due to high voltage across the cell membrane
Electroporation	Cell membranes are disrupted through a rapid effect of current passing through cellular tissue Denatured proteins within the lipid bilayer lose their 3-dimensional structure and distort existing pores or form pathologic intramembrane pores resulting in homeostatic changes of intracellular contents and cell death

debridement is crucial to preventing infection but often leaves a wound that requires free tissue transfer for stable coverage of the vital structures. The success of the free flap closure is dependent on that adequate debridement. Nonviable tissue left behind may get infected and may compromise the patency of the anastomosis and the flap tissue viability.

Elevation of the extremity is helpful to facilitate venous return before and after surgeries. Splinting the hand in the safe position with metacarpophalangeal joints in flexion and the interphalangeal joints in extension is important to avoid a dysfunctional burn claw hand deformity.[3] Early hand therapy also plays a significant role in the early management to avoid stiffness and joint contractures. Complex wound care to keep underlying tissues clean and viable is also essential to maintain exposed structures from infection and desiccation. Temporizing wounds using skin substitutes or negative pressure wound therapy should be considered until the patient or the wound is ready for definitive flap closure.[4]

OPERATIVE CONSIDERATIONS

Timing of the microsurgical reconstruction of a burned hand requires careful planning. The patient must be stable to endure a prolonged surgery. The surgeon must decide if the reconstruction of the burned hand should be performed acutely or in a delayed fashion. Early reconstruction with a free flap may sometimes be the only way to attempt hand salvage. Performing early microsurgical reconstruction also provides the benefits of early wound closure, early mobility and decreased hospitalization. Pan and colleagues[5] reported a series of 38 patients who received a free fasciocutaneous flap transfer for reconstruction of burned hands with 100% flap survival; 32 of those reconstructions were performed within the first 21 days of care. Jabir and colleagues recently published data of a series of 23 free flaps used for acute burn reconstruction where despite a morbidity of approximately 25%, every free flap survived. On the other hand, other large series reporting microsurgical reconstruction of the burned hand suggest that flap failure is higher in the acutely reconstructed patient as compared with those undergoing delayed reconstruction. This theory is based on a less stable physiologic milieu caused by a global release of inflammatory mediators, tissue edema, vessel damage, and potential contamination, reducing the chances of free flap survival.[6] Shen and colleagues provide data on a group of 70 cases, where 54 flaps were performed early and had a flap failure rate of 17%, while 16 flaps

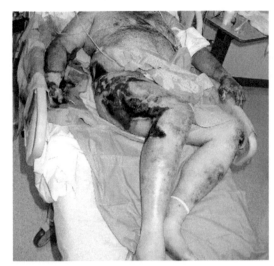

Fig. 2. Electric burn injury with entry point on right thigh and exit point on right wrist.

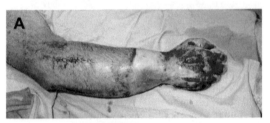
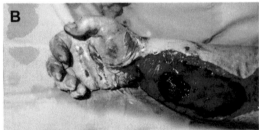

Fig. 3. Right hand electrical burn injury after initial debridement of the (A) dorsum and (B) volar aspects of the hand and forearm.

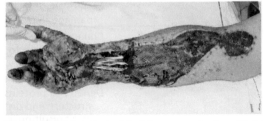

Fig. 4. Right hand electrical burn required multiple debridements until all tissue was declared viable.

were performed in a delayed fashion with no flap failure.[7] Abramson and colleagues reported a series of 45 free flaps in burn reconstruction, of which 12 flaps were performed within 96 hours and the rest in a delayed fashion; there was a flap failure rate of 4% also found only within the acute period.[8] In another large series, Sauerbier and colleagues also demonstrated a flap failure rate of 12% that was highest when performed within 5 and 21 days after trauma, and with no flap failure occurring during delayed reconstructions.[9] Their higher failure rate was attributed to the hostile tissue environment during peak proinflammatory windows.

Observations of pathologic changes that occur on the vessels following thermal or electric injuries suggest that there is damage to the tunica media and endothelium, vascular occlusion, aneurysmal formation with thrombosis, segmental narrowing of major extremity vessels, and marked decrease in the density of small nutrient vessels, thus strengthening the recommendation to perform the microvascular anastomosis outside the zone of injury. This is particularly relevant in electrical injuries in which the zone of injury may be extensive and may require the use of interposition vein grafts. Although vascular imaging may assist in determining vessel availability, Shen and colleagues claimed that appreciation of patency is often obscured by artifacts and technical errors, and that intraoperative direct inspection under the microscope is a direct and reliable method to assess vessel integrity.[7]

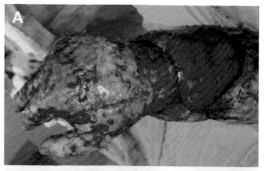
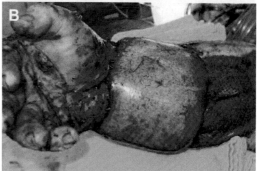

Fig. 6. Complete coverage of the (A) dorsal and (B) volar wrist was obtained.

Many principles of the management of electrical burns to the upper extremity are identified in the case presented in **Figs. 2–9**. The patient sustained a 40% total body surface area (TBSA) third-degree

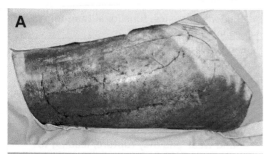
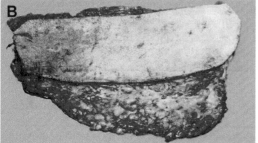

Fig. 5. (A) The nonburned left thigh of the patient was used to obtain a (B) left fasciocutaneous anterolateral thigh free flap for coverage.

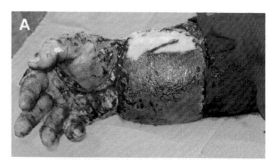
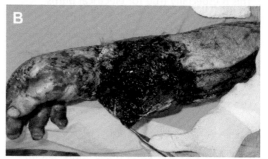

Fig. 7. (A) Early postoperative complication. Upon exploration, (B) the anastomosis site performed initially within the zone of injury was noticed to be blown out.

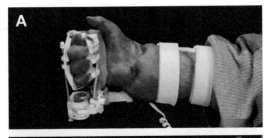

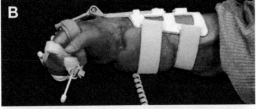

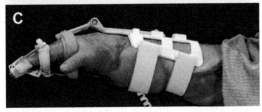

Fig. 8. Flap was salvaged with a vein graft to perform anastomosis outside the zone of injury. (*A–C*) Aggressive hand therapy initiated.

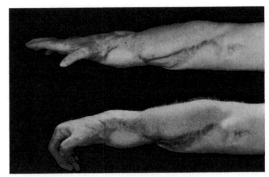

Fig. 9. Postoperative result demonstrating a healed wound with adequate range of motion.

electrical burn. The deepest burn was noted at an exit site of the right wrist. Early fasciotomies decompressed the limb, permitting continued perfusion. Burn debridement involved skin excision in most of the areas involved and muscle excision around the wrist including the pronator quadratus. Multiple debridements were performed until all tissue was viable. The patient's condition prevented early flap closure of the exposed extensor and flexor tendons and underlying exposed bone. Once the patient was off pressors for hemodynamic instability, the free anterolateral

Table 3	
Tips to promote successful outcomes in the microsurgical management of hand and upper extremity burns	
Tip	**Rationale**
Match tissue types	Bulky flaps are less functional than thin pliable flaps
Use fascial or fasciocutaneous flaps when secondary procedures are expected under the flap.	Easy elevation Muscle flaps may be very fibrotic, not easy to elevate and may not cover the wound after elevation due to swelling
The anastomosis should be performed outside the zone of trauma if possible This is especially true for electrical burns	Traumatized vessels are unreliable and are prone to clot formation Vessels around electrical burns are damaged and weak and may rupture, leading to hemorrhage and flap loss or limb loss
Fascial flaps allow easy gliding of exposed tendons	Adhesions are less common with fascia
Tendon grafts or transfers can be performed at the same time as the free flap	Early motion permitted to decrease stiffness and contractures
Use spare parts when available	Amputated tissue may be a repository of extra tissue such as nerves, tendons, bone, or skin that can be used as a graft or vascularized tissue transfer
Early range of motion of digits, wrist, elbow, and shoulder	An anastomosis and newly inset flaps are not a contraindication to early motion Immobilization leads to stiffness and to contractures

thigh flap provided the enormous amount of tissue required to cover the circumferential wrist wound. Extra fascia was taken to wrap around the desiccated tendons. A fasciocutaneous flap was chosen, because secondary tenolysis and tendon and nerve grafts were anticipated at a later date. The early postoperative period was complicated by a vascular rupture as the anastomosis blew out. The initial anastomosis was within the zone of injury. The salvage vein graft was taken to an area outside of the electrical exit site, and the flap was salvaged. Early aggressive therapy and many secondary procedures permitted a functional outcome and return to work for the patient. This case highlights many of the tips identified in **Table 3**:

- Early fasciotomy and debridement
- Second looks and multiple debridements, because electrical burns have progressive necrosis of muscle
- Flap closure when the patient is stable
- Performing the anastomosis outside the zone of injury to avoid complications

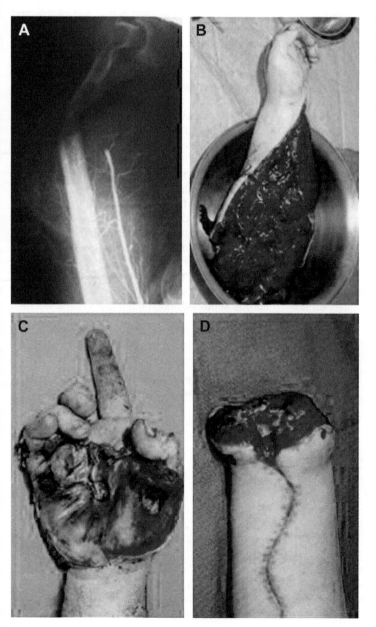

Fig. 10. (*A, B*) Patient enrolled on a rollover motor vehicle collision (MVC) with bilateral upper extremity injuries including a prolonged avascular left upper extremity that required amputation at the arm and (*C, D*) a severe deep right hand burn that required amputation at a distal forearm.

- Fasciocutaneous flaps when secondary procedures are anticipated
- Early therapy

Reconstructive Options

There is a wide variety of well-described free tissue transfer options available to reconstruct the complex burned hand and upper extremity. These include muscular flaps, musculocutaneous flaps, fascial flaps and fasciocutaneous flaps, vascularized tendons or bones, and composite flaps. Any flap could be potentially thinned, pre-expanded, prefabricated, prelaminated, or made chimeric. Complex reconstructive efforts have also included microsurgery involving targeted muscle reinnervation and vascularized composite allotransplantation. The selection of the reconstructive method is mainly based on the characteristics of the remaining viable tissues and the extent of the injury. Salvage of the burned hand and restoring function are the main priorities; nevertheless, sometimes patients with extensive grade 4 burns benefit more from an early amputation.[10] Patients who lose the hand may be considered for myoelectric or body-powered prosthetics, targeted muscle reinnervation, or transplantation. Most burned hands are amenable for salvage and can be reconstructed with microsurgical transfer of flaps. Selection of the flap will depend on the desired tissue composition needed for reconstruction, the size of the wound, the necessary pedicle length to reach outside zone of injury, body habitus, and comorbidities. Donor flap selection is often challenging in the burn patient, as other areas that have sustained burn injuries are not viable options for tissue transfer. The same limitation plays a role when considering skin grafting of the free flap. Sometimes amputated tissue may be a repository of extra tissue spare parts such as nerves, tendons, bone, or skin that can be used as a graft or vascularized tissue transfer (Figs. 10–12).[11] When possible, discussing the surgeon's flap preference with the patient may lead to better-perceived cosmetic outcomes.

The desired tissue composition of the flap needed for reconstruction of the hand is selected depending on what structures are injured. There are marked anatomic and functional differences between the dorsum, the palm, and the digits that need to be individually addressed. The skin of the dorsum of the hand is thin and pliable and provides supple coverage to the immediately underlying extensor tendons and bones. This area is routinely covered with fascial and fasciocutaneous flaps. Flap options for the hand dorsum include the contralateral radial forearm flap, anterolateral thigh fascia or fasciocutaneous flap, lateral arm fascia or fasciocutaneous flap, serratus fascia (Figs. 13 and 14), dorsal thoracic fascia, gracilis flap with skin graft, scapular fascia or fasciocutaneous flap (Fig. 15), temporoparietal fascial flap, or a thinned deep inferior epigastric artery perforator flap.[12] Larger flaps for other areas on the upper extremity may include the latissimus muscle, parascapular flap, transverse rectus abdominis myocutaneous flap, and rectus abdominus flap. Considerations can be given to thinning the flap before inset.[13]

The palm of the hand is formed of glabrous, thick, hairless skin anchored through complex fibrous septa. Although most palm burns will heal

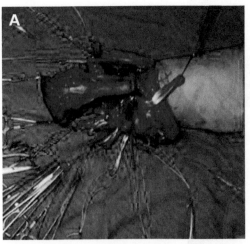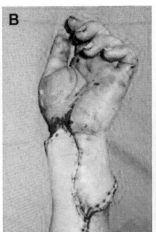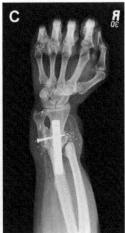

Fig. 11. Utilizing the concept of spare parts, this patient's viable amputated left hand was replanted to the right distal forearm stump. (A) Initial structures matching function are identified and (B) the hand replanted in a reverse configuration (C) with a single bone forearm to permit pronation and supination.

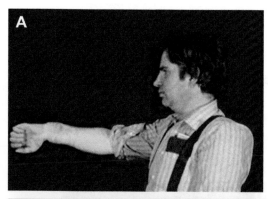

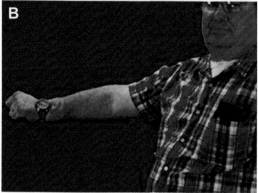

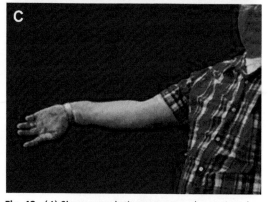

Fig. 12. (*A*) Since completing recovery, the patient has been able to perform his daily routine. At an older age, the patient continues with adequate range of motion on (*B*) pronation and (*C*) supination.

with conservative treatment, when the palm requires healthy vascularized tissue flap options should include fasciocutaneous flaps with similar characteristics. Uygur and colleagues[14] reported remarkable results providing sensate thin glabrous skin for burned hand palm reconstruction with minimal donor morbidity using the medial pedis perforator flap. Medial plantar flap has also been used for thicker and smaller areas of the palm or digits that require reconstruction.[15] In selective

cases, a free flap may be used to salvage a finger. Hung and colleagues[16] reported a series of 16 free flaps for digit reconstruction with 100% flap survival using different free groin fasciocutaneous or osteocutaneous flaps, and free contralateral dorsal metacarpal artery flap. When the thumb skin is circumferentially burned, one may recur to a toe wrap around free flap if the feet are not injured.[17] When the severity of the burn results in finger loss, pollicization or toe transfer can be reliably performed. Kim and colleagues[18] reported satisfactory results in 15 cases of toe tissue transfer for reconstruction of digits damaged by electrical burns.

When tendon reconstruction is needed, immediate or delayed tendon reconstruction with either grafts or transfers is appropriate, although immediate reconstruction is preferred to start early motion (**Fig. 16**). Immediate reconstruction as a composite flap with the accompanying tendon is an option if the donor site is available.[11]

Despite appropriate initial management, burned patients frequently develop hand contractures that may require microsurgical reconstruction. Skin contractures are frequently addressed with local tissue rearrangement and skin grafts. When this is not possible due to the extensive nature of the defect's exposed structures, free flap coverage is indicated. The first web space is particularly prone to severe contracture and often requires fasciocutaneous flaps for reconstruction, most commonly the lateral arm flap (**Fig. 17**). When a contraction has caused joints to become stiff, one must ensure the contracted joint is released prior to insetting of the flap. This often requires capsulotomies, volar plate release, checkrein ligament release, intrinsic muscle release, and tenolysis. Postoperative care usually includes joint immobilization until flap viability is confirmed, at which point early passive and active range of motion hand therapy is initiated. Excellent flap survival with good outcomes has been reported by multiple groups using arterialized venous flaps, dorsalis pedis flaps, posterior interosseous flaps, radial forearm flaps, free medial pedis perforator flaps, anterolateral thigh flaps, and free thin DIEP flaps.[12,14,19–21]

Severely burned hands may result in loss of the entire hand. Options to restore function have been rapidly evolving throughout the last decades. Conventional prosthetic technology requires that existing musculature control the prosthetic device. Body-powered systems employ cables driven by muscle motion to directly affect movement in the prosthetic. Myoelectric devices work more intuitively, as intact musculature is wired to control the terminal device. First reported in 2004,

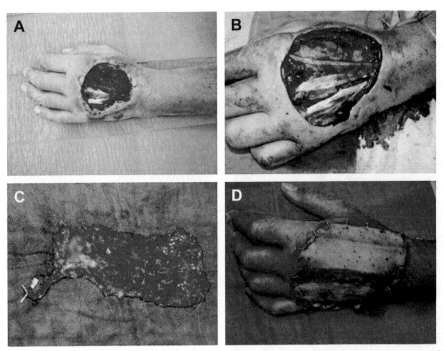

Fig. 13. (A) 42 year old woman with a left hand dorsum soft tissue defect following a burn injury. (B) The hand underwent debridement until healthy tissues were reached. (C) A free serratus fascia was used to reconstruct the defect of the dorsum of the hand (D) followed by immediate placement of a split-thickness skin graft.

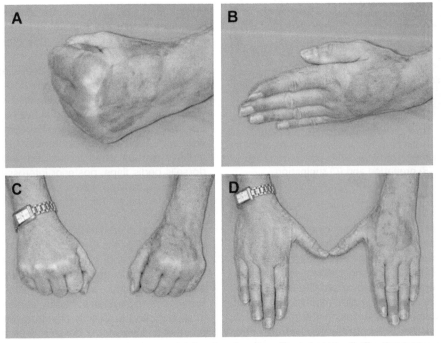

Fig. 14. The same patient 1 year postoperatively showing functionally and aesthetically pleasing results on (A) flexion of the hand, (B) extension of the hand, and when compared with the (C, D) contralateral hand.

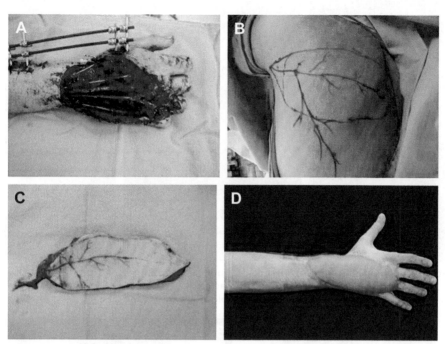

Fig. 15. (*A*) A 21-year-old man sustained a right hand dorsum road rash burn during an MVC. The left scapula flap was selected for reconstruction. (*B*) Donor flap was marked and (*C*) obtained free style for microsurgical reconstruction. (*D*) The hand extension function remains intact along with a good cosmetic result.

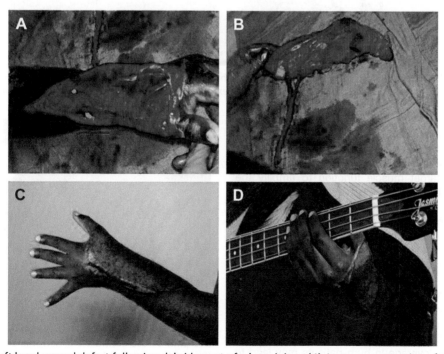

Fig. 16. Left hand wound defect following debridement of a burn injury. (*A*) Acute reconstruction of the thumb extensor function was performed with a transfer of the extensor indices proprius to the extensor pollicis longus. (*B*) The anterolateral thigh flap was selected as a free tissue transfer (*C*) to cover the entire defect. (*D*) The patient is satisfied, as he healed well and is able to perform his daily activities with normal hand function.

358

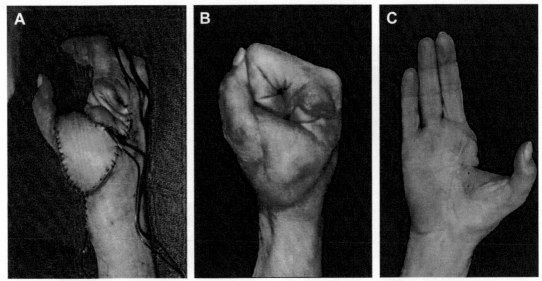

Fig. 17. Patient with a right hand first web space contracture following burn reconstruction that led to amputation of the index finger. (*A*) She underwent excision of contracted tissues followed by coverage with a free ipsilateral lateral arm flap. She healed adequately and (*B*) is now able to make a fist and (*C*) abduct and extend her thumb.

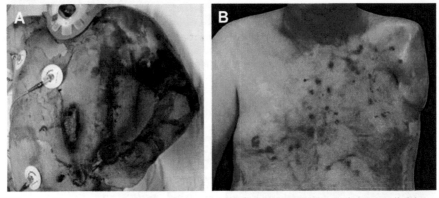

Fig. 18. (*A*) 56-year-old man with full thickness burns to his left upper extremity and chest wall. (*B*) 4 months after serial debridements and amputation of the left upper extremity at the level of the glenohumeral joint.

targeted muscle reinnervation (TMR) became one of the most important advancements in prosthetic rehabilitation (**Figs. 18–20**). TMR uses nerve transfers to retarget muscle function to amplify the signaling from residual nerves, allowing intuitive control of the prosthetic. This improves the utility of the prosthetic device and allows patients to integrate the prosthetic into their self-image.[22]

Vascularized composite allotransplantation (VCA) has become a rapidly advancing therapeutic option for reconstruction of complex hand burns (**Figs. 21–23**). VCA facilitates the goal of replacing like with like, however with the burden of immunosuppression for graft acceptance. Recent studies indicate that the use of cadaveric skin allotransplantation providing temporary coverage in burn patients may lead to an initial sensitization, leading to an acquired ability of the immune system to react to foreign human leukocytes (HLAs) by producing antibodies and

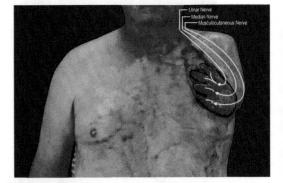

Fig. 19. Superimposed diagram of the appearance of the muscle flaps 7 days after undergoing targeted muscle reinnervation procedure showing the operative plan to use contralateral serratus anterior free flap with nerve repairs of median, musculocutaneous, and ulnar nerves to the branches of the long thoracic nerve to separate slips of the serratus anterior muscle.

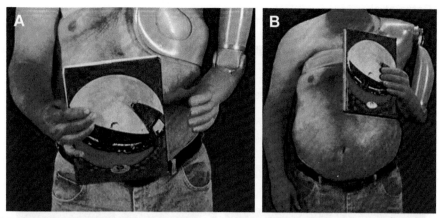

Fig. 20. (A) Patient demonstrating elbow flexion and open grasp (B) and elbow flexion and closed grasp with the prosthesis.

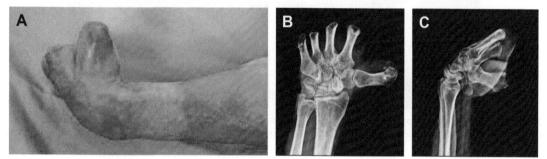

Fig. 21. (A) Gross appearance of a pretransplant left dominant hand with transmetacarpal amputations and a fixed flexion deformity of the wrist. (B) Anteroposterior and (C) lateral radiographs.

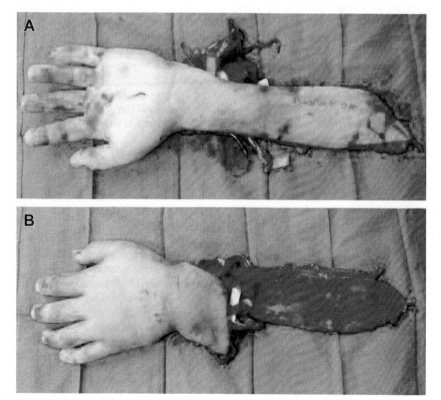

Fig. 22. (A) Volar and (B) dorsal views of a donor left hand allograft with a volar forearm fasciocutaneous extension prior to transplantation.

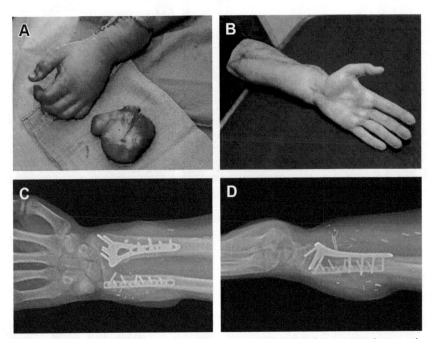

Fig. 23. (*A*) Postoperative appearance of immediately transplanted hand with amputated stump shown for comparison. (*B*) Gross appearance 1 year after hand transplantation with (*C*) posteroanterior and (*D*) lateral view radiographs.

developing memory cells. This may contribute as a major factor for acute graft rejection, suggesting VCA may be sought as an early strategy to obtain definitive reconstruction avoiding procedures triggering HLA antibody formation. When sensitization has occurred, one may consider desensitization treatment options such as immunoadsorption and plasma exchange to eliminate anti-HLA and anti-A/B antibodies in the patient's plasma, proteosomal inhibitors to indirectly reduce the alloantibody production, splenectomy to eliminate a major source of B-cells and plasma cells, and intravenous immunoglobulins (IVIG) and/or anti-B cell agents. Desensitized patients do have an increased risk to severe infections and malignancy.[23]

SUMMARY

The patient with burned hands requires complex care. When planning microsurgical reconstruction of the burned hand and upper extremity, one must take into account special considerations pertaining to burned patients. With adequate early management and careful planning and selection of the reconstructive technique, microsurgical reconstruction of the burned hand is safely performed with good functional and aesthetic outcomes.

REFERENCES

1. Karanas YL, Buntic RF. Microsurgical reconstruction of the burned hand. Hand Clin 2009;25(4):551–6.

2. Saaiq M, Zaib S, Ahmad S. Early excision and grafting versus delayed excision and grafting of deep thermal burns up to 40% total body surface area: a comparison of outcome. Ann Burns Fire Disasters 2012;25(3):143–7.

3. Fufa DT, Chuang SS, Yang JY. Prevention and surgical management of postburn contractures of the hand. Curr Rev Musculoskelet Med 2014; 7(1):53–9.

4. Neumeister MW, Brown RE. Mutilating hand injuries: principles and management. Hand Clin 2003;19(1): 1–15, v.

5. Pan CH, Chuang SS, Yang JY. Thirty-eight free fasciocutaneous flap transfers in acute burned-hand injuries. Burns 2007;33(2):230–5.

6. Jabir S, Frew Q, El-Muttardi N, et al. A systematic review of the applications of free tissue transfer in burns. Burns 2014;40(6):1059–70.

7. Shen TY, Sun YH, Cao DX, et al. The use of free flaps in burn patients: experiences with 70 flaps in 65 patients. Plast Reconstr Surg 1988;81(3):352–7.

8. Abramson DL, Pribaz JJ, Orgill DP. The use of free tissue transfer in burn reconstruction. J Burn Care Rehabil 1996;17(5):402–8.

9. Sauerbier M, Ofer N, Germann G, et al. Microvascular reconstruction in burn and electrical burn injuries of the severely traumatized upper extremity. Plast Reconstr Surg 2007;119(2):605–15.

10. Schulze SM, Weeks D, Choo J, et al. Amputation following hand escharotomy in patients with burn injury. Eplasty 2016;16:e13.

11. Russell RC, Neumeister MW, Ostric SA, et al. Extremity reconstruction using nonreplantable tissue ("spare parts"). Clin Plast Surg 2007;34(2):211–22, viii.

12. Chew BK, Chew DY, Kirkpatrick JJ, et al. The free thin DIEP flap in microsurgical reconstruction of severe hand contractures following burn injury. J Plast Reconstr Aesthet Surg 2008;61(10): 1266–7.

13. Adani R, Tarallo L, Marcoccio I, et al. Hand reconstruction using the thin anterolateral thigh flap. Plast Reconstr Surg 2005;116(2):467–73.

14. Uygur F, Duman H, Ulkür E, et al. Chronic postburn palmar contractures reconstruction using the medial pedis perforator flap. Ann Plast Surg 2008;61(3): 269–73.

15. Huang QS, Wu X, Zheng HY, et al. Medial plantar flap to repair defects of palm volar skin. Eur J Trauma Emerg Surg 2015;41(3):293–7.

16. Hung MH, Huang KF, Chiu HY, et al. Experience in reconstruction for small digital defects with free flaps. Ann Plast Surg 2016;76(Suppl 1):S48–54.

17. Kempný T, Lipový B, Hokynková A, et al. Wrap-around flap in urgent thumb reconstruction after high-voltage electrical injury. Burns 2012;38(7): e20–3.

18. Kim HD, Hwang SM, Lim KR, et al. Toe tissue transfer for reconstruction of damaged digits due to electrical burns. Arch Plast Surg 2012;39(2): 138–42.

19. Woo SH, Seul JH. Optimizing the correction of severe postburn hand deformities by using aggressive contracture releases and fasciocutaneous free-tissue transfers. Plast Reconstr Surg 2001; 107(1):1–8.

20. Misani M, Zirak C, Hau LT, et al. Release of hand burn contracture: comparing the ALT perforator flap with the gracilis free flap with split skin graft. Burns 2013;39(5):965–71.

21. Uygur F, Duman H, Celiköz B. Use of free anterolateral thigh perforator flap in the treatment of chronic postburn palmar contractures. Burns 2008;34(2): 275–80.

22. Agnew SP, Ko J, De La Garza M, et al. Limb transplantation and targeted reinnervation: a practical comparison. J Reconstr Microsurg 2012;28(1):63–8.

23. Klein HJ, Schanz U, Hivelin M, et al. Sensitization and desensitization of burn patients as potential candidates for vascularized composite allotransplantation. Burns 2016;42(2):24.

Heterotopic Ossification Following Upper Extremity Injury

 CrossMark

Shailesh Agarwal, MD, Shawn Loder, BS, Benjamin Levi, MD*

KEYWORDS

- Heterotopic ossification • Burn injury • Elbow • Upper extremity

KEY POINTS

- Heterotopic ossification (HO) is the formation of ectopic bone within or involving soft tissues, including joint spaces, nerve, and/or muscle.
- HO occurs in patients following trauma, and often develops in the elbows of patients with severe burn injuries, even without direct injury to this anatomic site.
- HO causes restricted motion and subsequent joint contractures, chronic pain, and open wounds.
- Diagnostic approaches to HO are limited primarily to clinical presentation and radiography.
- Prophylactic measures against HO include nonsteroidal antiinflammatory drugs and radiotherapy, although these may have adverse consequences with imperfect outcomes.

INTRODUCTION

Heterotopic ossification (HO) is the pathologic formation of extraskeletal bone within soft tissues or joints. HO occurs in 2 patient populations: those who have severe trauma and those who have genetic mutations in the bone morphogenetic protein (BMP) signaling pathway. The latter are a minority of patients with an extremely debilitating disease process, representing approximately 500 individuals nationwide. However, patients with trauma, including musculoskeletal injury, spinal cord injury (SCI)/traumatic brain injury (TBI), and burns represent a much larger population of patients at risk for HO. Patients with any of these injuries may develop HO in the upper extremities, even if the extremities are uninjured from the initial trauma.

HO presents a substantial barrier to patient recovery after major trauma, burns, and surgical procedures. These patients have often already undergone procedures related to the initial traumatic insult, and may present 6 or more months later with signs that indicate HO, including localized pain or discomfort, reduced range of motion, and open wounds. However, current therapeutic modalities are limited in their ability to prevent HO, and surgical excision to remove the osseous lesion is unable to address chronic sequelae of HO, such as pain and joint contractures. Furthermore, even after successful excision, patients are at risk for recurrence because of the local inflammation caused by surgery.

The elbow is the most common anatomic location of HO in patients with burns, even in the

Disclosures: B. Levi was supported by funding from National Institutes of Health/National Institute of General Medical Sciences grant K08GM109105-0, Plastic Surgery Foundation, the Association for Academic Surgery Roslyn Award, American Association for the Surgery of Trauma Research & Education Foundation Scholarship, and American College of Surgeons Clowes Award. S. Agarwal was supported by the Coller Society Research Fellowship, NIH Loan Repayment Program, National Institutes of Health, F32AR06649901A1, and Plastic Surgery Foundation.
Section of Plastic Surgery, University of Michigan, 1500 East Medical Center Drive, Ann Arbor, MI 48109, USA
* Corresponding author. 1150 West Medical Center Drive, MSRB2 A574, Ann Arbor, MI 48109.
E-mail address: blevi@umich.edu

Hand Clin 33 (2017) 363–373
http://dx.doi.org/10.1016/j.hcl.2016.12.013
0749-0712/17/© 2016 Elsevier Inc. All rights reserved.

absence of burns to the upper extremity.[1–3] However, diagnosis of HO at this site can be particularly challenging, because the elbow can become stiff after trauma because of prolonged inactivity or direct injury. Cognitive decline caused by prolonged sedation can further compromise successful rehabilitation in these patients.[4] Although there are several surgical approaches to remove HO in the upper extremity, none is able to completely restore preinjury function.[5]

EPIDEMIOLOGY AND RISK FACTORS

HO occurs in patients following musculoskeletal injury and extensive burns. A recent review of nearly 3000 patients with burn injuries from 6 high-volume centers found that 3.5% of patients developed HO.[6] Included patients were 18 to 64 years old with total body surface area (TBSA) greater than 20%; 65 years old or older with TBSA 10% or greater; or any patients with burn injury to face/neck, hands, or feet.[6] Patients with the highest odds of developing HO had greater than 30% TBSA burns and patients with upper extremity burns requiring grafting had nearly 100 times higher odds of developing HO. Overall, elbow HO has been reported to occur in 0.1% to 3.3% of patients with burns.[7–9] A systematic review of reports describing excision of HO in the elbow found that 28% (174 out of 626) of cases were in patients with burns, 55% (343 out of 626) of cases were in patients with trauma, and 17% (109/626) were in patients with TBI.[10] Studies of patients with burns have found the elbow to be the most commonly involved joint, with formation approximately 3 months after the initial injury.[1–3] These findings provide further evidence that HO may form in the elbow after a variety of injuries.

In patients with elbow fractures, those who underwent surgery more than 1 week after injury or had mobilization of the elbow delayed by more than 2 weeks were at the highest risk for HO, with 7% (55 out of 786) of patients developing HO.[11] Another review of 124 patients with elbow fractures found clinically relevant HO, defined as being class 2 or greater using the Hastings and Graham classification scheme, in 21% (26 out of 124) of patients.[12]

HO is also reported in the lower limbs of patients with polytrauma, including blast injuries, as in those sustained by military members. A review of injured military personnel with amputations found that more than 60% of the 213 residual limbs had HO.[13] A separate study by the same group found that TBI was associated with HO, as was an increased injury severity score ($\geq$16; odds ratio, 2.2; $P<.05$).[13,14] More than 20% of patients with

SCI have been reported to develop HO.[15,16] Increased systemic inflammation, local spasticity, and prolonged immobilization all place these patients at higher risk, and both preclinical and clinical studies are investigating how controlling these sequelae of trauma may reduce or eliminate HO.[17]

In addition, patients who have had elective orthopedic operations are also at risk for HO, particularly those who have had total hip arthroplasty (THA). One study cited more than 40% of patients developing some form of ectopic bone after THA.[18] More recent studies have reported HO rates ranging from 26% to 58% in THA patients.[19–21] The predictably higher rate of HO in these patients has prompted investigators to test prophylactic measures such as nonsteroidal antiinflammatory drugs (NSAIDs) or radiation therapy to prevent HO or its recurrence, as described later.[22–33]

DIAGNOSIS
Examination

Because of the central role of the elbow in upper extremity movement, HO at this site can cause substantial disability. Signs include limited range of motion, arthritis, pain, stiffness, and swelling. Concomitant symptoms of ulnar nerve compression at the elbow can occur requiring detailed sensory and motor examination of the upper extremity in the ulnar nerve distribution. This examination should include evaluation of 2-point discrimination, documentation of Wartenberg or Froment signs, examination of the intrinsic muscles for atrophy, and testing for Tinel sign over the cubital tunnel.[34] Delayed conduction on nerve conduction studies can provide additional objective data regarding the severity of nerve compression.

Current Imaging Techniques

At present a conclusive diagnosis of HO is based on radiographic imaging. Patients may present with clinical signs or symptoms prompting radiograph imaging (**Fig. 1**). Ectopic bone on radiograph can aid in determining the appropriate approach for excision. Importantly, radiographic imaging modalities are able to detect only the ossified lesion. These imaging modalities do not identify patients who are developing early cartilage deposits that later undergo ossification, nor are they able to identify patients who are at the highest risk for developing HO before even cartilage formation. Therefore, at the time when patients have presented with clinical signs or symptoms prompting radiographic evaluation, the major therapeutic option available to patients is surgical

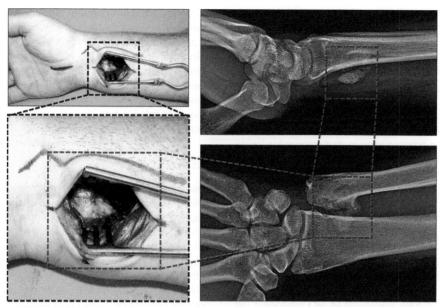

Fig. 1. Operative views and radiography showing HO present in the soft tissue of the wrist.

excision, which is ablative and does not restore function. Radiotherapy or NSAID therapy, which are currently studied for prophylaxis, have not been shown to reduce the size of ossified lesions.

MRI may provide further information regarding the relationship between the ossified lesion and surrounding soft tissue structures. Proximity to nerves can be instructive in determining the risks of surgical excision, and in surgical planning. MRI also allows the identification of surrounding areas of inflammation based on T2 hyperintensity, which indicates edema.

Experimental Imaging Techniques

Alternative techniques for detecting HO lesions before ossification are now in preclinical and clinical investigation. Identification of HO before ossification may allow prophylactic measures to be instituted, such as radiotherapy or NSAIDs, which do not typically affect ossified lesions. One of these modalities is single-photon emission computed tomography (SPECT), which is able to correlate metabolic activity using radioisotope uptake with the presence of osseous lesions (**Fig. 2**). Areas of early HO may be nonossified but have high metabolic activity, indicated by increased uptake of the radioisotope.[35,36] Studies are now underway to determine whether SPECT can guide extent of surgical excision, or whether evidence of metabolic activity can guide therapeutic intervention. Ideally, imaging to identify highly metabolic foci before ossification may provide a prophylactic window. However, this technology

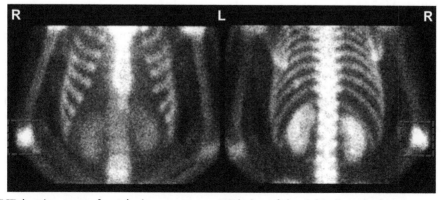

Fig. 2. SPECT showing areas of uptake in a preosseous HO lesion of the right elbow (*red box*).

requires specialized imaging protocols, is time consuming, and does not provide real-time information to guide surgery.

Another clinically available imaging modality that may be useful for the identification of HO is ultrasonography. One study reported that ultrasonography was able to identify HO even before the development of clinical signs.[37] A recent case report describes the use of ultrasonography to identify a heterogeneous, hypervascular lesion that eventually developed into HO. Ultrasonography was even able to identify the lesion 2 weeks before bone scan showed characteristic intense metabolic activity.[37] The changes identified by ultrasonography may represent cartilage that precedes HO, and is identifiable by ultrasonography in other musculoskeletal conditions.[38] Our laboratory is currently studying how ultrasonography findings correspond with specific histologic features during HO formation. Ultimately, a noninvasive point-of-care approach to HO diagnosis, as provided by ultrasonography, would facilitate in-office evaluation of at-risk patients.

Experimental imaging techniques are also being studied in the laboratory for their ability to elucidate tissue changes before ossification. Raman spectroscopy is one such imaging modality that is able to identify spectral changes associated with collagen and early mineral deposition; 2 critical components of osseous lesions (**Fig. 3**).[39] Using a mouse model of HO, the authors found that Raman spectroscopy was able to detect changes associated with HO up to 2 weeks before radiographic evidence in a mouse model.[39] Raman spectroscopy does not require administration of radiotracers and is not invasive, providing another opportunity for point-of-care diagnosis in the office.[40,41] Furthermore, the development of algorithms that

can interpret spectroscopic readings may obviate challenges associated with user expertise as required for ultrasonography.

In addition, despite the numerous imaging modalities that are available clinically, none have been standardized for HO imaging. Some surgeons prefer to rely on physical examination and wait until edema has decreased and scars have optimized before intervention.[4]

PREVENTION

The approach to patients at risk for HO involves both prevention and surgical excision (**Fig. 4**). Because of the variable frequency of HO after trauma, and the potential adverse effects associated with preventive therapy, routine prophylaxis against HO is not standard practice for patients with trauma.

NSAIDs have been shown to be effective for both primary prevention of HO and secondary prevention (after excision) of recurrent HO.[22–28] NSAIDs are thought to prevent HO by reducing inflammation and simultaneously reducing signaling through the BMP pathway. Recent literature suggests that cellular components of the inflammatory response to trauma, including macrophages and neutrophils, can induce osteogenic differentiation through their production and secretion of BMP ligands. Clinical studies have shown that NSAIDs reduce HO after THA procedures.[33,42,43] In a retrospective review of 152 patients who underwent surgical excision for posttraumatic elbow HO, 30.7% (23 out of 75) of untreated patients and 10% (8 out of 77) of celecoxib-treated patients experienced recurrence within 3 months after surgery. These findings persisted at 9 months after injury, when 57% of untreated patients and 26% of celecoxib-treated

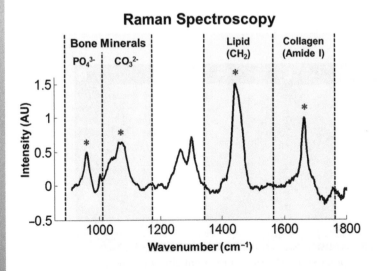

Raman Spectroscopy

Fig. 3. Raman spectroscopy identifies distinct peaks for mineral, lipid, and protein in early/developing HO lesions. AU, arbitrary units. AU, arbitrary units. *Indicates spectral peaks depicting the designated composition. (*Modified from* Peterson JR, Okagbare PI, De La Rosa S, et al. Early detection of burn induced heterotopic ossification using transcutaneous Raman spectroscopy. Bone 2013;54(1):30; with permission.)

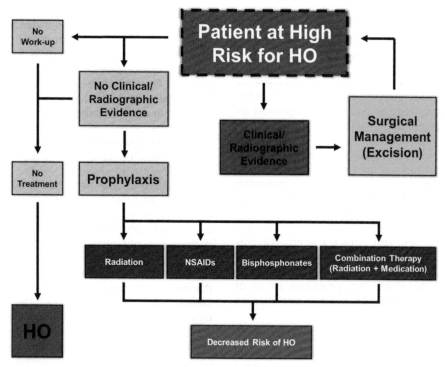

Fig. 4. An approach to surgical and nonsurgical management of HO.

patients had developed recurrence.[44] The protocol reported in that study was daily celecoxib (200 mg) administered for a total of 28 days after surgery.[45] However, use of NSAIDs has consequences, because they may increase the risk of gastrointestinal bleeding, which is already increased in patients with severe musculoskeletal or neurologic injury; proton pump inhibitors can reduce the risk of gastrointestinal bleeding. Furthermore, musculoskeletal injury often includes some component of normal bone injury, such as fractures; however, NSAIDs and selective cyclooxygenase (COX)-2 inhibitors have been shown to reduce fracture healing in patients and animal models.[46,47] The mechanism by which NSAIDs reduce fracture healing remains unclear, although it may be a mechanism similar to its effect on HO: reduced inflammation and BMP signaling. Overall, studies have shown that NSAIDs are a more cost-effective approach to HO prevention than radiotherapy, and do not have inferior results.[28,48]

Radiation therapy has also been extensively studied as a preventive strategy for patients and can be administered either preoperatively or postoperatively.[9,28–33,49–53] With respect to upper extremity HO, radiation has been shown to be effective in the reduction of HO recurrence after initial excision.[9,51,52] One study found that, of 11 cases of elbow HO in patients with burns who underwent excision and radiation therapy within 24 hours after excision, only 1 elbow developed recurrence, with no reported wound-healing complications.[9] Another study reported recurrence in 10% (n = 19) of elbows that underwent initial HO excision with radiation therapy administered within 48 hours after surgery.[50] In another report of 20 patients with excised HO and radiation therapy, 2 (10%) developed recurrent lesions.[52] A recurrence rate of 8% (3 out of 36) was described in another group of patients who had received postoperative radiation therapy after elbow HO excision.[51] These findings suggest that radiation therapy is well tolerated in the perioperative period and that the risk of recurrence after excision with radiation prophylaxis is near 10%. These findings compare favorably with rates of 30% described in other studies without prophylaxis.

In addition, bisphosphonates have been studied for the prevention of HO. Initial double-blinded studies showed a significant reduction in HO after trauma with etidronate treatment.[54] A retrospective review found that patients with burns treated with etidronate had a higher incidence of HO compared with patients who were untreated.[55] In another report, no patients (n = 5) who underwent surgical excision of HO had recurrence after intravenous infusion with the bisphosphonate pamidronate.[56] Treatment was not associated with adverse effects such as osteomalacia or osteoporosis.

SURGICAL MANAGEMENT
Indications

Surgical excision remains a central aspect of HO management, because patients often present after a radiographically identifiable lesion forms. Patients may present with signs or symptoms concerning for HO, including joint arthritis causing pain or restricted motion. Patients may also present with signs of sensory or motor disruption consistent with ulnar nerve disruption. The indications for operative intervention vary among surgeons, but include arthritis with loss of motion more than 30° and pain at the end of arc.[5] Contraindications to operative intervention include inadequate soft tissue envelope, loss of motor function at the elbow that precludes return of function, and inability to perform postexcision rehabilitation.[5]

Approach

Both open and arthroscopic procedures have been described for HO excision. In general, an open approach is recommended for patients with prior fractures or in the setting of prior procedures in which nerve anatomy can be aberrant. Open procedures are also preferred when a large joint contracture needs to be released and soft tissue coverage is necessary, as is often the case in patients who present late. Nerve involvement is best addressed with an open procedure in which decompression of the nerve can be performed.

The surgical approach for open excision has been described through a posterior midline incision to gain access to both the lateral and medial aspects of the elbow and minimize risk to cutaneous nerve branches.[4,57] An incision shifted slightly medially may reduce the risks of wound-healing complications and allow for ulnar nerve decompression; a lateral approach may also minimize wound-healing complications but does not provide access to the ulnar nerve.[58] Other surgeons prefer 2 separate incisions located medially and laterally.[5] Patients with burn injury directly involving the elbow should have incisions placed over the most durable skin that allows access to the elbow.[57] In all instances, thick skin flaps should be raised to avoid skin necrosis and reduce injury to cutaneous nerves during elevation.

Operative Techniques

Restricted flexion may indicate impingement by anterior osteophytes and a tight posterior capsule, whereas loss of extension may be caused by involvement of posterior osteophytes and anterior capsule tightness. Separation of HO from native bone requires identification of a tissue plane, although this may be difficult to identify in some patients. An osteotome or rongeur can be used to separate joined structures, although care must be taken to avoid disrupting the normal bone surface.[57] When anterior HO is removed, the underlying capsule is usually involved and needs to be released, which is not always the case with posterior HO.[57]

Medially, the ulnar nerve is identified, traced proximally and distally freeing it from the scar of the HO, and transposed anteriorly into subcutaneous tissues. Ulnar nerve injury has been reported in these patients, although it is difficult to determine whether this is always caused by excision, or by the underlying disorder.[45] Identification of the nerve well proximal to the elbow joint decreases risk of ulnar nerve injury.[4] The ulnar nerve may be encased in heterotopic bone, requiring careful dissection. The nerve can then be transposed anteriorly into the subcutaneous tissues.[57] Laterally, the posterior interosseous branch of the radial nerve is identified and protected. The radial nerve proper is usually well protected; however, when anterolateral HO is present, the radial nerve can be identified between the brachialis and brachioradialis.[4] The median nerve and brachial artery are usually not encased in HO. However, during dissection of the anterior musculature, the median nerve must be protected.

The anterior or posterior capsule should then be released depending on the patient's primary restriction (extension, anterior; flexion, posterior). Soft tissue coverage may be required for patients with burns if a scar contracture is also released at the same time. Coverage of important structures can be performed using brachioradialis or flexor carpi ulnaris muscle flaps followed by skin grafting.

At the end of the procedure, the elbow is gently manipulated to confirm improved passive range of motion. This manipulation should be done carefully to avoid further injury in a fresh surgical field. Patients are then placed in a dorsal Orthoplast splint overnight with range-of-motion exercises initiated within 24 hours afterward. A complete neurovascular examination should be performed postoperatively to confirm preserved function of all 3 major nerve branches.

Rehabilitation

Rehabilitation protocols vary among published reports. Some advocate early continuous passive motion with additional use of static progressive or dynamic splints after a month postexcision.[58,59] Care must be taken not to perform aggressive range of motion to avoid reinstating the inflammation that was responsible for the heterotopic bone in the first place. Studies are underway to better understand the role of immobilization and range of motion on burn-induced HO as well as postresection HO development.

Outcomes

Preinjury function is rarely restored with HO excision, although range of motion and contractures are generally improved. Most series are single-center case reports and report an improvement of 50° to 110° in arc of motion.[57,60–62] Complications include infection, nerve injury, and recurrence. One systematic review included 33 studies with 626 elbows and reported a mean improvement in arc of motion of 67° (range, 13°–131°).[10] They further stratified data by initial injury type, including trauma, burn, and traumatic brain injury; patients with trauma had the best mean improvement in motion (109°), whereas patients with burns and patients with TBI had reduced improvements (88° and 75° respectively). Fourteen percent of patients (41 out of 299) required reoperation because of residual stiffness from recurrent HO,[31] infection,[5] ulnar fracture,[2] ulnar nerve dysfunction,[2] and brachial artery rupture.[1,10] Because of the risks of postexcision stiffness and HO recurrence, postoperative management is critical to patient recovery. A systematic review of more than 600 elbows that underwent HO excision found a recurrence rate of 20%.[10]

BASIC SCIENCE RESEARCH
Animal Models

HO occurs in a variety of clinical scenarios, which has led to the development of several animal models for preclinical investigation. HO in these models is generally assessed using radiographic means, including radiographs or micro–computed tomography (microCT) scanning. Our laboratory regularly uses the burn/tenotomy model, in which a mouse receives hind-limb Achilles tendon transection and dorsal 30% TBSA burn injury.[63–65] This model is intended to replicate the polytrauma often observed in patients who develop HO. Therapeutic approaches to reduce inflammation caused by the burn injury alone are sufficient to reduce the volume of HO on microCT. In this model, HO forms through endochondral ossification, similar to human HO (**Fig. 5**). Therapeutics such as COX-2 inhibitors that are in clinical investigation also reduce HO in this model (**Fig. 6**).[65]

Military personnel with blast injuries are also at high risk for HO. A group of researchers at the naval academy has developed a rat model of HO in which the hind limb is exposed to high-energy blast followed by transfemoral amputation and bacterial inoculation. These extensive injuries are similar to the conditions experienced by wounded military personnel; in this rat model, HO forms at the site of the transfemoral amputation.[66,67]

Patients with TBI or SCI are also at high risk for developing HO in the hips. Recently, one group found that mice with spinal cord transection develop HO in the gluteal musculature after local injection of cardiotoxin, a chemical agent that induces myonecrosis.[68] Mice that receive cardiotoxin without spinal cord transection do not develop HO. Further studies are required to understand how the spinal cord transection mediates HO formation, and whether this effect is caused by local versus systemic inflammation caused by the SCI.

Other models of HO that have been used include local implantation of BMP-impregnated sponges and transgenic mice with hyperactive BMP receptor activity.[69] BMP-impregnated sponges do not reproduce the clinical scenario encountered by patients with trauma, but may be representative of HO in patients with BMP implants. In addition, transgenic mice with hyperactive BMP receptor activity are used as models of fibrodysplasia ossificans progressiva (FOP). FOP is a genetic condition in which patients develop progressive, painful ectopic osseous lesions after minor trauma. A causative mutation in the type I BMP receptor ACVR1 has been identified in these patients; transgenic mice with this mutated ACVR1 transgene develop HO after local activation of the mutation and injection of cardiotoxin.[70]

These models underscore the variety of clinical scenarios in which HO can develop, ranging from patients with burn and trauma, as in patients who develop upper extremity HO, and those who have genetic mutations. Importantly, genetic mutations or polymorphisms are not thought to underlie the HO seen in patients with trauma.

Therapeutics Under Laboratory Investigation

The animal models described earlier are being evaluated for experimental treatments against trauma-induced HO. The first series of compounds being evaluated are inhibitors of the BMP signaling pathway. These therapeutics, including LDN-193189, are kinase inhibitors that target the type I BMP receptor ACVR1/ALK2.[65,70] The authors have shown efficacy in the burn/tenotomy model, and mechanistic studies to improve

Condensation   Chondrification   Ossification

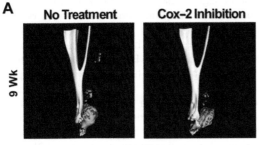

Fig. 5. Histologic progression of HO in a mouse model recapitulates the process of endochondral ossification.

targeting and therapy delivery are in progress.[65] Drugs with improved specificity for BMP receptors are also being designed using LDN-193189 as a structural analogue.

Another series of drugs under investigation are the retinoic acid receptor gamma agonists.[69] These drugs have been shown to block or reduce HO in models of recombinant BMP2 delivery, and

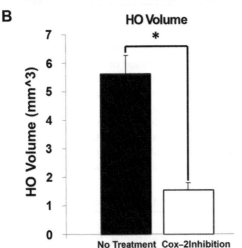

Fig. 6. COX-2 inhibitors decrease the formation of HO in a murine burn-trauma model. (*A*) Representative 3-D microCT images. (*B*) Quantification of HO volume. *p<0.05. (*Adapted from* Peterson JR, De La Rosa S, Eboda O, et al. Treatment of heterotopic ossification through remote ATP hydrolysis. Sci Transl Med 2014;6(255):255ra132. *Reprinted with* permission from AAAS.)

in the transgenic mouse model described earlier. Retinoid signaling is an inhibitor of chondrogenesis, an essential early histologic phase of HO. Although promising, these therapeutics should be used with caution in patients with burns given their detrimental effect on wound healing.

Another group of drugs under investigation are inhibitors of hypoxic signaling. Hypoxia-inducible factor-1α (HIF-1α) is a mediator of hypoxic signaling that upregulates vascular endothelial growth factor to induce angiogenesis. Recently, HIF-1α has been recognized as a mediator of chondrogenesis as well, possibly through activation of the chondrogenic transcription factor SOX9. The authors have recently shown that inhibitors of HIF-1α are able to reduce or block HO after burn/tenotomy and in a transgenic mouse model of hyperactive BMP receptor.[63]

One of the challenges associated with prevention of trauma-induced HO is patient selection. Not all patients who have been in major trauma develop HO, and therefore administering therapeutics indiscriminately risks adverse effects. There is a need to synthesize techniques for early diagnosis with therapies that prevent progression of the lesion. In addition, further studies are required to evaluate the impact of these diseases on overall wound healing. As the clinical appreciation of HO and associated risk factors improves and the laboratory investigations into therapies advance, a directed approach to preventing HO in high-risk populations is anticipated using targeted, effective, and safe drugs.

SUMMARY

HO presents a substantial barrier to rehabilitation for patients with severe burns or trauma. Although surgical excision is a mainstay of management for this condition, this is unable to address the chronic sequelae of HO, including chronic pain, joint contractures, nerve dysfunction, and open wounds. Current therapeutic modalities are aimed at excision and the prevention of recurrence using NSAIDs or radiation therapy. Research is now focused on identifying alternative strategies to prevent the initial occurrence of HO through NSAIDs and novel inhibitors of the BMP signaling pathway.

ACKNOWLEDGMENTS

Collaborate with Boehringer Ingleheim on project not discussed here. We have filed a patent application for the new use of Rapamycin in heterotopic ossification. IP has not yet been licensed.

REFERENCES

1. Orchard GR, Paratz JD, Blot S, et al. Risk factors in hospitalized patients with burn injuries for developing heterotopic ossification–a retrospective analysis. J Burn Care Res 2015;36(4):465–70.
2. Pontell ME, Sparber LS, Chamberlain RS. Corrective and reconstructive surgery in patients with postburn heterotopic ossification and bony ankylosis: an evidence-based approach. J Burn Care Res 2015; 36(1):57–69.
3. Medina A, Shankowsky H, Savaryn B, et al. Characterization of heterotopic ossification in burn patients. J Burn Care Res 2014;35(3):251–6.
4. Ring D, Jupiter JB. Operative release of complete ankylosis of the elbow due to heterotopic bone in patients without severe injury of the central nervous system. J Bone Joint Surg Am 2003;85-A(5):849–57.
5. Adams JE. Elbow contracture and heterotopic ossification. In: Weiss AP, editor. Textbook of hand and upper extremity surgery. Chicago: The American Society for Surgery of the Hand; 2013.
6. Levi B, Jayakumar P, Giladi A, et al. Risk factors for the development of heterotopic ossification in seriously burned adults: a National Institute on Disability, Independent Living and Rehabilitation Research burn model system database analysis. J Trauma Acute Care Surg 2015;79(5):870–6.
7. Elledge ES, Smith AA, McManus WF, et al. Heterotopic bone formation in burned patients. J Trauma 1988;28(5):684–7.
8. Evans EB, Smith JR. Bone and joint changes following burns; a roentgenographic study; preliminary report. J Bone Joint Surg Am 1959;41-A(5):785–99.
9. Maender C, Sahajpal D, Wright TW. Treatment of heterotopic ossification of the elbow following burn injury: recommendations for surgical excision and perioperative prophylaxis using radiation therapy. J Shoulder Elbow Surg 2010;19(8):1269–75.
10. Veltman ES, Lindenhovius AL, Kloen P. Improvements in elbow motion after resection of heterotopic bone: a systematic review. Strategies Trauma Limb Reconstr 2014;9(2):65–71.
11. Bauer AS, Lawson BK, Bliss RL, et al. Risk factors for posttraumatic heterotopic ossification of the elbow: case-control study. J Hand Surg 2012; 37(7):1422–9.e1-6.
12. Hong CC, Nashi N, Hey HW, et al. Clinically relevant heterotopic ossification after elbow fracture surgery: a risk factors study. Orthop Traumatol Surg Res 2015;101(2):209–13.
13. Potter BK, Burns TC, Lacap AP, et al. Heterotopic ossification following traumatic and combat-related amputations. Prevalence, risk factors, and preliminary results of excision. J Bone Joint Surg Am 2007;89(3):476–86.
14. Potter BK, Forsberg JA, Davis TA, et al. Heterotopic ossification following combat-related trauma. J Bone Joint Surg Am 2010;92(Suppl 2):74–89.
15. Reznik JE, Biros E, Marshall R, et al. Prevalence and risk-factors of neurogenic heterotopic ossification in traumatic spinal cord and traumatic brain injured patients admitted to specialised units in Australia. J Musculoskelet Neuronal Interact 2014;14(1):19–28.
16. Wittenberg RH, Peschke U, Botel U. Heterotopic ossification after spinal cord injury. Epidemiology and risk factors. J Bone Joint Surg Br 1992;74(2): 215–8.
17. Citak M, Suero EM, Backhaus M, et al. Risk factors for heterotopic ossification in patients with spinal cord injury: a case-control study of 264 patients. Spine 2012;37(23):1953–7.
18. Maloney WJ, Krushell RJ, Jasty M, et al. Incidence of heterotopic ossification after total hip replacement: effect of the type of fixation of the femoral component. J Bone Joint Surg Am 1991;73(2): 191–3.
19. Back DL, Smith JD, Dalziel RE, et al. Incidence of heterotopic ossification after hip resurfacing. ANZ J Surg 2007;77(8):642–7.
20. Amstutz HC, Beaule PE, Dorey FJ, et al. Metal-on-metal hybrid surface arthroplasty: two to six-year follow-up study. J Bone Joint Surg Am 2004;86-A(1):28–39.
21. Treacy RB, McBryde CW, Pynsent PB. Birmingham hip resurfacing arthroplasty. A minimum follow-up of five years. J Bone Joint Surg Br 2005;87(2):167–70.
22. Rath E, Warschawski Y, Maman E, et al. Selective COX-2 inhibitors significantly reduce the occurrence of heterotopic ossification after hip arthroscopic surgery. Am J Sports Med 2016;44(3):677–81.
23. Oni JK, Pinero JR, Saltzman BM, et al. Effect of a selective COX-2 inhibitor, celecoxib, on heterotopic ossification after total hip arthroplasty: a case-controlled study. Hip Int 2014;24(3):256–62.
24. Vasileiadis GI, Sioutis IC, Mavrogenis AF, et al. COX-2 inhibitors for the prevention of heterotopic ossification after THA. Orthopedics 2011;34(6):467.
25. Xue D, Zheng Q, Li H, et al. Selective COX-2 inhibitor versus nonselective COX-1 and COX-2 inhibitor

in the prevention of heterotopic ossification after to- tal hip arthroplasty: a meta-analysis of randomised trials. Int Orthop 2011;35(1):3–8.

26. Grohs JG, Schmidt M, Wanivenhaus A. Selective COX-2 inhibitor versus indomethacin for the preven- tion of heterotopic ossification after hip replacement: a double-blind randomized trial of 100 patients with 1-year follow-up. Acta Orthop 2007;78(1):95–8.

27. Beckmann JT, Wylie JD, Kapron AL, et al. The effect of NSAID prophylaxis and operative variables on heterotopic ossification after hip arthroscopy. Am J Sports Med 2014;42(6):1359–64.

28. Vavken P, Dorotka R. Economic evaluation of NSAID and radiation to prevent heterotopic ossification af- ter hip surgery. Arch Orthop Trauma Surg 2011; 131(9):1309–15.

29. Seegenschmiedt MH, Makoski HB, Micke O, German Cooperative Group on Radiotherapy for Benign Dis- eases. Radiation prophylaxis for heterotopic ossifica- tion about the hip joint–a multicenter study. Int J Radiat Oncol Biol Phys 2001;51(3):756–65.

30. Seegenschmiedt MH, Keilholz L, Martus P, et al. Pre- vention of heterotopic ossification about the hip: final results of two randomized trials in 410 patients using either preoperative or postoperative radiation ther- apy. Int J Radiat Oncol Biol Phys 1997;39(1):161–71.

31. Seegenschmiedt MH, Goldmann AR, Martus P, et al. Prophylactic radiation therapy for prevention of het- erotopic ossification after hip arthroplasty: results in 141 high-risk hips. Radiology 1993;188(1):257–64.

32. Pellegrini VD Jr. Radiation prophylaxis of heterotopic ossification. Int J Radiat Oncol Biol Phys 1994;30(3): 743–4.

33. D'Lima DD, Venn-Watson EJ, Tripuraneni P, et al. Indomethacin versus radiation therapy for hetero- topic ossification after hip arthroplasty. Orthopedics 2001;24(12):1139–43.

34. Virk MS, Rodner CR. History and physical examina- tion. In: Weiss AP, editor. Textbook of hand and up- per extremity surgery. Chicago: The American Society for Surgery of the Hand; 2013.

35. Lima MC, Passarelli MC, Dario V, et al. The use of SPECT/CT in the evaluation of heterotopic ossification in para/tetraplegics. Acta Ortop Bras 2014;22(1):12–6.

36. Lin Y, Lin WY, Kao CH, et al. Easy interpretation of heterotopic ossification demonstrated on bone SPECT/CT. Clin Nucl Med 2014;39(1):62–3.

37. Lin SH, Chou CL, Chiou HJ. Ultrasonography in early diagnosis of heterotopic ossification. J Med Ultra- sound 2014;22(4):222–7.

38. Podlipska J, Guermazi A, Lehenkari P, et al. Com- parison of diagnostic performance of semi- quantitative knee ultrasound and knee radiography with MRI: Oulu Knee Osteoarthritis Study. Sci Rep 2016;6:22365.

39. Peterson JR, Okagbare PI, De La Rosa S, et al. Early detection of burn induced heterotopic ossification

using transcutaneous Raman spectroscopy. Bone 2013;54(1):28–34.

40. Harris M, Cilwa K, Elster EA, et al. Pilot study for detection of early changes in tissue associated with heterotopic ossification: moving toward clinical use of Raman spectroscopy. Connect Tissue Res 2015;56(2):144–52.

41. Crane NJ, Polfer E, Elster EA, et al. Raman spectro- scopic analysis of combat-related heterotopic ossifi- cation development. Bone 2013;57(2):335–42.

42. Romano CL, Duci D, Romano D, et al. Celecoxib versus indomethacin in the prevention of heterotopic ossification after total hip arthroplasty. J Arthroplasty 2004;19(1):14–8.

43. Tozun R, Pinar H, Yesiller E, et al. Indomethacin for prevention of heterotopic ossification after total hip arthroplasty. J Arthroplasty 1992;7(1):57–61.

44. Sun Y, Cai J, Li F, et al. The efficacy of celecoxib in pre- venting heterotopic ossification recurrence after open arthrolysis for post-traumatic elbow stiffness in adults. J Shoulder Elbow Surg 2015;24(11):1735–40.

45. Lee EK, Namdari S, Hosalkar HS, et al. Clinical re- sults of the excision of heterotopic bone around the elbow: a systematic review. J Shoulder Elbow Surg 2013;22(5):716–22.

46. Spiro AS, Beil FT, Baranowsky A, et al. BMP-7- induced ectopic bone formation and fracture heal- ing is impaired by systemic NSAID application in C57BL/6-mice. J Orthop Res 2010;28(6):785–91.

47. Bauer DC, Orwoll ES, Fox KM, et al. Aspirin and NSAID use in older women: effect on bone mineral density and fracture risk. Study of Osteoporotic Fractures Research Group. J Bone Miner Res 1996;11(1):29–35.

48. Vavken P, Castellani L, Sculco TP. Prophylaxis of het- erotopic ossification of the hip: systematic review and meta-analysis. Clin Orthop Relat Res 2009; 467(12):3283–9.

49. Citak M, Grasmucke D, Cruciger O, et al. Heterotopic ossification of the shoulder joint following spinal cord injury: an analysis of 21 cases after single-dose radia- tion therapy. Spinal Cord 2016;54(4):303–5.

50. Mishra MV, Austin L, Parvizi J, et al. Safety and effi- cacy of radiation therapy as secondary prophylaxis for heterotopic ossification of non-hip joints. J Med Imaging Radiat Oncol 2011;55(3):333–6.

51. Robinson CG, Polster JM, Reddy CA, et al. Postop- erative single-fraction radiation for prevention of het- erotopic ossification of the elbow. Int J Radiat Oncol Biol Phys 2010;77(5):1493–9.

52. Heyd R, Buhleier T, Zamboglou N. Radiation therapy for prevention of heterotopic ossification about the elbow. Strahlenther Onkol 2009;185(8):506–11.

53. Cipriano C, Pill SG, Rosenstock J, et al. Radiation therapy for preventing recurrence of neurogenic het- erotopic ossification. Orthopedics 2009;32(9).

54. Stover SL, Hahn HR, Miller JM 3rd. Disodium etidro- nate in the prevention of heterotopic ossification

following spinal cord injury (preliminary report). Paraplegia 1976;14(2):146–56.

55. Shafer DM, Bay C, Caruso DM, et al. The use of eidronate disodium in the prevention of heterotopic ossification in burn patients. Burns 2008;34(3):355–60.

56. Schuetz P, Mueller B, Christ-Crain M, et al. Amino-bisphosphonates in heterotopic ossification: first experience in five consecutive cases. Spinal Cord 2005;43(10):604–10.

57. Ring D, Jupiter JB. Operative release of ankylosis of the elbow due to heterotopic ossification. Surgical technique. J Bone Joint Surg Am 2004;86-A(Suppl 1):2–10.

58. Lindenhovius AL, Linzel DS, Doornberg JN, et al. Comparison of elbow contracture release in elbows with and without heterotopic ossification restricting motion. J Shoulder Elbow Surg 2007;16(5):621–5.

59. Brouwer KM, Lindenhovius AL, de Witte PB, et al. Resection of heterotopic ossification of the elbow: a comparison of ankylosis and partial restriction. J Hand Surg 2010;35(7):1115–9.

60. Baldwin K, Hosalkar HS, Donegan DJ, et al. Surgical resection of heterotopic bone about the elbow: an institutional experience with traumatic and neurologic etiologies. J Hand Surg 2011;36(5):798–803.

61. Gaur A, Sinclair M, Caruso E, et al. Heterotopic ossification around the elbow following burns in children: results after excision. J Bone Joint Surg Am 2003;85-A(8):1538–43.

62. Salazar D, Golz A, Israel H, et al. Heterotopic ossification of the elbow treated with surgical resection: risk factors, bony ankylosis, and complications. Clin Orthop Relat Res 2014;472(7):2269–75.

63. Agarwal S, Loder S, Brownley C, et al. Inhibition of Hif1alpha prevents both trauma-induced and genetic heterotopic ossification. Proc Natl Acad Sci U S A 2016;113(3):E338–47.

64. Peterson JR, Eboda ON, Brownley RC, et al. Effects of aging on osteogenic response and heterotopic ossification following burn injury in mice. Stem Cells Dev 2015;24(2):205–13.

65. Peterson JR, De La Rosa S, Eboda O, et al. Treatment of heterotopic ossification through remote ATP hydrolysis. Sci Transl Med 2014;6(255):255ra132.

66. Polfer EM, Hope DN, Elster EA, et al. The development of a rat model to investigate the formation of blast-related post-traumatic heterotopic ossification. Bone Joint J 2015;97-B(4):572–6.

67. Pavey GJ, Qureshi AT, Hope DN, et al. Bioburden increases heterotopic ossification formation in an established rat model. Clin Orthop Relat Res 2015;473(9):2840–7.

68. Genet F, Kulina I, Vaquette C, et al. Neurological heterotopic ossification following spinal cord injury is triggered by macrophage-mediated inflammation in muscle. J Pathol 2015;236(2):229–40.

69. Shimono K, Tung WE, Macolino C, et al. Potent inhibition of heterotopic ossification by nuclear retinoic acid receptor-gamma agonists. Nat Med 2011;17(4):454–60.

70. Yu PB, Deng DY, Lai CS, et al. BMP type I receptor inhibition reduces heterotopic [corrected] ossification. Nat Med 2008;14(12):1363–9.

Postburn Contractures of the Elbow and Heterotopic Ossification

 CrossMark

Mary Claire Manske, MD[a],*, Douglas P. Hanel, MD[b]

KEYWORDS

- Elbow contracture • Burn contracture • Heterotopic ossification • Surgical intervention

KEY POINTS

- The elbow is among the most common joints to develop contracture following burn injuries and usually becomes contracted in a flexed position.
- Elbow ankylosis reduces the working area that the hand can reach by 90%.
- Functionally limiting elbow contractures most frequently result from deep burns involving the skin, subcutaneous tissue, tendon, muscle joint capsule, and bone.
- The elbow joint is particularly susceptible to heterotopic ossification, especially at the ulnohumeral joint, which causes a rigid block to motion that is recalcitrant to nonoperative intervention.
- Surgical intervention is aimed at releasing or excision of all pathologic structures limiting motion and should include an ulnar nerve transposition to prevent postoperative ulnar nerve palsy and maximize.

INTRODUCTION

As critical care medicine and the survivorship of patients with severe and life-threatening injuries continue to improve, patients and health care providers are faced with the challenge of managing the long-term sequelae of these severe injuries. This challenge is particularly evident in the care of patients with devastating burn injuries, whose mortality has decreased from 24% in the 1970s to 7% in the early 2000s. This improved survivorship is due to the development of dedicated burn centers.[1–3] However, with increased survival come increased substantial morbidity and disability as a consequence of these injuries. Among the most common and debilitating sequelae of burn injuries are joint contractures. They develop in approximately one-third of burn patients[4–6] and limit the joint motion necessary to perform activities of daily living, occupational obligations, and recreational pursuits. Upper extremity contractures constitute most burn contractures (72%), with the elbow being among the most commonly involved joints (34%).[4] Despite appropriate wound care, physical therapy, and early surgical intervention in the acute setting, functionally limiting elbow contractures still occur and often require additional surgical management.

This article reviews the pathophysiology and pathoanatomy of postburn contractures of the elbow as well as the clinical evaluation, treatment, and outcomes of these challenging deformities, with a particular emphasis on elbow contractures resulting from involvement of subcutaneous structures and heterotopic ossification.

[a] Hand and Microvascular Surgery, Department of Orthopedic Surgery, Harborview Medical Center, University of Washington, 325 Ninth Avenue, Seattle, WA 98102, USA; [b] Hand and Upper Extremity Surgery, Department of Orthopedic Surgery, Harborview Medical Center, University of Washington, 325 Ninth Avenue, Seattle, WA 98102, USA
* Corresponding author.
E-mail address: mclairemanske@gmail.com

Hand Clin 33 (2017) 375–388
http://dx.doi.org/10.1016/j.hcl.2016.12.014
0749-0712/17/© 2017 Elsevier Inc. All rights reserved.

PATHOPHYSIOLOGY OF CONTRACTURE DEVELOPMENT

The propensity of a burn wound to develop a contracture is influenced by several factors, including severity of injury (both depth and extent) and the duration of wound healing.

Severity of Soft Tissue Injury

Depth of tissue injury

The risk and severity of scarring and contracture are in part determined by the depth of the burn injury, which is classified into 4 broad categories (**Table 1**).[7]

Superficial and superficial partial thickness burns involve the epidermis or the epidermis and papillary (superficial) dermis, respectively. Because the dermal appendages are intact, these injuries are capable of regenerative healing due to the migration of keratinocytes from the dermal appendages as well as collage deposition from the superficial fibroblasts from the papillary dermis. Consequently, these wounds reliably heal with little to no scarring in 5 to 14 days and do not result in contractures.[7,8] By contrast, deep partial-thickness and full-thickness burns injure the reticular dermis (deep dermal layer), including the dermal appendages, and are incapable of skin regeneration.[9–11] In contrast to superficial burns, deep injuries heal by scar formation from deep dermal fibroblasts. In comparison to the superficial dermal fibroblasts in the papillary dermis, the deep dermal fibroblasts from the reticular dermis produce more collagen[12]; proliferate more slowly[13]; have less collagenase[14]; and produce more α-smooth muscle actin compared with superficial fibroblasts.[8] In this regard, deep dermal fibroblasts resemble fibroblasts found in hypertrophic scar, which is observed in 32% to 94% of burn injuries.[11,15–17] Moreover, with increased burn depth, signaling pathways initiating the conversion of fibroblasts to myofibroblasts (associated with wound contracture and hypertrophic scar) are activated.[11] Thus, injuries involving the deep dermis often lead to the development of dense, hypertrophic scarring, which can result in joint deformity, especially when the burned tissue lies directly over a joint.

Fourth-degree burn injuries are those that penetrate into the subcutaneous tissue and underlying structures, including muscles, tendons, joints, and bones. In addition to the contracture resulting from skin involvement, fibrosis of myotendinous structures, scarring of the joint capsule, and formation of heterotopic bone contribute to the development of more severe joint deformity and limitations in range of motion.

Heterotopic ossification, a condition in which mature lamellar bone develops in tissue that does not normally ossify, is an uncommon but debilitating complication of burn injuries, occurring in 1% to 3% of patients.[18] Although the cause and pathogenesis of heterotopic ossification have not been completely elucidated, postburn ectopic bone formation has been associated with greater depth of injury,[19] increased time to wound coverage,[20] the number of ventilator days, the number of trips to the operating room,[21] and greater than 20% total body surface area (TBSA) burned, in particular, arm and forearm burns that require grafts.

EXTENT OF BURN INJURY

Burn injury size has been correlated with contracture development. Both TBSA of burned tissue and TBSA requiring skin grafting are predictors of contracture development.[4] Although greater than 20% TBSA involved by burn injury is often cited as the threshold for increased risk of contracture development, functionally limiting joint contractures have been reported in patients with as little as 8% TBSA involved.[22] In addition to the risk of developing contractures, increased TBSA requiring skin graft is associated with the *severity*

Table 1 Depth of burn injury			
Degree	**Depth**	**Layers Affected**	**Healing Time**
First degree	Superficial	Epidermis only	Within 7 d
Second degree A	Superficial partial	Papillary dermis	1–3 wk
Second degree B	Deep partial	Reticular dermis	>3 wk
Third	Full thickness	Full thickness of dermis, may extend into subcutaneous fat	Does not heal spontaneously
Fourth		Subcutaneous fat, muscle, tendon, joint (variable)	Does not heal spontaneously

Modified from Evers LH, Bhavsar D, Mailänder P. The biology of burn injury. Exp Dermatol 2010;19(9):778.

of contracture development,[4] reflecting the cumulative effect of depth and breadth of burn injury.

The association between TBSA and contracture development is likely multifactorial, because greater TBSA is found in conjunction with other indicators of injury severity that are also risk factors for contracture development, including inhalational injury, depth of burn injury, duration of immobilization, and duration of hospitalization. Nevertheless, there may also be a cellular basis for this association, as larger burns (increased TBSA) are strongly correlated with myofibroblast development; larger burn wounds have a higher percentage of contractile myofibroblasts, which are known to cause wound contraction and hypertrophic scarring.[16]

DURATION OF HEALING AND TIME TO WOUND COVERAGE

Another factor affecting scar and contracture development is the duration of healing. Burn wounds heal in 3 phases: inflammatory, proliferative, and remodeling. All but the duration of these phases is variable and modifiable. Factors that prolong inflammatory and proliferative phases result in increased scarring and contracture development.

Depth of Injury

Deep partial thickness and full thickness injuries are associated with an extended duration of inflammation and proliferation compared with more superficial burns.[11] This prolonged inflammatory phase results from delayed apoptosis of fibroblasts and myofibroblasts, which leads to imbalanced and excessive collagen deposition, wound contraction, and hypertrophic scarring.[23]

Infection

Infection also prolongs the inflammatory phase. Several mechanisms contribute to this, including the increase in inflammatory cells required to fight the infection, and the ability of infection to convert superficial wounds to partial- or full-thickness wounds. Finally, active infection delays time to definitive wound coverage.[18]

Tension

An additional factor extending the inflammation and cellular proliferation is excessive wound tension. Nearly all deep burn wounds have some element of skin tension resulting from wound contracture and deficiency of skin, for which early physical therapy is often indicated. However, when the soft tissue envelope is unstable, aggressive physical therapy leads to skin breakdown, prolonged inflammation, and a vigorous scar response.[18] In addition, increased tension on wounds causes mechanical stimuli that induce the conversion of fibroblasts to myofibroblasts. Myofibroblasts are associated with wound contraction and hypertrophic scars.[11]

Early Wound Coverage

Early wound coverage has been reported to decrease the duration of inflammation, induce fibroblast apoptosis, and reduce the incidence and severity of scarring.[24,25] Moreover, early wound coverage decreases the risk of infection and decreases the incidence of heterotopic bone formation.[20] Consequently, in the acute phase of burn injuries, surgical intervention (often with excision of deeply burned tissue and skin grafting or flap coverage) is often used to treat deep burn wounds, because these are unlikely to heal spontaneously in less than 2 to 3 weeks. Early wound coverage takes tension off the injured tissue by replacing it with healthy tissue, decreases the risk of infection, and, in the case of skin grafting, shifts the mechanism of healing from healing by secondary intention to healing by primary intention by migration of keratinocytes from intact dermal appendages in the interstices of the skin graft.

PATHOANATOMY OF POSTBURN ELBOW CONTRACTURES

The elbow is among the most common joints affected by postburn contractures, second only to the shoulder, and most commonly results in limited flexion-extension arc of motion. Deformity in this plane of motion results from several anatomic factors, including the following:

- The relative strength of the elbow flexors compared with the elbow extensors (limits extension)
- The tendency to hold the elbow flexed in a position of comfort following injury (limits extension)
- Involvement of the antecubital fossa causes scarring of the anterior elbow structures (limits extension)
- Heterotopic bone formation involving the ulnohumeral joint (limits both flexion and extension)

Because of the numerous functional structures in the elbow, patients with deep burn injuries to the upper extremities develop elbow contractures from the involvement of several structures, including hypertrophic skin scarring, fibrosis of musculotendinous structures, thickening of the joint capsule, and heterotopic ossification. For reasons that have not been elucidated, the elbow joint is particularly susceptible to heterotopic ossification and is the most commonly involved joint when periarticular ectopic ossification develops.[22,26,27] Postburn heterotopic ossification about the elbow most commonly affects the ulnohumeral joint, usually along the posteromedial aspect in close proximity to the ulnar nerve and may cause ulnar nerve dysfunction.[26] Although ectopic ossification may develop in joints distant from the site of burn injuries, periarticular ossification severe enough to cause functionally limiting joint motion usually occurs in association with areas of deep burns, wounds complicated by hypertrophic scarring, prolonged immobilization, wound infection, delayed wound closure, and recurring local trauma (including aggressive passive range of motion).[26]

PREOPERATIVE EVALUATION
History

Preoperative evaluation begins by determining a patient's principal concern. Patients with postburn elbow contractures typically present with stiffness and limited range of motion of the elbow affecting activities of daily living. Pain may be present at the end range of motion secondary to tension on contracted tissue, but typically is not present in the midarc of motion. In addition, patients with postburn elbow contractures secondary to heterotopic ossification often report elbow swelling, a palpable mass, or symptoms of ulnar nerve dysfunction (numbness, parasthesias, clumsiness with the hand, hand weakness, atrophy).[26] If not spontaneously reported by the patient, providers should specifically inquire about neurologic symptoms, including numbness, paresthesias, and motor weakness, to determine the presence of peripheral nerve compression.

In addition to the patient's concerns, a thorough understanding of the original injury, including the mechanism of thermal injury (flame, contact, electrical), extent of burn injury (TBSA involved, inhalation injury), and previous treatments, including physical therapy and surgical procedures (prior skin graft or flap coverage), allows surgeons to determine the structures involved in the contracture development, establish an appropriate treatment plan to address all elements of abnormality, anticipate intraoperative findings, and avoid complications. In addition, any history of neurologic deficit, both peripheral and central, is important to elucidate because it may influence surgical treatment or the ability to participate in postoperative rehabilitation. In particular, surgeons should

inquire about paresthesias or motor deficits that may indicate a compressive peripheral neuropathy. Finally, the patient's occupation, recreational activities, and postoperative goals should be discussed to determine their expectations and functional demands as well as to establish realistic postoperative goals.

Examination

On clinical examination, the clinician should assess the status of the soft tissue envelope and note the location of previous scars, skin grafts, and flaps. It may be helpful to classify skin contractures as described by Cartotto and colleagues[28] (linear or diffuse) or as described by Stern and colleagues[29] (simple band, complex band, diffuse scar, or limited scar), because this aids in surgical planning and has prognostic implications. In addition, the quality of the surrounding tissue should be assessed to determine options for reconstruction of soft tissue deficits, if required.

Palpation of the burned area is used to determine the depth of tissue involvement and distinguish superficial contractures from deep contractures. Superficial contractures are identified by the presence of soft pliable subcutaneous tissues underlying the thickened hypertrophic skin.[18] In contrast, deep tissue contractures resulting from subcutaneous fibrosis, contracted tendons and muscle, and joint capsule thickening are distinguished by the immobility of the subcutaneous tissues on palpation and firmer endpoint with forced passive extension. In cases of periarticular ectopic ossification causing limited motion, there is often a hard stop to passive motion and severe joint contraction, with or without the presence of a palpable bony prominence or mass.[18]

A goniometer should be used to quantify both active and passive flexion and extension as well as forearm pronation and supination. Finally, it is important to perform and document a thorough neurovascular examination, principally to assess ulnar nerve function, and to compare postoperative findings with the preoperative evaluation. Sensation should be objectively documented with 2-point discrimination or monofilament testing. Motor function should be quantified on a 5-point scale. If sensory or motor dysfunction is present on examination, electrodiagnostic studies should be obtained before surgery.

Additional Studies

In cases of suspected heterotopic ossification, anteroposterior (AP), lateral, and oblique radiographs of the elbow and AP and lateral radiographs of the forearm should be obtained to identify the extent of ectopic ossification and determine whether the ossification is mature, as indicated by well-defined cortical margins (**Fig. 1**).

An axial computed tomographic (CT) scan of the elbow and forearm with coronal and sagittal reformatted images is used to define the location of heterotopic ossification and aids in surgical planning. Three-dimensional reconstructions of CT imaging can be helpful, but are not routinely required. Bone scans are not helpful; they will be positive for years after burn trauma and provide no information that will direct treatment.

If there are concerns about the integrity of the blood supply to the soft tissue envelope or a pedicle interposition flap is being considered, Doppler ultrasound, angiography, or vascular studies of the elbow and proximal forearm may be obtained to determine if the surgical plan is viable.

Unless there is concern for infection, the authors do not routinely obtain tests to assess infection or inflammatory status (complete blood count, erythrocyte sedimentation rate, C-reactive protein, joint aspiration). They do obtain preoperative laboratory tests for the patient undergoing prolonged general anesthesia.

TREATMENT
Nonoperative

For patients with elbow contractures caused principally by soft tissue scarring, physical therapy is an appropriate initial treatment. Interventions provided by a therapist include the following:

- Pressure garments for edema control
- Silicone for scar softening
- Splinting, static, and/or dynamic
- Active and gentle passive range-of-motion exercises

With elbow contractures resulting from heterotopic ossification, stretching, splinting, and range-of-motion exercises are rarely effective in improving range of motion and, instead, may exacerbate scarring, pain, and patient frustration.[18] Although edema control and scar softening are recommended, the authors do not advocate a prolonged course of stretching and range-of-motion exercises in patients with heterotopic ossification limiting motion.

Operative

Indications and contraindications
Surgery is indicated for elbow contractures causing functional limitations, including superficial contractures that persist despite nonoperative interventions and deep contractures resulting from deep tissue fibrosis or ectopic ossification that are not amenable to physical therapy. Normal elbow arc of motion is from 0° (full extension) to 145° flexion, although most activities of daily living are performed within an arc of motion from 30° to 130°.[30] Any decrease in this 100° functional arc of motion should prompt consideration of surgical intervention (**Fig. 2**).

Surgery may be contraindicated in several situations. Operative intervention should not proceed in the setting of active infection. Surgery addressing heterotopic ossification is more often dictated by scar maturation than ossification of heterotrophic bone. The authors do not think that failure of mature ossification, as demonstrated by the presence of

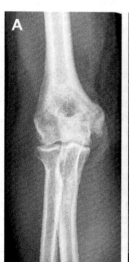
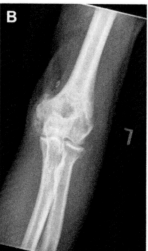
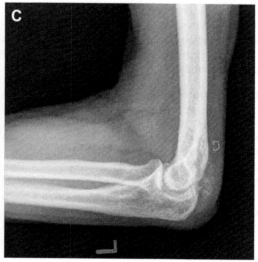

Fig. 1. (*A–C*) Radiographs demonstrating posteromedial heterotopic ossification involving the ulnohumeral joint in a patient with left upper extremity burn injury.

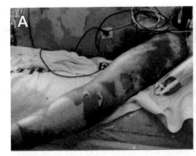
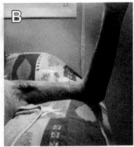
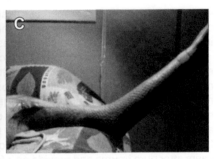

Fig. 2. (*A*) Acute left upper extremity full-thickness burns. (*B, C*) Preoperative limitations in flexion and extension in a patient with an elbow contracture following a burn injury involving greater than 60% TBSA.

well-rounded cortical edges and cessation of progressive expansion on radiographs, is a contraindication to excision. They do recognize that in the setting of burn care, very few patients come to their service with immature ectopic bone. Additional contraindications to surgery include inability to participate in postoperative rehabilitation, comorbid medical conditions precluding surgery, and symptoms insufficiently bothersome to warrant surgery.

Timing of surgical intervention
The timing of surgical intervention depends on the structures involved in the contracture.

Superficial contractures The timing of surgery for contractures secondary to skin contraction or hypertrophic scarring is controversial. Traditionally, many surgeons have recommended waiting until the scar tissue has fully matured and improvements with physical therapy have plateaued, usually about 9 to 12 months following the injury.[31] Others have advocated for earlier intervention, based on evidence of similar outcomes in patients undergoing early release (less than 1 year following injury) compared with later release (>1 year) and no adverse consequence of earlier surgical intervention.[32] Indications for early surgical interventions include unstable wounds or scars under significant tension that cause scar hypertrophy or secondary contractures.

Deep contractures Early surgical intervention is recommended for elbow contractures resulting from fibrosis of deep structures (muscle, fascia, tendons) or heterotopic ossification, because these are often recalcitrant to therapy. In particular, patients with elbow contractures secondary to heterotopic ossification should undergo surgical intervention as soon as the ossification is mature on radiographs (corticated margins, stable size, and appearance on serial radiographs), to prevent secondary contractures of adjacent soft tissues. This maturation of the ossification may occur as early as 4 months following injury. Similarly, patients with ulnar nerve dysfunction secondary to

compression by soft tissue contracture or heterotopic ossification should also undergo early surgical intervention to prevent permanent neurologic deficit.

SURGICAL INTERVENTION

Surgical intervention is aimed at releasing all pathologic structures impairing motion and covering soft tissue defects. In addition, procedures that increase elbow extension should include anterior transposition of the ulnar nerve, to prevent secondary tension on the nerve following elbow release.

Factors guiding surgical intervention include depth of injured tissue (ie, degree of burn injury), breadth of involved tissue (linear vs diffuse), the quality of the surrounding tissue, and severity of joint contracture (>or <50% of motion) (**Fig. 3**).[33]

Superficial Linear Contractures

A superficial linear contracture is a well-defined narrow band of scar surrounded by adjacent pliable tissue. Isolated scar bands causing mild contracture (less than 50% loss of range of motion) are amenable to procedures that lengthen the contracted tissue by rearranging the local tissue to allow unaffected tissues to break up the scar, such as a Z-plasty, V-Y advancement, or one of their variants.[33] Z-plasties may safely be used in scarred skin so long as full-thickness flaps of skin and subcutaneous tissue are raised; rounded (rather than pointed) tips of the flaps are designed, and flaps are not closed under tension.[28] Often, linear scars across the antecubital fossa are not amenable to a single large ("classic") Z-plasty because the flaps are too large.[34] However, a compound Z-plasty, consisting of multiple Z-plasties in a series, results in lengthening similar to a single large Z-plasty. With smaller flaps, there is less tension on the individual flaps, and less transverse shortening. The 4-flap or 5-flap Z-plasty is particularly useful to re-create the concavity of the antecubital fossa. Alternatively, when there is supple, pliable skin on one side of a narrow scar

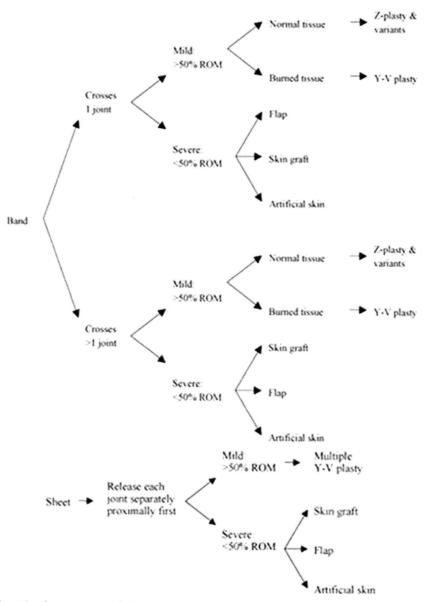

Fig. 3. An algorithm for treatment of elbow contracture release. ROM, range of motion. (*Modified from* Hudson DA, Renshaw A. An algorithm for the release of burn contractures of the extremities. Burns 2006;32(6):667–8; with permission.)

contracture, a three-fourth Z-plasty may be used, in which the longitudinal band is divided and a local flap of mobile supple tissue is interposed.[28]

Alternatives to Z-plasty scar reconstruction include V-Y advancement and its modifications, such as the double-reverse V-Y advancement, V-M plasty, V-W plasty.[35] More complicated local tissue arrangement, such as the 7 flap-plasty, trapeze flap-plasty, or rhomboid flap,[18] are technically more demanding in their design but may provide better effacement of contracture webbing and improve the contour of the antecubital fossa.

When superficial linear contractures result in severe limitations in elbow range of motion, local tissue rearrangement is rarely sufficient to restore motion and cover the soft tissue deficit. In these situations, thick skin grafts, local or distant flap coverage, or artificial skin is typically required.

Superficial Diffuse Contractures

Diffuse superficial contractures of the elbow are broader than linear contractures, forming sheets of scar across the antecubital fossa and beyond.

Because of the more extensive surface area involved, release of even mild contractures (<50% loss of motion) results in a large soft tissue defect that cannot be closed completely with local tissues.

These contractures are best managed with division of the contracture and soft tissue coverage of the resultant skin defect. Depending on the configuration of the contracted skin, serial Z-plasties, multiple V-Y advancements, or a transverse incision with a dart (or fishtail) incision at the end can be made across the point of maximal tension. The location of the incision may be modified to accommodate local anatomy and, in severe or especially broad contractures, more than one incision may be required.[28]

The technique for soft tissue coverage is influenced by the dimensions of the wound, exposure of vital structures (neurovascular structures, tendon, joint), availability of uninjured local tissue, and surgeon preference. Options for coverage are listed in **Table 2**.

Deep Contractures

Deep contractures result from scarring and fibrosis deep to the dermis and often involve heterotopic ossification of the periarticular tissue. The goal of surgical intervention is to excise all impediments to elbow motion and minimize risk of recurrence. Although the specific surgical techniques vary based on the abnormality to be

addressed, the potential anatomic components of deep contracture release include the following:

1. Release of skin contractures and hypertrophic scar
2. Biceps tendon lengthening and myotomy of fibrosed musculature
3. Anterior and posterior joint capsule release
4. Excision of heterotopic bone
5. Decompression and transposition of the ulnar nerve
6. Assess elbow stability and repair/reconstruct collateral ligaments if necessary
7. Soft tissue coverage as needed

SURGICAL TECHNIQUE OF DEEP CONTRACTURE RELEASE
Patient Positioning

The patient is positioned supine on a well-padded operating table. Either a general anesthetic or brachial plexus block may be used. The limb is abducted from the torso and placed on a hand table. If the shoulder is mobile, external rotation provides access to the medial and anterior elbow while internal rotation allows access to the posterior and lateral elbow.

The extremity is then prepped and draped from the fingertips to the axilla. The authors prefer not to use a tourniquet, because it limits tissue mobilization, causes venous engorgement during prolonged cases, obscures small vessel bleeding, and causes reactive hyperemia when the tourniquet is deflated. Rather, they inject the planned incision with local anesthetic mixed with 1/200,000 epinephrine after the limb is prepped, which provides excellent hemostasis when the injection is performed approximately 20 minutes before skin incision.

Incision

Like all such cases, the choice of skin incision is influenced by the location of heterotopic ossification, previous incisions, and skin graft scars. Ideally, existing incisions are incorporated into the surgical approach, but in those cases where there is circumferential scarring, medial and lateral incisions are centered on the midaxis of the arm and forearm. The incision is started at the easily palpated epicondyles and extended proximally along the shaft of the humerus and distally along the anterior to the ulna medially and 2 to 3 cm anterior to the ulna laterally.

In the event of previous soft tissue coverage of the elbow, skin grafts may be incised or raised after they are well-healed; free and pedicled flaps may be safely raised as early as 2 to 3 months

Table 2 Options for soft tissue coverage following elbow contracture release	
Skin graft	Full thickness
	Split thickness
Local fascial, fasciocutaneous, or axial pedicle flaps	Random 3:1 fasciocutaneous
	Radial artery
	Ulnar artery
	Posterior interosseous artery
	Lateral arm flap
	Medial arm flap
Local muscle flap	Flexor carpi ulnaris
	Brachioradialis
Regional pedicled flap	Latissimus dorsi
	Serratus anterior
	Extended lateral arm
Free tissue transfer	Anterolateral thigh
	Gracilis
	Rectus abdominus
	Contralateral radial forearm
	Latissimus dorsi

following tissue transfer as long as they are well healed, although the authors avoid making incisions over the axial vessel of a pedicled or free flap.

In those cases where the scarring is so supple that mobilization will allow direct closure or so severe that coverage will require pedicled or free flaps, a posterior skin incision is a utilitarian approach that provides circumferential access to the medial, lateral, anterior, and posterior elbow. Most commonly, the heterotopic ossification is localized to the posteromedial elbow, in which case, a posteromedial incision over the course of the ulnar nerve is used (**Fig. 4**). An anterior approach to the elbow for heterotopic ossification excision may be used when there is an existing soft tissue defect anteriorly, which will be addressed at the time of contracture release or for elbow contractures resulting from isolated anterior elbow abnormality with no evidence of abnormality elsewhere.

Posterior Approach

The posterior approach begins with a longitudinal skin incision along the posterior arm, curving the incision just medial or lateral to the olecranon tip, extending distally along the subcutaneous border of the ulnar. Full-thickness medial and lateral skin flaps are elevated from the triceps fascia and to the extensor fascia along the subcutaneous border of the ulna distally with care to identify and protect the ulnar nerve medially.

Medial Heterotopic Bone Excision

Using the incision described above, the ulnar nerve is identified proximally in the arm outside of the zone of scarring and ossification and followed distally through the cubital tunnel and 2 heads of flexor carpi ulnaris. All constricting structures are released, including heterotopic ossification that may be encasing the nerve (**Fig. 5**), using Freer elevators, synovial and Kerrison

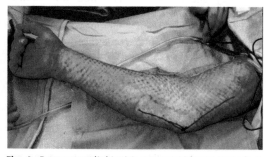

Fig. 4. Posteromedial incision to provide access to heterotopic ossification involving the ulnohumeral joint causing limited motion and ulnar nerve dysfunction.

rongeurs, and osteotomes. The nerve is then mobilized from the cubital tunnel. The medial intermuscular septum is identified and traced along its attachment to the humerus and excised. Crossing vessels are either suture ligated or cauterized. The interval between the brachialis and anterior elbow capsule with its associated ectopic ossification is developed; the median nerve and brachial artery are protected, and the ectopic bone is removed. As the flexor-pronator mass is elevated from the medial epicondyle and proximal ulna, care should be taken to preserve the medial collateral ligament (MCL) if possible, especially the anterior band, which lies deep the flexor capri ulnaris. Doing so prevents elbow instability; in chronic severe contractures, release of the posterior band of the MCL may be indicated.

Contracted anterior capsule should be excised with the heterotopic bone. When the coronoid fossa is encountered, it should be cleared of fat and synovium. As the excision proceeds radially, the radial nerve is at risk in the depth of the exposure; if lateral heterotopic ossification requires excision, a lateral approach should be used so that the radial nerve can be identified and protected during ectopic bone excision.

Any procedure that results in increased elbow flexion should include an anterior transposition of the ulnar nerve. The ulnar nerve is encased in scar, and improved elbow motion risks increased traction on the ulnar nerve postoperatively. If a submuscular ulnar nerve transposition is performed, the median nerve must be exposed. The median nerve is exposed by isolating the medial intermuscular septum and identifying the median nerve along the anterior and superior surface of the septum. The nerve is followed distally to the antecubital fossa. Another approach to the median nerve is to find it in the antecubital fossa. The lacertus fibrosis is identified and incised in line with the leading edge of the pronator teres until the biceps tendon is encountered. With blunt finger dissection, the pulse of the brachial artery is palpated and the median nerve is identified medial to the artery. Frequently, the anterior investing fascia of the arm is densely scarred and incised along the course of the median nerve.

Tendon and Muscle Release

The fascia of the biceps and brachialis muscle is often fibrosed and released with several transverse incisions through the anterior epimysium. Tenolysis of the biceps tendon should be performed if there are adhesions limiting motion. If this does not improve elbow extension, steplengthening of the biceps tendon and/or a

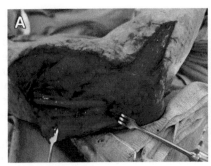 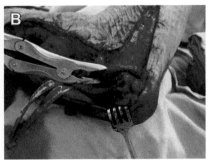

Fig. 5. (*A*) Ulnar nerve encased in heterotopic ossification. (*B*) Excision of heterotopic ossification surrounding the ulnar nerve.

brachialis myotomy may be performed. Rarely, full motion may not be achieved because of the contracture of the neurovascular structures.

Lateral Exposure

If the heterotopic ossification involves the lateralmost aspect of the radiocapitellar joint, a lateral column approach proximally and Kocher or Kaplan approach distally are used to expose the elbow joint. In the proximal aspect of the surgical field, the brachioradialis and extensor carpi radialis longus are identified and elevated from the supracondylar ridge and lateral epicondyle to expose the underlying brachialis. The radial nerve can be identified and protected through this exposure. In densely scarred tissue, the radial nerve may not be easily identified in these intervals. To locate the nerve, the posterior surface of lateral intermuscular septum is identified at the lateral epicondyle and followed proximally by carefully releasing the triceps muscle off the septum. Branches of the radial nerve (lateral brachial cutaneous nerve, posterior antebrachial cutaneous nerve) are identified as they cross the septum and traced back to the radial nerve as it pierces the septum between 6 and 10 cm proximal to the lateral epicondyle.

The capsule is incised along the anterior border of the lateral ulnar collateral ligament, and the proximal fibers of the supinator are elevated subperiosteally. As long as the dissection remains subperiosteal, the posterior interosseous nerve is protected within the substance of the supinator as it crosses the radial neck 3 to 4 cm distal to the radiocapitellar joint.

As heterotopic bone is encountered, the capsule and heterotopic bone are excised in continuity. Dissection proceeds medially until the coronoid is encountered. The authors find it helpful to place a blunt right-angled retractor in the interval between the brachialis muscle and the underlying capsule to allow direct visualization of the heterotopic ossification and minimize the risk of neurovascular injury.

Posterior Exposure

When needed, the posterior elbow is approached from the lateral side by elevating the triceps from the lateral column and posterior humerus. With care to preserve the triceps insertion on the olecranon, the interval between the triceps and posterior joint capsule is developed with blunt elevator. Care should be taken not to injure the radial nerve, which crosses the posterior humerus 11 cm proximal to the lateral epicondyle, when using a blunt elevator to release the triceps off the distal humerus. The posterior capsule and heterotopic ossification are excised from the olecranon fossa. If necessary, the posteromedial elbow can be approached by working on the medial side of the triceps and incising the posterior band of the MCL to access the medial side of the posterior elbow joint.

Closure

Before wound closure, elbow stability should be assessed. If either the medial or the lateral collateral ligaments were released during the procedure, they should be reconstructed with tendon allograft (palmaris or plantaris) and secured with suture anchors or bone tunnels. Of particular importance are the anterior band of the MCL and the ulnar lateral collateral ligament. If stability cannot be restored with ligament reconstruction, mechanical joint fixation with either an internal or an external joint fixator should be considered.

After thorough irrigation, a closed suction drain is placed. In addition, continuous infusion pumps delivering local anesthetic may be placed to augment postoperative pain control, but the authors do not use them. Muscle attachments are repaired to bone with suture passed through interosseous tunnels or suture anchors. The ulnar nerve should be transposed anterior in a subcutaneous or submuscular fashion. Skin should not be closed under tension. In those cases where midaxial incisions have been used successfully, the wounds can be closed, and it should be noted that the tension of the wound closure is not affected by elbow position. If a posterior or anterior incision has been used, then excessive stress will lead to wound disruption in flexion in the case of a posterior wound and in extension with an anterior wound. This excessive stress is quite obvious at the time of closure and, when encountered, will require the surgeon to perform local flaps, pedicled flaps and, in the most severe cases, free tissue transfer to accommodate the elbow release.

A sterile soft dressing is applied to the wound; the limb is immobilized in a resting splint, and motion exercises are started on the first day postoperatively (**Fig. 6**).

POSTOPERATIVE MANAGEMENT

Range-of-motion exercises are initiated on the first postoperative day. Pain is palliated with regional anesthesia delivered to the brachial plexus using indwelling catheter infusion for 2 days. Continuous passive motion is used for those 2 days. When the block has worn off, active and active-assisted range-of-motion exercises are initiated. Static progressive splints are used and are worn continuously for 2 weeks except when performing exercises. After 2 weeks, nighttime splinting in the position of the greatest loss of motion replaces alternating flexion and extension splints. Strengthening exercises are initiated a 6 weeks postoperatively. Splinting and exercises are continued for 6 months postoperatively, after which there does not appear to be any improvement in range of motion. Anecdotally, however, patients often report that even though their range of motion does not quantitatively improve beyond 6 months, their strength, ease of motion, and functional gains continue for up to 2 years.

Both pharmacologic and radiologic treatments have been described to decrease the risk of recurrent ectopic ossification. Patients without a history of gastrointestinal ulcers or renal disease are prescribed ketorolac 30 mg intravenously every 8 hours for 24 hours (3 doses). The authors do not prescribe oral nonsteroidal anti-inflammatory medications, such as indomethacin, postoperatively, given their high potential for gastrointestinal and renal complications and low rate of patient tolerance and compliance.

Perioperative radiation therapy is limited to select patients with recurrent ectopic ossification. The authors do not recommend routine use of radiation in patients undergoing first time resection, especially patients that require skin grafts or flap coverage for wound closure. In the rare incidence that radiation therapy is considered, a discussion of the risk and benefits is conducted, including wound breakdown, neuritis, lymphedema, and remote risk of postradiation sarcoma. When indicated, they use a single 700-cGy dose of external beam radiation within 36 hours of surgery.

OUTCOMES AND COMPLICATIONS

Overall, the outcomes of elbow contracture release and heterotopic ossification in burn patients are quite good (**Fig. 7**). In a systematic review by Veltman and colleagues,[36] all patients with postburn elbow contractures who underwent elbow release with heterotopic bone excision experienced substantial improvement in their range of motion. Patients with complete ankylosis of the elbow had a mean improvement of 79° following this procedure, and patients with partial limitation of their range of motion improved by an average of 75°. Postoperatively, patients had a mean arc of motion of 88°, from 31° to 119°.

Moreover, the authors compared the outcomes of heterotopic bone excision in burn patients with trauma and closed head injury patients and found that the cause of heterotopic bone did not influence the long-term outcome after excision and contracture release. These findings are contrary

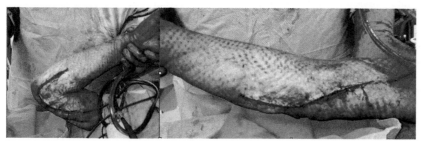

Fig. 6. Intraoperative elbow flexion and extension immediately following heterotopic ossification excision and elbow release.

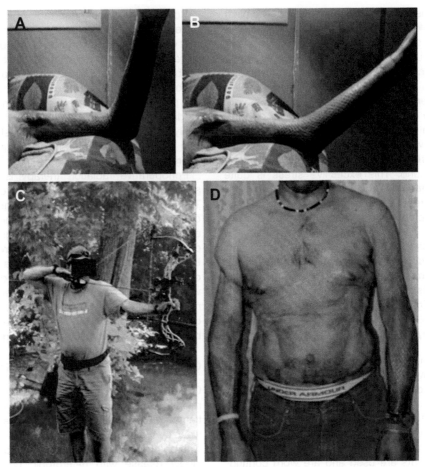

Fig. 7. (*A*) Preoperative flexion. (*B*) Preoperative extension. (*C*, *D*) Postoperative function.

to a previous reports by Lee and colleagues,[37] who found that burn injury patients had a significantly greater increase in range of motion (84°) compared with trauma (63°) or head injury (70°) patients. In either study, the improvement in function bodes well for burn patients with limited elbow motion and willingness to undergo release of their stiff elbows.

Few studies report patient-rated outcomes following heterotopic bone excision. However, one systematic review reported that the Mayo elbow performance score following heterotopic ossification excision was 85.4 in burn patients, compared with 86.4 in trauma patients, both of which correspond to a "good" outcome.[37]

In another series evaluating factors associated with greater improvements in range of motion postoperatively, the authors found that patients who underwent simultaneous ulnar nerve transposition experienced significantly greater postoperative range of motion compared with those who did not undergo ulnar nerve transposition (80° improvement vs 50°).[38]

Complications

The rate of postoperative complications in burn patients undergoing elbow release has been reported as 17%, which is similar to the complication rate in trauma and closed head injury patients.[37,38] Reported complications include recurrent ectopic ossification, ulnar nerve dysfunction, elbow instability, and deep infection. A systematic review of complication rates following elbow release and ectopic bone excision in all patients undergoing this procedure (including but not limited to burn patients) reported recurrent heterotopic ossification (20%), wound infections (12%), and ulnar nerve dysfunction (11%) as the most common complications.[36]

A minority of patients require additional surgery following ectopic bone excision for postburn elbow contractures (5%).[36] When additional surgeries were required, they were performed for residual stiffness due to recurrent heterotopic bone, ulnar nerve dysfunction, and infection.

SUMMARY

Postburn contractures of the elbow are an uncommon but debilitating sequelae of severe burn injuries, resulting from thermal injury to both deep and superficial tissues. When periarticular heterotopic bone forms in association with burn injuries, severe and rigid contractures may develop that prohibit basic functions of daily living and are often refractory to nonoperative intervention. Surgical intervention is aimed at releasing or excising all pathologic anatomy limiting elbow motion. In properly indicated patients, surgical intervention results in substantial improvement in elbow motion, allowing patients to return to activities of daily living, employment, and recreational activities.

REFERENCES

1. Tompkins RG, Burke JF, Schoenfeld DA, et al. Prompt eschar excision: a treatment system contributing to reduced burn mortality: a statistical evaluation of burn care at the Massachusetts General Hospital (1974-1984). Ann Surg 1986;204:272–81.

2. Ryan CM, Schoenfeld DA, Thorpe WP, et al. Objective estimates of the probability of death from burn injuries. N Engl J Med 1998;338:362–6.

3. Tompkins RG. Survival from burns in the new millennium: 70 years experience from a single institution. Ann Surg 2015;261(2):263–8.

4. Schneider JC, Holavanahalli R, Helm P, et al. Contractures in burn injury: defining the problem. J Burn Care Res 2006;27(4):508–14.

5. Richard R, Miller S, Staley M, et al. Multimodal versus progressive treatment techniques to correct burn scar contractures. J Burn Care Rehabil 2000; 21:506–12.

6. Dobbs ER, Curreri PW. Burn: analysis of results of physical therapy in 681 patients. J Trauma 1972; 12:242–8.

7. Evers LH, Bhavsar D, Mailänder P. The biology of burn injury. Exp Dermatol 2010;19:777–83.

8. Zhu Z, Ding J, Shankowsky HA, et al. The molecular mechanism of hypertrophic scar. J Cell Commun Signal 2013;7(4):239–52.

9. Tiwari VK. Burn wound: how it differs from other wounds? Indian J Plast Surg 2012;45(2):364–73.

10. Goel A, Shrivastava P. Post-burn scars and scar contractures. Indian J Plast Surg 2010;43(Suppl)): S63–71.

11. Chiang RS, Borovikova AA, King K, et al. Current concepts related to hypertrophic scarring in burn injuries. Wound Repair Regen 2016;24(3):466–77.

12. Ali-Bahar M, Bauer B, Tredget EE, et al. Dermal fibroblasts from different layers of human skin are heterogeneous in expression of collagenase and types I and III procollagen mRNA. Wound Repair Regen 2004;12(2):175–82.

13. Feldman SR, Trojamowska M, Smith EA, et al. Differential responses of human papillary and reticular fibroblasts to growth factors. Am J Med Sci 1993; 305(4):203–7.

14. Wang J, Dodd C, Shankowsky HA, et al. Deep dermal fibroblasts contribute to hypertrophic scarring. Lab Invest 2008;88(12):1278–90.

15. Lawrence JW, Mason ST, Schomer K, et al. Epidemiology and impact of scarring after burn injury: a systematic review of the literature. J Burn Care Res 2012;33(1):136–46.

16. Tredget EE, Levi B, Donelan MB. Biology and principles of scar management and burn reconstruction. Surg Clin North Am 2014;94(4):793–815.

17. Bombaro KM, Engrav LH, Carrougher GJ, et al. What is the prevalence of hyper-trophic scarring following burns? Burns 2003;29:299–302.

18. Kung TA, Jebson PJ, Cederna PS. An individualized approach to severe elbow burn contractures. Plast Reconstr Surg 2012;129(4):663–73.

19. Medina A, Shankowsky H, Savaryn B, et al. Characterization of heterotypic ossification in burn patients. J Burn Care Res 2014;35(3):251–6.

20. Klein MB, Logsetty S, Costa B, et al. Extended time to wound closure is associated with increased risk of heterotopic ossification of the elbow. J Burn Care Res 2007;28:447–50.

21. Levi B, Jayakumar P, Giladi A, et al. Risk factors for the development of heterotopic ossification in seriously burned adults: a National Institute on Disability, Independent Living and Rehabilitation Research burn model system database analysis. J Trauma Acute Care Surg 2015; 79(5):870–6.

22. Chen HC, Yang JY, Chuang SS, et al. Heterotopic ossification in burns: our experience and literature reviews. Burns 2009;35:857–62.

23. Gauglitz GG, Korting HC, Pavicic T, et al. Hypertrophic scarring and keloids: pathomechanisms and current and emerging treatment strategies. Mol Med 2011;17:113–25.

24. Rudolph R. Inhibition of myofibroblasts by skin grafts. Plast Reconstr Surg 1979;63:473–80.

25. Garbin S, Pittet B, Montandon D, et al. Covering by a flap induces apoptosis of granulation tissue myofibroblasts and vascular cells. Wound Repair Regen 1996;4:244–51.

26. Pontell ME, Sparber LS, Chamberlain RS. Corrective and reconstructive surgery in patients with postburn herterotopic ossification and bony ankylosis: an evidence-based approach. J Burn Care Res 2015; 36(1):57–69.

27. Munster AM, Bruck HM, Johns LA, et al. Heterotopic calcification following burns: a prospective study. J Trauma 1972;12(12):1071–4.

28. Cartotto R, Cicuto BJ, Kiwanuka HN, et al. Common postburn deformities and their management. Surg Clin North Am 2014;94(4):817–37.

29. Stern PJ, Law EJ, Benedict FE, et al. Surgical treatment of elbow contractures in postburn children. Plast Reconstr Surg 1985;76(3):441–6.

30. Morrey BF, Askew LJ, Chao EY. A biomechanical study of normal functional elbow motion. J Bone Joint Surg Am 1981;63:872–7.

31. Wainwright DJ. Burn reconstruction: the problems, the techniques, and the applications. Clin Plast Surg 2009;36:687–700.

32. Greenhalgh DG, Gaboury T, Warden GD. The early release of axillary contractures in pediatric patients with burns. J Burn Care Rehabil 1993; 14:39–42.

33. Hudson DA, Renshaw A. An algorithm for the release of burn contractures of the extremities. Burns 2006;32:663–8.

34. Hove CR, Williams EF, Rodgers BJ. Z-plasty: a concise review. Facial Plast Surg 2001;17(4):289–94.

35. Askar I. Double reverse V-Y-plasty in postburn scar contractures: a new modification of V-Y-plasty. Burns 2003;29:721–5.

36. Veltman ES, Lindenhovius ALC, Kloen P. Improvements in elbow motion after resection of heterotopic bone: a systematic review. Strategies Trauma Limb Reconstr 2014;9(2):65–71.

37. Lee EK, Namdari S, Hosalkar HS, et al. Clinical results of the excision of heterotopic bone around the elbow: a systematic review. J Shoulder Elbow Surg 2013;22:716–22.

38. Salazar D, Golz A, Israel H, et al. Heterotopic ossification of the elbow treated with surgical resection: risk factors, bony ankylosis, and complications. Clin Orthop Relat Res 2014;472(7):2269–75.

Outcomes Assessment After Hand Burns

Shepard P. Johnson, MBBS[a], Kevin C. Chung, MD, MS[b],*

KEYWORDS

- Burns • Hand • Outcomes • WHO-ICF

KEY POINTS

- Improving the quality of care of hand burns requires accurate assessments of functional disabilities and clinical outcomes.
- Despite the availability of several hand and burn outcomes measures instruments, few have been validated in hand burn patients.
- The International Classification of Functioning Disability and Health Core Sets for Hand Conditions should be the standard guide for assessing hand burn outcomes.
- Currently, a comprehensive assessment of hand burn outcomes requires a generic health-related quality of life questionnaire complemented by hand- or burn-specific instruments.
- Further research is needed to validate outcomes instruments in hand burn populations.

INTRODUCTION

Hand burn injuries can result in devastating functional impairments with biological, social, and psychological consequences that limit community and professional reintegration, and can hamper quality of life.[1–7] Improving the quality of hand burn injury management requires accurate measurement of functional disabilities and treatment outcomes. This is accomplished through outcome assessments that provide information on the effectiveness of clinical interventions, rehabilitation, and treatments.[8–11] Furthermore, as United States health care policies transition to value-based insurance models, outcomes assessments are increasingly being applied to evaluate quality and cost-effectiveness of health care.[4,8–11]

Hand burn outcomes measures focus on both the systemic impact of injuries, with health-related quality of life (HRQL) assessments, as well as disease-specific disabilities such as appearance, movement, and symptomology (eg, pain).[4,6,12] Although no universal outcomes instruments exist to evaluate hand burn injuries comprehensively, the availability and quality of assessments are improving. Formally, descriptive outcomes and objective mechanical measures were implored to evaluate the success of a surgical approach or rehabilitation program.[8,12] Through an appreciation of environmental, personal, and psychosocial health influences on health outcomes, health care professionals now emphasize the clinical relevance of assessments that evaluate

Disclosure Statement: The authors have nothing to disclose.

Research reported in this publication was supported by the National Institute of Arthritis and Musculoskeletal and Skin Diseases of the National Institutes of Health under Award Number 2 K24-AR053120-06 (Dr K.C. Chung). The content is solely the responsibility of the authors and does not necessarily represent the official views of the National Institutes of Health.

[a] Department of Surgery, Saint Joseph Mercy Ann Arbor, 5333 McAuley Drive, Suite 2111, Ypsilanti, MI 48197, USA; [b] Section of Plastic Surgery, Department of Surgery, The University of Michigan Health System, 2130 Taubman Center, SPC 5340, 1500 East Medical Center Drive, Ann Arbor, MI 48109-5340, USA
* Corresponding author.
E-mail address: kecchung@umich.edu

Hand Clin 33 (2017) 389–397
http://dx.doi.org/10.1016/j.hcl.2016.12.011

subjective measures through patient-reported outcomes (PRO).[8,13–18]

The biopsychosocial approach to evaluating functional disabilities has been promoted by the World Health Organization (WHO), and their efforts to standardize outcomes assessments through the International Classification of Functioning Disability and Health (ICF) framework.[19] Although numerous outcomes assessment instruments are available to investigate burn or hand injuries, few have been validated in the subpopulation of hand burns. Current literature efforts in hand burn injury outcomes are dedicated to understanding how comprehensively and accurately instruments assess the outcomes outlined in the WHO-ICF.[19–22] This article provides an overview on the purpose, availability, and application of outcomes assessments in hand burns.

INTERNATIONAL CLASSIFICATION OF FUNCTIONING DISABILITY AND HEALTH

The ICF is a comprehensive classification of health and health-related domains and is the WHO framework for measuring health and disability at the individual and population levels.[19] This framework helps to conceptualize a patient's quality of life by relating the function and disability of an individual in the context of environment, personal, and disease-related factors (Fig. 1).[19–21] The specific domains evaluated by the WHO-ICF include body structure, body function, activity, and participation. The ICF provides a "foundation and a common framework allowing all conditions to be compared using a common metric—the impact on the functioning of the individual," and should be used clinically for "functional status assessment, goal setting and treatment planning and monitoring, as well as outcome measurement."[19]

Using the WHO-ICF framework is an important step toward standardizing health outcomes measures. To facilitate this process, current and future outcomes instruments should be defined by what WHO-ICF domains/subdomains they evaluate. This will allow clinicians to effectively monitor specific WHO-ICF domains and identify outcomes that are deficient within the biopsychosocial model. In 2011, Rudolf and colleagues[20] published a paper outlining the formal consensus process of developing the ICF Core Sets for Hand Conditions that "provides the basic international standard of what should be measured and reported to describe functioning and disability of patients with hand conditions." Included in this document is the brief WHO-ICF Core Set for Hand Conditions (Table 1) that provides a minimal standard of outcomes to describe functioning and is a valuable tool to improve hand burn outcomes measures.

PATIENT-REPORTED OUTCOMES

PROs have become an important adjunct in the assessment of the WHO-ICF domains. PROs are a recognized and standardized method of reporting a patients' perspective on treatment benefits, and may be the outcome most important to patients. PROs are reports coming directly from patients about how they function or feel in relation to a health condition and its treatment.[8,13,15–17] They are now widely used as clinician-based outcomes to gain further knowledge on domains such as "symptoms, functioning, health perception, satisfaction, and [HRQL]."[23] This is in contrast with traditional objective outcomes measures, such as functional metrics (eg, range of motion [ROM], grip strength, degree of contracture), morbidity, and other physiologic markers, that fail to accurately assess HRQL and psychosocial domains.[7,12,24]

PROs facilitate a more complete understanding of the functioning and disability caused by health conditions as described by the WHO-ICF. For

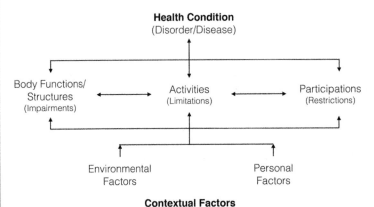

Fig. 1. The International Classification of Functioning Disability and Health (ICF) is a classification of health and health-related domains, and is the World Health Organization (WHO) framework for measuring health and disability at the individual and population levels. (*From* Meirte J, van Loe'y NE, Maertens K, et al. Classification of quality of life subscales within the ICF framework in burn research: identifying overlaps and gaps. Burns 2014;40(7):1354; with permission.)

Table 1
Brief international classification of functioning, disability and health - core set for hand conditions by the World Health Organization

ICF Category	Title
Body functions	
b152	Emotional functions
b265	Touch function
b270	Sensory functions related to temperature and other stimuli
b280	Sensation of pain
b710	Mobility of joint functions
b715	Stability of joint functions
b730	Muscle power functions
b760	Control of voluntary movement functions
b810	Protective functions of the skin
Body structures	
s120	Spinal cord and related structures
s720	Structure of shoulder region
s730	Structure of upper extremity
Activities and participation	
d230	Carrying out daily routine
d430	Lifting and carrying objects
d440	Fine hand use
d445	Hand and arm use
d5	Self-care
d6	Domestic life
d7	Interpersonal interactions and relationships
d840-d859	Work and employment
Environmental factors	
e1	Products and technology
e3	Support and relationships
e5	Services, systems and policies

Data from Rudolf KD, Kus S, Chung KC, et al. Development of the International Classification of Functioning, Disability and Health Core Sets for Hand Conditions – results of the World Health Organization international Consensus Process. Disabil Rehabil 2012;34(8):681–93.

example, the Patient and Observer Scar Assessment Scale (POSAS) is an outcome instrument that includes PROs, such as pain, itching, appearance, and overall opinion on burn scars.[25] This provides subjective insight that is unattainable by traditional, objective measures. Although PROs are beneficial to the evaluation of hand burns, the available literature suggests that current PRO instruments incompletely evaluate all the WHO-ICF domains.[3,7,17,21]

In a recent systematic review, Coenen and colleagues[17] evaluated the ability of PRO measures used in the field of hand injuries to capture the WHO-ICF domains of function and environment. They assessed 8 available outcomes instruments, such as the Michigan Hand Outcomes Questionnaire (MHQ) and The Disabilities of the Arm, Shoulder, and Hand Score (DASH), and provided comprehensive tables to summarize the second-level WHO-ICF outcomes that are adequately measured by each instrument.[17,26–28] For example, the authors found that both the MHQ and DASH are suitable instruments to evaluate "Activities and participations: b134 Sleep functions." Coenen and colleagues[17] concluded that, although the functioning aspects stated by the patients are captured partially by questionnaires, the WHO-ICF environment and body structure domains are often disregarded in current PRO measures.

CLINOMETRIC PROPERTIES

Before using an outcomes questionnaire, the appropriateness of the instrument must be demonstrated through a statistical analysis of its clinometric properties.[8,29–31] These properties, as well as the practicality (eg, user friendliness of questionnaires), should be considered before selecting an instrument for clinical or research purposes. Furthermore, clinometric properties vary by study population and setting and, therefore, the appropriateness of an instrument may not be applicable across all cultures or age groups.[29–33] As a result of the paucity of information on clinometric properties of outcome instruments used in hand burn patients, selecting an instrument can be difficult. A basic understanding of the metrics that determine the quality of outcomes assessments is required to select the correct instrument for a given system, disease, patient population, or study question (**Table 2**).[8,13,29–31]

In response to the lack of standardization of outcomes instruments in medical literature, Mokkink and colleagues[32,33] published the COSMIN study (COnsensus-based Standards or the selection of health Measurement INstruments), which provides guidelines on evaluating the methodological quality of studies on health status measurement instruments. Likewise, in the pursuit of transparency on the quality of instruments, the Patient Reported Outcomes Measurement Information System (PROMIS) was created to provide a bank of tested questionnaires and their ability to measure specific outcome domains.[34] Although substantial efforts remain to identify validated, comprehensive

Table 2
Clinometric properties help to determine the quality of an outcomes assessment instrument

Clinometric	Description
Validity	Descriptive term used to mean that an instrument accurately reflects the concept that it is intended to measure.
Content validity	Subjective assessment of the comprehensiveness of an instrument and how adequately items cover an area that needs to be assessed.
Criterion validity	Demonstrates how a new scale correlates with a gold standard. This validity is not applied in outcomes research because no reference standard can be defined to compare to each patient's individual assessment of outcomes.
Reproducibility	Measures reliability and it refers to the extent to which repeated administration of an instrument to a stable population yields the same results.
Responsiveness	Reflects the ability to detect change, and is frequently defined as the minimally important change (or minimal clinically important difference) from the perspective of the patient or their provider. The level of change in an instrument score must reflect a true change in the condition (not test–retest errors).
Interpretability	The degree to which one can assign qualitative meaning to an instrument's quantitative scores.
Feasibility	The ease to which an outcome assessment instrument can be applied in the clinical setting.

Data from Refs.[8,13,29–31]

outcome assessment instruments, we provide an overview of common approaches to assessing outcomes in hand burns.

ASSESSING OUTCOMES

To standardize hand burn outcomes research, outcomes should be categorized within the WHO-ICF Core Sets for Hand Conditions (**Fig. 2**). The researcher can then identify the most appropriate instruments available to assess these outcomes. The WHO emphasizes the importance of measuring all WHO-ICF domains to accurately report disabilities related to a disease; therefore, both global and hand-specific instruments are often indicated. Last, given the absence of a perfect outcome measure instrument, the limitations of instruments used and the WHO-ICF components not assessed within a study, should be disclosed.

HAND BURN OUTCOMES

Falder and colleagues[2] originally proposed 7 core domains to comprehensively assess outcomes after burn injuries, including skin, neuromuscular function, sensory and pain, psychological function, physical role function, community participation and perceived quality of life. With the introduction of the WHO-ICF Core Sets for Hand Conditions, a more robust, structured list of outcomes exists.[19,20] Both proposals strive for a holistic assessment of

burn outcomes, but this is currently not attainable with a single outcomes measuring tool. Furthermore, clinicians may prefer to investigate a specific outcome of interest, such as functionality, aesthetics, or scarring characteristics, when evaluating a burn injury patient. In this regard, having unique outcome measuring instruments can be both necessary and complimentary.

Global Outcomes Measures

Measuring HRQL is the leading outcome in burn care research.[21,24] To fully understand the impairments of burn injuries, isolated or multiple, the systemic impact of the injury should be considered.[21,35–38] This concept is supported by the WHO, which defines quality of life as "an individual's perception of their position in life in the context of the culture and value systems.... It is a broad ranging concept affected in a complex way by the person's physical health, psychological state, personal beliefs, social relationships, and their relationships to salient features of their environment."[39]

The Short Form-36, Sickness Impact Profile, European Quality of Life 5 Dimensions, and the brief Burn Specific Health Scale (BSHS-B) are frequently used generic HRQL questionnaires in burn research.[40–44] The BSHS-B is disease-specific, self-rated questionnaire developed to assess the quality of recovery after a burn injury.[43,44] This instrument is likely more relatable to patients with hand burns, because the

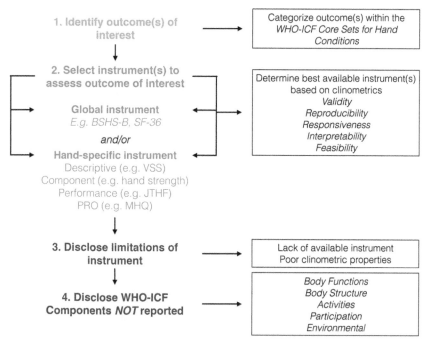

Fig. 2. Assessing outcomes in hand burn research involves (1) identifying outcomes of interest and categorizing these within the WHO-ICF Core Sets for Hand Conditions, (2) selecting appropriate global and/or hand-specific outcome measure instruments, (3) identifying the limitations of the instruments chosen, and (4) identifying deficiencies in assessing the WHO-ICF domains to accurately report disabilities related to a disease. BSHS-B, Burn Specific Health Scale-Brief; JTHF, Jebsen-Taylor Hand Function Test; MHQ, Michigan Hand Outcomes Questionnaire; SF-36, Short Form-36; VSS, Vancouver Scar Scale; WHO-ICF, World Health Organization-The International Classification of Functioning Disability and Health.

measurement includes the outcomes of heat sensitivity and hand function (to measure fine motor skills).[21,44] Although generic HRQL questionnaires provide a global assessment of function and disability, 2 systematic reviews by Meirte and colleagues[21] and Cieza and Stucki[45] have found that contextual factors (eg, environmental, personal, and social factors), body function, and mental function are poorly evaluated. For examples, social support, a well-recognized adjunct to coping with and recovering from burn injuries, is often incompletely assessed.[21,45] Similarly, personal factors that influence function and quality of life (eg, age, gender, and educational level) are often overlooked or underappreciated.

Meirte and colleagues[21] found that generic HRQL questionnaires fail to sufficiently evaluate all WHO-ICF domains and, therefore, recommend adjunct outcome assessments to appreciate the impact of burns. Additionally, Van Baar and colleagues[3] concluded that available outcome assessments do not provide sufficient information to estimate the functional consequences of burns. Functional outcomes often assessed include mental health, self-care, domestic life, education, and work status. Less attention is afforded to the

consequences of burns on body structure, movement, and skin, domains that can be dramatically affected by hand burns.[3,21]

Hand-Specific Outcomes Measures

The ICF Core Sets for Hand Conditions serves as the standard of what should be measured and reported to describe disabilities in hand burn patients.[19,20] This framework provides a unified language to identify, monitor, and communicate outcomes in patients. Although the WHO-ICF Core Sets for Hand Conditions was recently introduced, there are an abundance of hand-specific outcome instruments that predate this standardization. Currently, there is no agreed upon best method for assessing hand function after burn injuries, because there is little information on how accurately WHO-ICF domains are assessed with available instruments.[12,17]

Hand outcome assessments may include descriptive, component measures (eg, ROM), performance measures (eg, objective dexterity tests), or PROs (eg, questionnaires).[7] Unfortunately, few outcomes instruments are validated in hand burns. Lin and colleagues[7] found in their systematic

review that no burn-specific hand function outcomes measures exists, and that the applicability,
reliability, validity and responsiveness of hand
function measures in patients with hand burns
needs further investigations.

Descriptive outcomes measures

Clinicians have used descriptive outcomes to
define burn injuries and evaluate therapeutic interventions. One approach is to use deformity de-
scriptions, such as webspace contracture, dorsal
skin contracture, and boutonniere deformity, to
categorize and describe disabilities from hand
burns.[12] Likewise, the number of contractures,
severity of contractures, and total body surface
area of burn requiring grafting have all been used
to quantify the severity of burn injuries.[46] This
descriptive approach lacks standardization and
is hampered by subjectivity, and has limited usefulness compared with more current, robust
instruments.

Scar scales are an alternative descriptive option
that has garnered substantial attention in the burn
literature.[47,48] Because burn injuries often lead to
soft tissue disfigurements, describing the appearance of burns is frequently used to assess burn
severity, rehabilitation, and effectiveness of therapeutic interventions. Burn scar scales provide an
objective assessment of descriptive parameters
including appearance (eg, vascularization and
pigmentation) and physical characteristics (eg,
height, texture, and pliability). Additionally, some
burn scar scales have added PRO to assess patient symptoms (eg, pain, pruritus) and opinions
of appearance.[24,25,47–49]

The Vancouver Scar Scale (VSS) and the
POSAS are 2 commonly used instruments applied
in the burn and scar literature.[25,49] Although both
scales have been used to assess hand burn outcomes, they have not been validated in this population.[50,51] Tyack and colleagues[47] reviewed the
clinometric properties of 18 commonly used burn
scar scales and found that the POSAS had high
reliability but indeterminate validity, whereas the
VSS was investigated rigorously but had indeterminate quality clinometric properties. In a separate
systematic review, Van der Wal and colleagues[30]
found that the POSAS was the highest quality
scale, because it includes a comprehensive list
of scar features, incorporates patient's opinion,
and has superior internal consistency and reliability when compared with the VSS. Despite
these findings, both instruments are used routinely
in burn injury research. For example, Hultman and
associates[52] used the VSS to demonstrate
improvement in the signs of symptoms of hypertrophic burn scars with use of laser therapies.

Component outcomes measures

ROM deficits are common in hand burn injuries
secondary to joint contractures, hence, the
intrigue in using this as a surrogate outcome for
hand function.[12,53] Unfortunately, the measurement of ROM is not standardized and studies
have not shown a clear correlation between
ROM and functional performance improvement.[12]
Similarly, objective physical measures (eg, hand
strength and endurance) have been used as
hand burn outcomes. Clifford and colleagues[54]
evaluated grip strength dynamometry and found
that it is a reliable and valid outcomes measure
for burn-affected upper limb strength. The authors
concluded that grip strength allows clinicians to
quantify impairments that contribute to loss of
hand function. Unfortunately, it is difficult to interpret how component measures translate to
disability and daily activity impairment. Therefore,
these assessment instruments should be used in
conjunction with more dynamic outcome measure
such as the BSHS-B.

Performance outcomes measures

Performance tests assess hand function with specific and standardized tasks. Unlike descriptive
outcomes, performance test are designed to
assess activity limitations and participation restric-
tions in patients with hand function problems by
simulating activities of daily life.[4–8] For example,
the Jebsen-Taylor Hand Function Test (JTHF)
evaluates hand movements such as writing and
picking up objects, and has been used to evaluate
outcomes in burn patients.[7,55,56] These outcomes
measures aid in the evaluation of hand dexterity,
functional sensibility, daily tasks, and strength,
but are limited by the absence of the patient's
perspective on disabilities.

In 2009, Van de Ven-Stevens and coworkers[4]
published a systematic review of the clinometric
properties of available performance outcomes
hand instruments to assess limitations in activities
(as defined by the WHO-ICF as "the execution of a
task or action by an individual"). This study was
not limited to burn patients, but provided insight
into the shortcomings of performance assessments. Twenty-three instruments were reviewed,
including performance outcomes measures such
as pegboard tests, manipulating objects, and single task objectives. Although some outcomes
measures performed well, none of the instruments
had a uniformly positive rating in all clinometric
properties.

Patient-reported outcomes measures

The addition of PRO measure instruments has
made the biopsychosocial approach to outcomes

assessment attainable, by providing insight on how functional limitation are influenced by psychological and social factors.[17-20] The MHQ and DASH are 2 of the most common self-reported outcome measures used in upper extremity disorders. They are questionnaires that provide comprehensive feedback on a patients' perception of their overall hand function, activities of daily living, symptoms (eg, pain), social activities, work, sleep, aesthetics, and patient satisfaction.[26,27] Currently, as with the performance outcomes measures, the clinometric properties of most instruments are largely inconclusive to support their validity in hand burn outcomes. Wu and colleagues[5] did evaluate an abbreviated version of the DASH (the QuickDASH) in upper limb burn injury patients and found positive conclusions on the validity, repeatability and responsiveness of the instrument to assess change in functional levels in this patient population.

OUTCOMES DATABASES

Equally important to identifying and measuring outcomes related to hand burns is the organized collection of population data. Aggregating large volumes of patient outcome information into databases facilitates research endeavors aimed at improving the care of patients and comparing the effectiveness of interventions.[57] Electronic databases (eg, administrative claims databases) are powerful resources that allow for observational studies that are large, low cost, fast, and provide insight into how current health care practices affect outcomes.[57] Identifying the most pertinent hand outcomes to measure and include in large databases is an important component to the future of outcomes assessments in hand burn injuries.

The Burn Model System (BMS) National Database, established by The National Institute on Disability, Independent Living, and Rehabilitation Research, is the largest multicenter, longitudinal database on burn outcomes.[58] This database describes the functional and psychosocial recovery of burn patients, and was created with the purpose of improving the care of burn survivors.[58] Several outcomes instruments are collected by the BMS, predominantly global assessment measures, including the Short Form-36 and BSHS. Although the JTHF test was previously included in the BMS National Database, there is currently no hand-specific outcomes instrument. This database has been used to investigate a wide range of burn-related outcomes, including contractures related to burns, risk factors for heterotopic ossification in seriously burned adults, and satisfaction with life after burns.[59-61] Studies focused on

hand burns are feasible with the BMS, but the addition of hand-specific outcomes instruments, such as the MHQ, would enable more informative investigations.

SUMMARY

The WHO has provided a foundation for the field of hand surgery to effectively evaluate outcomes in hand disorders with the introduction of the ICF Core Sets for Hand Conditions. This paves the way for clinicians and researchers to establish standardized approaches to measuring outcomes in specific hand disorders, including burn injuries. There exists an abundance of outcomes instruments within burn and hand literature, respectively, but identifying the most appropriately instruments to evaluate the biopsychosocial disabilities after hand burns remains unclear. Several systematic reviews indicate that a comprehensive assessment of hand burns requires a global assessment of health-related quality of life, via generic outcomes measures instruments, complemented by hand-specific outcome instruments. For example, Byrne and colleagues[51] studied fat grafting for burn reconstruction of the hand, and the authors used multiple instruments, including grip strength, ROM, DASH, MHQ, and the POSAS to describe function and disability outcomes. Further information is needed to conclude on the validity (and other clinometric properties) of instruments to assess the outcomes outlined within WHO-ICF framework in hand burn patients.

REFERENCES

1. Druery M, Brown T, Muller M. Long term functional outcomes and quality of life following severe burn injury. Burns 2005;31:692–5.
2. Falder S, Browne A, Edgar D, et al. Core outcomes for adult burn survivors: a clinical overview. Burns 2009;35:618–41.
3. van Baar ME, Essink-Bot ML, Oen IM, et al. Functional outcome after burns: a review. Burns 2006; 32:1–9.
4. van de Ven-Stevens LA, Munneke M, Terwee CB, et al. Clinimetric properties of instruments to assess activities in patients with hand injury: a systematic review of the literature. Arch Phys Med Rehabil 2009;90:151–69.
5. Wu A, Edgar DW, Wood FM. The QuickDASH is an appropriate tool for measuring the quality of recovery after upper limb burn injury. Burns 2007;33: 843–9.
6. Cowan AC, Stegink-Jansen CW. Rehabilitation of hand burn injuries: current update. Injury 2013;44: 391–6.

7. Lin SY, Chang JK, Chen PC, et al. Hand function measures for burn patients: a literature review. Burns 2013;39:16–23.

8. Giladi AM, Chung KC. Measuring outcomes in hand surgery. Clin Plast Surg 2008;35(2):239–50.

9. Choudhry NK, Rosenthal MB, Milstein A. Assessing the evidence for value-based insurance design. Health Aff (Millwood) 2010;29:1988–94.

10. Epstein AM. The outcomes movement–will it get us where we want to go? N Engl J Med 1990;323: 266–70.

11. Heras PC, Burke FD, Dias JJ, et al. Outcome measurement in hand surgery: report of a consensus conference. Br J Hand Ther 2003;8:70–80.

12. Kowalske K. Outcome assessment after hand burns. Hand Clin 2009;25:557–61.

13. [updated March 2011]. In: Higgins JPT, Green S, editors. Cochrane Handbook for Systematic Reviews of Interventions Version 5.1.0. The Cochrane Collaboration; 2011. Available at: handbook.cochrane.org. Accessed April 12, 2016.

14. Bindra RR, Dias JJ, Heras-Palau C, et al. Assessing outcome after hand surgery: the current state. J Hand Surg Br 2003;28:289–94.

15. Szabo RM. Outcomes assessment in hand surgery: when are they meaningful? J Hand Surg Am 2001; 26:993–1002.

16. Alderman AK, Chung KC. Measuring outcomes in hand surgery. Clin Plast Surg 2008;35:239–50.

17. Coenen M, Kus S, Rudolf KD, et al. Do patient-reported outcome measures capture functioning aspects and environmental factors important to individuals with injuries or disorders of the hand. J Hand Ther 2013;26:332–42.

18. Brettschneider C, Lühmann D, Raspe H. Informative value of Patient Reported Outcomes (PRO) in Health Technology Assessment (HTA). GMS Health Technol Assess 2011;7:Doc01.

19. World Health Organization (WHO). International classification of functioning, disability and health (ICF). Available at: http://www.who.int/classifications/icf/en/. Accessed April 11, 2016.

20. Rudolf KD, Kus S, Chung KC, et al. Development of the international classification of functioning, disability and health core sets for hand conditions – results of the World Health Organization international consensus process. Disabil Rehabil 2012;34(8): 681–93.

21. Meirte J, van Loey NEE, Maertens K, et al. Classification of quality of life subscales within the ICF framework in burn research: identifying overlaps and gaps. Burns 2014;40:1353–9.

22. Adkinson JM, Bickham RS, Chung KC, et al. Do patient- and parent-reported outcomes measures for children with congenital hand differences capture WHO-ICF domains? Clin Orthop Relat Res 2015; 473:3549–63.

23. Changulani M, Okonkwo U, Keswani T, et al. Outcome evaluation measures for wrist and hand: which one to choose? Int Orthop 2008;32:1–6.

24. van Loey NE, Van Son MJ. Psychopathology and psychological problems in patients with burn scars: epidemiology and management. Am J Clin Dermatol 2003;4:245–72.

25. Draaijers LT, Tempelman FR, Botman YA, et al. The Patient and Observer Scar Assessment Scale: a reliable and feasible tool for scar evaluation. Plast Reconstr Surg 2004;113:1960–5.

26. Chung K, Pillsbury M, Walters M, et al. Reliability and validity testing of the MICHIGAN HAND OUTCOMES QUESTIONNAIRE. J Hand Surg Am 1998; 23:575–87.

27. Hudak PL, Amadio PC, Bombardier C. Development of an upper extremity outcome measure: the DASH (disabilities of the arm, shoulder and hand). Am J Ind Med 1996;29(6):e602–8.

28. Beaton DE, Wright JG, Katz JN. Upper Extremity Collaborative Group. Development of the Quick-DASH: comparison of three item-reduction approaches. J Bone Joint Surg Am 2005;87(5): e1038–46.

29. McDowell I. Measuring health: a guide to rating scales and questionnaires. Oxford: Oxford University Press; 2006.

30. van der Wal M, Verhaegen P, Middelkoop E, et al. A clinimetric overview of scar assessment scales. J Burn Care Res 2012;33:e79–87.

31. Terwee CB, Bot SDM, Boer MR, et al. Quality criteria were proposed for measurement properties of health status questionnaires. J Clin Epidemiol 2007;60:34–42.

32. Mokkink LB, Terwee CB, Stratford PW, et al. Evaluation of the methodological quality of systematic reviews of health status measurement instruments. Qual Life Res 2009;18:313–33.

33. Mokkink LB, Terwee CB, Patrick DL, et al. The COSMIN study reached international consensus on taxonomy, terminology, and definitions of measurement properties for health-related patient-reported outcomes. J Clin Epidemiol 2010;63:737–45.

34. National Institute of Health. Patient Reported Outcomes Measurement Information Systems (PROMIS). Available at: http://www.nihpromis.org/. Accessed April 11, 2016.

35. Guyatt GH, Feeny DH, Patrick DL. Measuring health-related quality of life. Ann Intern Med 1993; 118:622–9.

36. Koller M, Lorenz W. Quality of life: a deconstruction for clinicians. J R Soc Med 2002;95:481–8.

37. Elsherbiny OEE, Salem MA, El-Sabbagh AH, et al. Quality of life of adult patients with severe burns. Burns 2011;37:776–89.

38. Wasiak J, McMahon M, Danilla S, et al. Measuring common outcome measures and their concepts

using the International Classification of Functioning. Disability and Health (ICF) in adults with burn injury: a systematic review. Burns 2011;37:913–24.

39. World Health Organization (WHO). Study protocol for the World Health Organization project to develop a Quality of Life assessment instrument (WHOQOL). Qual Life Res 1993;2:153–9.

40. Edgar D, Dawson A, Hankey G, et al. Demonstration of the validity of the SF-36 for measurement of the temporal recovery of quality of life outcomes in burns survivors. Burns 2010;36:1013–20.

41. Novelli B, Melandri D, Bertolotti G, et al. Quality of life impact as outcome in burns patients. G Ital Med Lav Ergon 2009;31:A58–63.

42. Oster C, Willebrand M, Dyster-Aas J, et al. Validation of the EQ-5D questionnaire in burn injured adults. Burns 2002;35:723–32.

43. Blalock SJ, Bunker BJ, DeVellis RF. Measuring health status among survivors of burn injury: revisions of the Burn Specific Health Scale. J Trauma 1996;36:508–15.

44. Kildal M, Andersson G, Fugl-Meyer AR, et al. Development of a brief version of the Burn Specific Health Scale (BSHS-B). J Trauma 2001;51:740–6.

45. Cieza A, Stucki G. Content comparison of health-related quality of life (HRQOL) instruments based on the international classification of functioning, disability and health (ICF). Qual Life Res 2005;14:1225–37.

46. Schneider JC, Holavanahalli R, Helm P, et al. Contractures in burn injury part II: investigating joints of the hand. J Burn Care Res 2008;29:606–13.

47. Tyack Z, Simons M, Spinks A, et al. A systematic review of the quality of burn scar rating scales for clinical and research use. Burns 2012;38:6–18.

48. Vercelli S, Ferriero G, Sartorio F, et al. How to assess postsurgical scars: a review of outcome measures. Disabil Rehabil 2009;31:2055–63.

49. Baryza MJ, Baryza GA. The Vancouver Scar Scale: an administrative tool and its inter-rater reliability. J Burn Care Rehabil 1995;16:535–8.

50. Haslik W, Kamolz LP, Lumenta DB, et al. The treatment of deep dermal hand burns: how do we achieve better results? Should we use allogenic keratinocytes or skin grafts. Burns 2010;36:329–34.

51. Byrne M, O'Donnell M, Fitzgerald L, et al. Early experience with fat grafting as an adjunct for secondary burn reconstruction in the hand: technique, hand function assessment and aesthetic outcomes. Burns 2016;42:356–65.

52. Hultman CS, Friedstat JS, Edkins RE, et al. Laser resurfacing and remodeling of hypertrophic burn scars: the results of a large, prospective, before-after cohort study, with long-term follow-up. Ann Surg 2014;260(3):519–29.

53. Barillo DJ, Harvey KD, Hobbs CL, et al. Prospective outcome analysis of a protocol for the surgical and rehabilitative management of burns to the hands. Plast Reconstr Surg 1997;100:1442–51.

54. Clifford MS, Hamer P, Phillips M, et al. Grip strength dynamometry: reliability and validity for adults with upper limb burns. Burns 2013;39:1430–6.

55. Jebsen RH, Taylor N, Trieschmann RB, et al. An objective and standardized test offhand function. Arch Phys Med Rehabil 1969;50:311–9.

56. Holavanahalli R, Helm P, Gorman A, et al. Outcomes after deep full-thickness hand burns. Arch Phys Med Rehabil 2007;88:30–5.

57. Johnson SP, Chung KC. Comparative effectiveness research in hand surgery. Hand Clin 2014;30(3):319–27.

58. Goverman J, Mathews K, Holavanahalli RK, et al. The National Institute on Disability, independent living, and rehabilitation research Burn Model System: twenty years of contributions to clinical service and research. J Burn Care Res 2017;38(1):e240–53.

59. Goverman J, Mathews K, Goldstein R, et al. Adult contractures in burn injury: a Burn Model System National Database Study. J Burn Care Res 2017;38(1):e328–36.

60. Goverman J, Mathews K, Nadler D, et al. Satisfaction with life after burn: a Burn Model System National Database Study. Burns 2016;42(5):1067–73.

61. Levi B, Jayakumar P, Giladi A, et al. A National Institute on Disability, independent living and rehabilitation research Burn Model System database analysis. J Trauma Acute Care Surg 2015;79(5):870–6.

International Disease Burden of Hand Burns
Perspective from the Global Health Arena

CrossMark

Daniel S. Corlew, MD, MPH[a,b,*], K.A. Kelly McQueen, MD, MPH[c,d]

KEYWORDS

- Burden of disease • Global surgery • Hand burns • Burn contractures

KEY POINTS

- Burn injuries to the hands are particularly disabling relative to burn injuries in general.
- This added significance of burn injuries to the hands is exacerbated in the developing world because of the lack of compensatory assistance devices or societal adjustments.
- Because of the specific and varied nature of hand burns, enumerating their contribution to global burden of disease (BoD) is difficult, but it seems that there are approximately 18 million living with hand burn injuries.
- Approximately half of surviving burn victims in low-income and middle-income countries (LMICs) have significant hand injuries.
- As appropriate attention and resources are given to surgical needs in LMICs, it is anticipated that more people will survive burn injuries and that more prevention and resolution of hand burn contractures will occur. The increased overall survival figures might paradoxically result in an increase in the BoD due to hand burns.

INTRODUCTION

With the possible exception of severely disfiguring burns to the face, burns to the hands are arguably the most devastating in terms of human productivity and utility. With little affected surface area, and sometimes little overall injury, burns to the hands can result in complete loss of the ability to perform the functions necessary to provide a livelihood for self and family and even to perform activities of daily living. Compounding these effects is the increased risk of sustaining burns to the hands – unlike the core of the body, to which the heat or chemical agent must reach the body to inflict harm, the hands often reach out to that agent in an effort to ward off injury, to assist others, or in the course of usual work, such as cooking, manufacturing jobs, motor vehicle accidents, and so forth.

Burn injuries are most often a function of poverty. For a variety of reasons, there is a strong correlation between the incidence of burn injury and poverty, both within the developed world and among the global population.[1–4] In the developing world, there are many reasons for this

Neither author has any disclosures.
[a] Resurge International, 145 Wolfe Road, Sunnyvale, CA 94086, USA; [b] St. Thomas Rutherford Hospital, 1700 Medical Center Parkway, Murfreesboro, TN 37129, USA; [c] Department of Anesthesiology, Vanderbilt Global Anesthesia Fellowship, Vanderbilt Anesthesia Global Health & Development, Vanderbilt Institute for Global Health, Vanderbilt University Medical Center, 1301 Medical Center Drive, MCE 3161C, Nashville, TN 37232, USA; [d] Department of Surgery, Vanderbilt Global Anesthesia Fellowship, Vanderbilt Anesthesia Global Health & Development, Affiliate Faculty, Vanderbilt Institute for Global Health, Vanderbilt University Medical Center, 1301 Medical Center Drive, MCE 3161C, Nashville, TN 37232, USA
* Corresponding author. 2111 Riverview Drive, Murfreesboro, TN 37129.
E-mail address: scorlew@post.harvard.edu

Hand Clin 33 (2017) 399–407
http://dx.doi.org/10.1016/j.hcl.2016.12.010

hand.theclinics.com

correlation, depending on degree of poverty, cultural characteristics and customs, rural versus urban locale, or other available health care. The use of open fires for cooking is a frequent cause, especially among smaller children (**Fig. 1**). Unmanaged seizure disorders result in numerous burn injuries in LMICs.[1] Exposed electrical wiring, including unauthorized attempts to tap into electrical grids driven by the desperation of poverty, is a frequent cause[5] and undoubtedly disproportionately affects the hands. Kerosene stoves, also associated with poverty in the developing world, are a common cause of major burn injuries.[5] The hands, of course, are usually handling the object of injury when the accident occurs.

BURNS OF THE HAND AND MEASURING THE BURDEN OF DISEASE

Assessing the BoD due to burns is difficult for several reasons. The overarching issue is the vast spectrum of injuries, both incident and prevalent, that fall under the category of "burns." Many people, even in the face of significant injuries, do not (or are unable to) seek medical care, so never appear in any database of health care provision. These people conceivably may be counted by field studies carried out in the slums and villages of LMICs, but the task is gargantuan and has not been done to date. The methodology of surveys, such as is done by the Monitoring and Evaluation to Assess and Use Results Demographic and Health Surveys (MEASURE DHS), is perhaps the best concept for such assessment but is complicated by the relatively small proportion of victims, even in high-prevalence countries. The overall task is further complicated by the complexity of

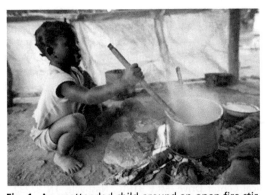

Fig. 1. An unattended child around an open fire stirring hot liquid with an instrument that could easily overturn the receptacle, spilling the hot liquid on the child. Loose clothing would have essentially completed the risk factors present in this situation. (*Photo by* Phil Borges for ReSurge International. Used with permission.)

possible injuries, which is magnified still more for hand burns. This is illustrated in the following hypothetical example.

A US worker sustains full-thickness burns to the dominant hand. After proper care, including débridement, grafting, aggressive hand therapy, and scar management, the patient is left with some tissue loss and with decreased range of motion of the thumb, index, and long fingers, such that she/he has a somewhat impaired dominant hand that may result in an alteration of duties in her/his former job. This patient is assessed through the American Medical Association *Guides to the Evaluation of Permanent Impairment*, which requires a lengthy assessment of loss of range of motion, sensation, and tissue loss to derive a reasonably precise valuation of impairment. The evaluation of this impairment is lengthy not necessarily because the US legal industry demands it but rather because the injury is complex, the functional effects on the hand are complex, and no abbreviated methodology can provide a true assessment of the injury.

In contrast, a rural villager in a sub-Saharan African country sustains the same injury. The care consists of little more than wound care directed by local custom and common sense (unless, of course, the patient has the misfortune of getting to a health care facility without basic burn expertise and the hand is immobilized for a prolonged period of time, resulting in complete loss of range of motion affecting the entire upper extremity). When the burn wound is finally healed, it likely has resulted in complete loss of reasonably normal use of the hand, but, regardless of the level of impairment, the only statistical representation of this patient in the summary measures of the Global Burden of Disease (GBD) study appears as a burn injury of less than 10% total body surface area (TBSA), with hand involvement, with long-term effects. The patient is postulated to have 98.8% utility in overall life for the rest of her/his life. This example is not pejorative toward the GBD in any way, because its goal is much more global in scope and it is constantly improving in its thoroughness,[6] but rather this is an indication of the difficulty of epidemiologically quantifying the nature of hand burns from a functional point of view.

The actual incidence and prevalence of burn injuries to the hands in the developing world are unknown. As the GBD study becomes increasingly sophisticated, this knowledge deficit presumably will decrease. The most recent iteration of the GBD study expanded the scope of assessment to 306 diseases and injuries in 188 countries,[7] and presumably each subsequent iteration will continue to expand into what is an almost infinite number of etiologies of human suffering. As noted in the previous example of the sequelae of a hand burn, the level of specificity required to provide optimal epidemiologic information for burn injuries is minute in the larger scheme of the GBD, even more so when specifically examining burns to the hands.

The GBD, first assessed in 1990, uses the disability-adjusted life year (DALY) as a metric to quantify the effect of injury or disease on the human condition. This is a vast improvement over simple mortality data as an evaluation of health but is more complex and subject to controversy than simply counting whether a person is alive or dead. The DALY is the sum of years of life lost (YLL) and years lost to disability (YLD) due to a particular problem. Although YLL is more straightforward, only requiring the determination that a person is alive or dead, YLD requires a valuation of life function and utility associated with a particular disease or injury. These disability weights (DWs) have been determined by progressively more sophisticated means[8–10] but understandably remain controversial[11–13] as they likely always will.

Disability-adjusted life years

DALYs = YLL + YLD

YLD = duration of disability × DW

DW ranges from 0 to 1 and is determined for each disease entity; 0 represents perfect health (or no disability) and 1 represents death (or total disability).

The first GBD considered burn injuries only in terms of 3 categories by TBSA: less than 20%, between 20% and 60%, and greater than 60% (the DWs were the same for the latter 2 categories),[14] the more recent version differentiated burns slightly more specifically, including the presence or absence of inhalational injury and acknowledging that burns involving the face, hands, or wrists warranted higher DWs.[9]

An assessment of the BoD for hand burns today essentially would deal exclusively with YLD. Although people undoubtedly have decreased life expectancy because of burns to the hands, as a general rule it is more reasonable to assume that those YLL would be attributed to some other aspect of the burn injury and those data would be lost in the enumeration of DALYs due specifically to hand burns. All of this, by definition, requires that anyone with "disability" in GBD terms,

or loss of function of the hands, has survived a burn injury.

Since disability due to hand burns presupposes survival of the burn injury, the overall improvement in burn survival anticipated in the LMIC setting in the wake of the report of *The Lancet* Commission on Global Surgery[15] and the added attention given to essential surgical needs[16,17] could be expected to increase rather than decrease the DALYs attributed to hand burns. The overall BoD due to burn injuries should decrease due to fewer deaths, counted in terms of YLL, but these surviving people are anticipated to have varying levels of disability, thereby having greater numbers of YLD. To mitigate this requires commensurate attention to the initial management of hand burns, with the goal of minimizing the contractures that so often accompany these injuries.

Poenaru and colleagues[18] contend that BoD for many surgical problems is better assessed in terms of incident and prevalent "met" need and "unmet" needs. Although they use the example of cleft lip and palate to illustrate their argument, burn injuries are also an appropriate example. In high-income countries (HICs), much potential mortality due to acute burn injuries is avoided, and much long-term impairment is avoided by instituting appropriate acute care, or meeting the incident met need. The prevalent met need is similarly addressed but is much smaller in HICs. In LMICs, however, the incident unmet need most commonly dwarfs the met need because of the many barriers to access, leading to the prevalent unmet need comprising a large proportion of the BoD due to burns. This concept is illustrated graphically in **Fig. 2**,[18] manifested at the human level by the many people living in LMICs with horrific burn contractures.

WHAT CAN BE SAID ABOUT THE BURDEN OF DISEASE DUE TO HAND BURNS IN LOW- AND MIDDLE-INCOME COUNTRIES IN 2017?

The most recent publication from the GBD study indicates that both the incidence of acute burns and the prevalence of chronic sequelae of burn injuries have decreased since 1990 (**Box 1**). Demographic changes in that time, both in longer life expectancy and in age distribution (an overall older populace), accentuate this decrease. This study found a 9.24% decrease in incidence (from 36.8 million to 33.4 million cases) but a 31.08% decrease when this was viewed as an age-standardized rate (from 653.9/100,000 to 450.6/100,000 population). In terms of prevalence of chronic sequelae, that is, longer-term problems associated with scarring and contractures, there was a 28.7% decrease in

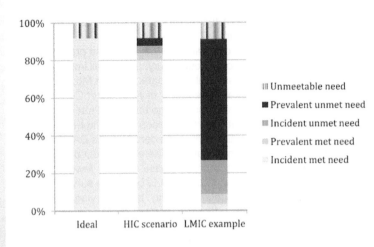

Fig. 2. Model disaggregation of surgical need in an ideal setting, in an HIC and in the current calculation for LMICs. (*From* Poenaru D, Ozgediz D, Gosselin RA. Burden, need, or backlog: a call for improved metrics for the global burden of surgical disease. Int J Surg 2014;12(5):484; with permission.)

age-standardized prevalence of cases compared with 1990 findings. There was a 36.8% decrease in age-standardized YLD in the same time period.[6]

Although the figures cited above apply to burn injuries overall, it is reasonable to assume that the proportion of injuries resulting in hand burns is similar. The literature in general does not address the specific incidence of hand burns,[4] but an idea of that proportion is needed. Over the past decade, the nongovernmental organization (NGO) ReSurge International has supported a burn-contracture reconstruction program in several LMICs. The program provides financial support on a per-patient basis for the surgical addressing of burn contractures. The greatest limitation of the usefulness of the data from that program in the assessment of the BoD is the selection of patients, because, by

definition, the only people included are those judged by the surgeons in the program to be appropriate candidates for reconstruction. This bias affects not only the numbers of people burned but also the demographic and epidemiologic characteristics. Many people in the catchment areas do not present for care, and others are not candidates for contracture release. Nevertheless, these data can give a glimpse into how hand burns may factor into the overall picture of burn injuries.

Between 2004 and 2012, 4302 patients in 8 countries were operated on under the auspices of this program (**Box 2**). The majority, 68%, were injured in open fire, most related to cooking. Another 16% were due to boiling liquid. Gender was almost equal, with 52% female and 48% male; 61% were age 15 or under. Of greatest interest, however, is that 52% of all burn injuries admitted for contracture release were burns of the wrist, hand, or digits. Another 10% were of the elbow (courtesy of ReSurge International, unpublished data, 2012. Available at: www.resurge.org). Again, the nature

---

Box 1
Summary of incidence and prevalence of burn injuries from Global Burden of Disease study

- Both the incidence of acute burns and the prevalence sequelae of burn injuries have decreased since 1990.

- Incidence decreased 9.24%, or when age-standardized, decreased from 654 to 451 per 100,000 population, or 31%.

- Age-standardized case prevalence decreased 28.7%.

- Age-standardized YLD prevalence decreased 36.8%.

Data from Vos T, Barber RM, Bell B, et al. Global, regional, and national incidence, prevalence, and years lived with disability for 301 acute and chronic diseases and injuries in 188 countries, 1990-2013: a systematic analysis for the Global Burden of Disease Study 2013. Lancet 2015;386(9995):743–800.

Box 2
Summary of patient characteristics in burn contracture reconstruction program

- 4302 between 2004 and 2012

- 68% open fire (cooking); 16% boiling liquid; 16% other causes

- 52% female; 48% male

- 61% age 15 or under

- 52% were burns of the wrist, hand, or digits

- 10% were burns of the elbow

Data from Resurge International, unpublished data, 2012.

of the bias of these data must be considered, but if it is accepted that 52% of the prevalent cases noted in the 2013 update of the GBD study[6] have hand injuries as a component, then there are more than 18 million people living with the sequelae of hand burn injuries, or more than 0.2% of the global population.

Jovic and colleagues[19] published a compendium of the surgical experience of a single plastic surgeon in Zambia over a 16-year period and found that 34.2% of the 5739 cases done were related to burns (**Box 3**). A review of the raw data of that study revealed that 52% of the burn cases involved the hand or elbow (43% hand and 9% elbow). This is approximately consistent with the findings in the program discussed previously. These hand burns represented 18% of the total cases done.[20]

With the association of burns with poverty, it is not surprising that the BoD due to burn injuries is highest in sub-Saharan Africa and South Asia. The high incidence of intentional burn injuries in some areas, both self-inflicted and from intentional assault, leads to a still higher prevalence of burns in India and some other South Asian countries. As the global economy improved over the past quarter century, however, so has the level of burn injuries. With millions of people in China having been brought out of poverty over this time, the BoD due to burns has seen a commensurate improvement.[21]

ADDRESSING THE BURDEN OF DISEASE DUE TO HAND BURNS

A comprehensive goal to decrease the BoD of hand burns in LMICs would include a country-wide prevention strategy with a public education campaign as well as greater access to appropriate care at all levels. This would start with better infrastructure and governmental activity, including better transportation, better safety net help for patients and families for prolonged loss of wages, better access to supplies for burn care in a referral

---

Box 3
Summary of Zambian study

- 5739 plastic surgery cases over 16 years
- 34.2% of these were burns
- 52% of burn cases were hand (43%) or elbow (9%)
- 18% of total plastic surgery cases were burns

Data from Jovic G, Corlew DS, Bowman KG. Plastic and Reconstructive Surgery in Zambia: epidemiology of 16 Years of Practice. World J Surg 2012;36(2):241–6.

---

hospital, more nursing care with training and experience in burn management, and more trained anesthesia and surgical personnel for these injuries. This would result in a major improvement in what Poenaru and colleagues[18] call incident met need, with the idea of decreasing the prevalent needs in the long term.[18,22]

Over the past decade, there has been increasing attention to the capacity of LMICs to provide necessary surgical services. Country-based surgical and anesthesia infrastructure surveys have informed the international literature as to the specific gaps and needs in surgical and safety equipment, essential medicines, and workforce.[23–38] These studies reveal the dearth of surgical capacity in many LMICs, perhaps more specifically in areas within LMICs that are most affected by a lack of resources. These studies also elucidate the issues of surgical safety that accompany deficient surgical infrastructure. Many LMICs have what seem to be appropriate concepts of a functional health care system that presumably has the capacity to avoid many of the hand contractures that are seen. On the ground, however, is found a lack of personnel at all levels of the health care spectrum and a lack of equipment and supplies.

Although these surveys did not reveal the actual surgical BoD, they did create a framework to describe unmet surgical need and the necessary details for improving access to surgery in LMICs. Weiser and colleagues recently provided an update of surgical volume around the world and additionally found that the most important correlative factor behind meeting needed surgical capacity is total expenditure on health within a country.[39]

With the advent of the Sustainable Development Goals[40] and The Lancet Commission on Global Surgery, concrete progress toward the scale up of surgical infrastructure by 2030 is not only proposed but also expected.[15,41] These improvements in LMICs provide for access to basic surgical care at the first level or most accessible referral hospital above that of the community primary health center. The common infrastructure required for the 44 surgical procedures deemed essential by the World Health Organization Global Initiative for Emergency and Essential Emergency Care[17,42] and described by the Disease Control Priorities Project[43] provides for initial hand burn management.

Prevention is the most cost-effective strategy for hand burns in LMICs but also a considerable challenge. Beyond prevention, however, the provision of public education related to the importance of early treatment could have an impact on the severity of many hand burns in LMICs.[44–46]

If access to comprehensive specialized surgical care is intimidating in many locales, a Haddon matrix assessment indicates that there are several interventions that can at least mitigate the disabling effects of many hand burns short of aggressive surgical care. Basic wound care is often a barrier to burn management in LMICs; this is an area of focus that has the potential to yield inexpensive gains in outcomes, especially for hand burns. Silver-based ointments and dressings may be ideal, but local alternatives, such as amniotic membrane, honey, banana leaf dressings, and exposure therapy, are well known to providers in LMICs.[47] Splinting also has special importance for hand burns, and local variation of the materials available for basic splinting are likely to insure that splinting is cost effective.[48]

In the acute setting, even for hand burns for which an optimally functional result truly can only be achieved by surgical intervention, proper wound care and splinting initially at the primary health care center can still improve the ultimate function. Although many providers require basic splinting education for hand burns, this investment in training for nurses, clinical officers, or technicians will help prevent or limit the crippling contractures all too common in LMICs. Focused educational efforts at this level of the health care system can facilitate this. The United Kingdom–based NGO Interburns[49,50] and the Australia-based NGO Interplast[51] have both conducted major educational efforts in all aspects of burn management in many LMICs, and it is possible that efforts such as those can start to filter down from the specialty centers to the less equipped but more accessible parts of health care systems.

WHAT IS KNOWN ABOUT POSTBURN RECONSTRUCTION IN LOW- AND MIDDLE-INCOME COUNTRIES?

Once established, contractures involving the hands can be difficult but often can be resolved or improved significantly with recreation of the original wound dimensions and a combination of local flaps and skin grafting, generally full thickness when feasible. As with most hand problems, postoperative management rivals the operation in terms of ultimate effectiveness of the intervention. The NGO International Women and Children's Burn Foundation[52] is one organization that has worked to establish rehabilitation centers for burn care in several LMICs and emphasizes the training of appropriate practitioners as well as making rehabilitative care economically feasible. Such focus on this aspect of care, including long-term economic feasibility, is critical to the amelioration of hand burn impairment in the developing world.

For reconstructive efforts in the face of established contracture, Agag and colleagues,[51] using the database from the ReSurge International program, discussed previously, found that better functionality for burns to the hand after reconstructive efforts was associated with the mechanism of the burn being hot liquid rather than open fire, with younger age, and with the time elapsed between the injury and presentation for reconstruction (**Box 4**).[53] Such information can be useful in planning surgical interventions, determining expectations, and patient selection, especially with limited resources.

Because of the frequent lack of available acute care for burn injuries in LMICs, the contractures that develop are often of far greater significance, and difficulty in management, than is seen in HICs. These represent the massive unmet prevalent need[18] in the developing world regarding burn care. Unfortunately, the actual burn injury that causes these devastating impairments often is only slightly more severe in terms of mechanism of injury or total physiologic manifestation than the ones that result only in 1-finger to 3-finger syndactyly. Only a few extra centimeters of injury separate these widely differing sequelae. Again, with current methodology in the measurement of the global BoD, there is no difference measured in these 2 degrees of injury, emphasizing the need for greater evaluation of this problem by those with specific interest in the effect of burn injuries on the hand.

As discussed elsewhere in this issue, (See Peter O. Kwan and Edward E. Tredget's article, "Biological Principles of Scar and Contracture"; and Matthew Brown and Kevin C. Chung's article, "Postburn Contractures of the Hand," in this issue) burn contractures simply illustrate the natural history of wound healing. In the absence of epithelial tissue, wounds contract to some degree but then epithelial edges seek other epithelial edges and a contracture is created. For upper extremity injuries, the least destructive form results in

---

Box 4
Contracture release was found to have better results

- When burn was due to hot liquid rather than open fire
- With younger age
- With less time elapsed between injury and release

Box 5
A few organizations with interest in burn injuries in low-income and middle-income countries

- International Society for Burn Injuries — worldburn.org
- National Academy of Burns–India — thenabi.org
- American Burn Association — www.ameriburn.org
- European Burns Association — www.euroburn
- College of Surgeons of East, Central and Southern Africa — COSECSA.org
- Bangladeshi Society of Burn Injuries
- Interburns — Interburns.org
- British Burn Association — britishburnassociation.org
- Australian and New Zealand Burns Association — anzba.org.au
- Acid Survivors Foundation — acidsurvivors.org
- International Women and Children's Burn Foundation — iwcbf.org
- World Health Organization — who.int

---

syndactyly, often with associated flexion contracture. With greater surface area affected and with greater depth of burn, totally disabling contractures of fingers, palm, wrist, and elbow can result. In areas of the world with limited resources for health care, however, the effects on the affected person are magnified, leading to a poverty trap[54] from which it can be extremely difficult to emerge.

SUMMARY

Burn injuries to the hands are a major health issue touching all aspects of life for those affected. As with almost all burns, the most vulnerable in global society are most affected, especially the very young and old in LMICs. These are problems correlated closely with poverty, and in some areas this is magnified by cultural issues. Enumerating the proportion of the global BoD due to hand burns is difficult for several reasons. First is the specificity of the injury in question — hands as a subset of burns, which are a subset of trauma, complicated by the exaggerated functional deficit per TBSA of burn that is inherent in hand injuries. Next is the point that burns result in a high prevalence of disease in addition to the incidence, because the effects of burns, especially hand burns, are generally long lasting, especially in LMICs where contractures can be the rule rather than the exception. Further complicating assessing the contribution of hand burns to the GBD is the wide variation in manifestation of these injuries. Although many disease processes can range in effect from quite mild to devastating, hand burns arguably do so as much as any other problem in the list of diseases and risk factors enumerated in the GBD.

Consequently, there are no specific, hard data from the developing world giving a picture of the extent of the BoD due to these injuries. By examining what is known about burn injuries in LMICs, however, it can be calculated that approximately half of all people who sustain significant burns and survive have hand injuries as a component. It can be further calculated that there may be approximately 18 million people living in the world today with significant impairment in their lives due to burns to the hands. Many, if not most, of the affected are children at the time of their injuries. Although some may ultimately receive some restorative care, improving their utility and productivity to some degree, many others will not. As more attention globally is paid to surgical needs, this number should increase over the next decade, providing some decrease in the prevalence of burn sequelae and, therefore, in the GBD due to hand burns (**Box 5**).

REFERENCES

1. Peck MD. Epidemiology of burns throughout the world. Part I: distribution and risk factors. Burns 2011;37:1087–100.
2. Ahuja RB, Bhattacharya S. Burns in the developing world and burn disasters. BMJ 2004;329:447–9.
3. Saisy S, Mostaque AK, Bari S, et al. Socioeconomic and cultural influence in the causation of burns in the urban children of Bangladesh. J Burn Care Rehabil 2001;22:269–73.
4. Forjouh SN. Burns in low- and middle-income countries: a review of available literature on descriptive epidemiology, risk factors, treatment, and prevention. Burns 2006;32:529–37.

5. Peck MD. Burns and fires from non-electric domestic appliances in low and middle income countries Part I. The scope of the problem. Burns 2008;34:303–11.

6. Charlson F, Erskine H, Ferrari A, et al. Global, regional, and national incidence, prevalence, and years lived with disability for 301 acute and chronic diseases and injuries in 188 countries, 1990-2013: a systematic analysis for the Global Burden of Disease Study 2013. Lancet 2015;386(9995):743–800.

7. Murray CJM, Barber RM, Foreman KJ, et al. Global, regional, and national disability-adjusted life years (DALYs) for 306 diseases and injuries and healthy life expectancy (HALE) for 188 countries, 1990–2013: quantifying the epidemiological transition. Lancet 2015;386:2145–91.

8. Salomon JA. New disability weights for the global burden of disease. Bull World Health Organ 2010; 88:879.

9. Salomon JA, Vos T, Hagan DR, et al. Common values in assessing health outcomes from disease and injury: disability weights measurement study for the Global Burden of Disease Study 2010. Lancet 2012;380:2129–43.

10. Salomon JA, Haagsma JA, Davis A, et al. Disability weights for the global burden of disease 2013 study. Lancet Glob Health 2015;3:e712–23.

11. Arnesen T, Nord E. The value of DALY life: problems with ethics and validity of disability adjusted life years. BMJ 1999;319:1423–5.

12. Anand S, Hanson K. Disability-adjusted life years: a critical review. J Health Econ 1997;16:685–702.

13. Gosselin RA, Ozgediz D, Poenaru D. A square peg in a round hole? Challenges with DALY-based "burden of disease" calculations in surgery and a call for alternative metrics,. World J Surg 2013;37:2507–11.

14. Mathers CD, Lopez AD, Murray CJL. The burden of disease and mortality by condition data, methods, and results for 2001. In: Lopez AD, Mathers CD, Ezzati M, et al, editors. Global burden of disease and risk factors. Washington, DC: The International Bank for Reconstruction and Development/The World Bank; 2006. p. 125.

15. Meara JG, Leather AJM, Hagander L, et al. Global surgery 2030: evidence and solutions for achieving health, welfare, and economic development. Lancet 2015;386(9993):569–624.

16. Shrime MG, Meara JG. How Surgery Can Fight Global Poverty. NY Times 2015. Available at: http://www.nytimes.com/2015/09/26/opinion/how-surgery-can-fight-global-poverty.html?. Accessed February 24, 2016.

17. Available at: http://www.who.int/surgery/global initiative/en/. Accessed April 7, 2015.

18. Poenaru D, Ozgediz D, Gosselin RA. Burden, need, or backlog: a call for improved metrics for the global burden of surgical disease,. Int J Surg 2014;12:483–6.

19. Jovic G, Corlew DS, Bowman KG. Plastic and Reconstructive Surgery in Zambia: Epidemiology of 16 Years of Practice. World J Surg 2012;36:241–6.

20. Personal review of raw data from Jovic 2012.

21. Institute for Health Metrics and Evaluation. Available at: http://vizhub.healthdata.org/gbd-compare/. Accessed February 24, 2016.

22. Ozgediz D, Poenaru D. The burden of pediatric surgical conditions in low and middle income countries: a call to action. J Pediatr Surg 2012;47:2305–11.

23. Weiser TG, Makary MA, Haynes AB, et al. Standardized metrics for global surgical surveillance. Lancet 2009;374:1113–7.

24. Bowman KG, Jovic G, Rangel S, et al. Pediatric emergency and essential surgical care in Zambian hospitals: a nationwide study. J Pediatr Surg 2013; 48:1363–70.

25. Notrica MR, Evans FM, Knowlton LM, et al. Rwandan surgical and anesthesia infrastructure: a survey of district hospitals. World J Surg 2011;35:1770–80.

26. Linden AF, Sekidde FS, Galukande M, et al. Challenges of surgery in developing countries: a survey of surgical and anesthesia capacity in Uganda's public hospitals. World J Surg 2012; 36(5):1056–65.

27. Zafar SN, McQueen KA. Surgery, Public Health, and Pakistan. World J Surg 2011;35:2625–34.

28. Vansell HJ, Schlesinger JJ, Harvey A, et al. Anaesthesia, surgery, obstetrics, and emergency care in Guyana. J Epidemiol Glob Health 2014;5(1):75–83.

29. Natuzzi ES, Kushner A, Jaqily R, et al. Surgical care in the Solomon Islands: a road map for universal surgical care delivery. World J Surg 2011;35:1183–93.

30. Kingham TP, Kamara TB, Cherian MN, et al. Quantifying surgical capacity in Sierra Leone: a guide for improving surgical care. Arch Surg 2009;144: 122–8.

31. Iddriss A, Shivute N, Bickler S, et al. Emergency, anaesthetic and essential surgical capacity in the Gambia. Bull World Health Organ 2011;89:565–72.

32. Spiegel DA, Choo S, Cherian M, et al. Quantifying surgical and anesthetic availability at primary health facilities in Mongolia. World J Surg 2011;35:272–9.

33. Penoyar T, Cohen H, Kibatala P, et al. Emergency and surgery services of primary hospitals in the United Republic of Tanzania. BMJ Open 2012;2(1): e000369.

34. Sherman L, Clement PT, Cherian MN, et al. Implementing Liberia's poverty reduction strategy: an assessment of emergency and essential surgical care. Arch Surg 2011;146:35–9.

35. Taira BR, Cherian MN, Yakandawala H, et al. Survey of emergency and surgical capacity in the conflict-affected regions of Sri Lanka. World J Surg 2010; 34:428–32.

36. Walker IA, Obua AD, Moulton F, et al. Paediatric surgery and anaesthesia in south-western Uganda: a

cross-sectional survey. Bull World Health Organ 2010;88:897–906.

37. Choo S, Perry H, Hesse AA, et al. Assessment of capacity for surgery, obstetrics, and anaesthesia in 17 Ghanaian hospitals using a WHO assessment tool. Trop Med Int Health 2010;15(9):1109–15.

38. LeBrun DG, Dhar D, Sarkar IH, et al. Measuring global surgical disparities: a survery of surgical and anesthesia infrastructure in Bangladesh. World J Surg 2013;37:24–31.

39. Weiser TG, Haynes AB, Molina G, et al. Size and distribution of the global volume of surgery in 2012. Bull WHO 2016;94:201F–9F.

40. Available at: http://www.un.org/sustainabledevelopment/sustainable-development-goals/. Accessed January 12, 2017.

41. Ng-Kamstra JS, Greenberg S, Abdullah F, et al. Global Surgery 2030: a roadmap for high income country actors. BMJ Glob Health 2016;1:e000011.

42. Mock C, Cherian M, Juillard C, et al. Developing priorities for addressing surgical conditions globally: Furthering the link between surgery and public health policy. World J Surg 2010;34:381–5.

43. Debas HT, Donkor P, Gawande A, et al, editors. Essential surgery. Disease control priorities, vol. 1, 3rd edition. Washington, DC: World Bank; 2015. p. 4–5. Table 1.1.

44. Mock C, Peck M, Peden M, et al. A WHO plan for burn prevention and care. Geneva (Switzerland): World Health Organization; 2008. Available at: http://whqlibdoc.who.int/publications/2008/9789241596299_eng.pdf. Accessed April 11, 2016.

45. Mashreky SH, Rahman A, Svanstrom L. Experience from community based childhood burn prevention programme in Bangladesh: Implication for low resource setting. Burns 2011;37:770–5.

46. Mock C, Peck M, Julliard C, et al. Burn prevention: success stories and lessons learned. Geneva (Switzerland): World Health Organization; 2011. Available at: http://apps.who.int/iris/bitstream/10665/97938/1/9789241501187_eng.pdf. Accessed April 11, 2016.

47. Gosselin RA, Charles A, Joshipura M, et al. Surgery and trauma care. In: Debas HT, Donkor P, Gawande A, et al, editors. Essential surgery. Disease control priorities, vol. 1, 3rd edition. Washington, DC: World Bank; 2015. p. 51.

48. Procter F. Rehabilitation of the burn patient. Indian J Plast Surg 2010;43(Suppl):S101–13. Available at: http://www.ijps.org/text.asp?2010/43/3/101/70730. Accessed April 11, 2016.

49. Available at: www.interburns.org. Accessed February 26, 2016.

50. Potokar T, Ali S, Chamania S, et al. A global overview of burn research highlights the need for forming networks with the developing world. Burns 2007;34(1):3–5.

51. Available at: www.interplast.org.au. Accessed February 26, 2016.

52. Available at: www.iwcbf.org. Accessed February 26, 2016.

53. Garcia LP, Huang A, Corlew DS, et al. A prospective review of 2506 burn contractures in developing countries: factors affecting improved function. Plast Reconstr Surg 2015;136(4 Suppl):147–8.

54. Banerjee AV, Duflo E. Poor economics: a radical rethinking of the way to fight global poverty. New York: Public Affairs; 2012.

Index

Note: Page numbers of article titles are in **boldface** type.

hand.theclinics.com

Printed and bound by CPI Group (UK) Ltd, Croydon, CR0 4YY

03/10/2024

01040383-0015